SECOND EDITION

Population Health

Creating a Culture of Wellness

Edited By

David B. Nash, MD, MBA
Founding Dean
Jefferson College of Population Health
Thomas Jefferson University
Philadelphia, PA

Raymond J. Fabius, MD
Co-founder and President
HealthNEXT
Philadelphia, PA

Janice L. Clarke, RN
Senior Medical Writer
Jefferson College of Population Health
Thomas Jefferson University
Philadelphia, PA

Alexis Skoufalos, EdD
Associate Dean for Strategic Development
Jefferson College of Population Health
Thomas Jefferson University
Philadelphia, PA

Melissa R. Horowitz
Project Director
Jefferson College of Population Health
Thomas Jefferson University
Philadelphia, PA

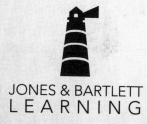

JONES & BARTLETT
LEARNING

World Headquarters
Jones & Bartlett Learning
5 Wall Street
Burlington, MA 01803
978-443-5000
info@jblearning.com
www.jblearning.com

Jones & Bartlett Learning books and products are available through most bookstores and online booksellers. To contact Jones & Bartlett Learning directly, call 800-832-0034, fax 978-443-8000, or visit our website, www.jblearning.com.

Substantial discounts on bulk quantities of Jones & Bartlett Learning publications are available to corporations, professional associations, and other qualified organizations. For details and specific discount information, contact the special sales department at Jones & Bartlett Learning via the above contact information or send an email to specialsales @jblearning.com.

08630-0

Production Credits

VP, Executive Publisher: David D. Cella
Publisher: Michael Brown
Associate Editor: Lindsey Mawhiney
Editorial Assistant: Nicholas Alakel
Production Manager: Tracey McCrea
Senior Marketing Manager: Sophie Fleck Teague
Art Development Assistant: Shannon Sheehan
Manufacturing and Inventory Control Supervisor:
  Amy Bacus

Composition: Cenveo Publisher Services
Cover Design: Scott Moden
Rights and Media Coordinator: Mary Flatley
Cover and Title Page Image: © Mikael Damkier/Shutterstock
Printing and Binding: Edwards Brothers Malloy
Cover Printing: Edwards Brothers Malloy

Library of Congress Cataloging-in-Publication Data
Population health: creating a culture of wellness / [edited by] David B. Nash, Raymond J. Fabius, Alexis Skoufalos, Janice Clarke, Melissa R. Horowitz. -- Second edition.
    p. ; cm.
Preceded by: Population health / David B. Nash ... [et al.]. c2011.
Includes bibliographical references and index.
ISBN 978-1-284-08630-0 (pbk.)
I. Nash, David B., editor. II. Fabius, Raymond J., editor. III. Skoufalos, Alexis, editor. IV. Clarke, Janice, 1943- , editor. V. Horowitz, Melissa R., editor.
[DNLM: 1. Delivery of Health Care—organization & administration--United States.
    2. Delivery of Health Care—economics—United States. 3. Disease Management—United States.
    4. Health Care Reform—United States. 5. Health Promotion—United States. W 84 AA1]
RA395.A3
362.1--dc23
                        2014042569

6048
Printed in the United States of America
19 18 17 16 15   10 9 8 7 6 5 4 3

DEDICATION

To Es, Leah, Rachel, and Jake—you make it all worthwhile.

—DBN

To all of my family, friends, colleagues, and mentors who have supported, encouraged, and taught me along my journey. In particular I want to dedicate this book to my wife, Sara, and my two sons, Michael and Daniel, and their wives, Laurie and Katie. Additionally I want to thank my dear friend David Nash for inviting me to collaborate with him on many projects over the years, including this effort.

—RJF

To Tom, for his unfailing support and love.

—AS

With love to Bill and our combined family, and thanks to Noah Webster.

—JLC

To Josh, Alex, David, and Sammy—your support and love mean the world to me. You inspire me every day.

—MRH

To our alumni and current and future students, who challenge us to address the ever-changing demands of health care.

Prior to July 1, 2015 the Jefferson College of Population Health was known as the
Jefferson School of Population Health.

CONTENTS

SECTION II: POPULATION HEALTH AND THE PATIENT

SECTION IV: BUSINESS

SECTION V: POPULATION HEALTH RESEARCH

FOREWORD TO SECOND EDITION

From volume to value, the spectrum of care, healthcare reform—these words have entered the everyday lexicon of patients, physicians, nurses, and hospital and health system CEOs. But philosophy and good intentions will not get us through the difficulties that currently exist in this twilight zone of health care, whereby we are undergoing a paradigm shift from a hospital-dominated, disease-driven economic model to one that rewards everyone in the system for helping the patients they serve become and remain healthy. The Patient Protection and Affordable Care Act (whatever your politics) serves as a clarion call to all of us who serve in or need the American healthcare system. The time to act is now; we can no longer afford the luxury of philosophical debate.

That call to action is answered by Dr. Nash and his colleagues in the second edition of a book that could not have come at a better time. Both the academic and street credentials of the authors should be motivating for anyone who cares about moving from healthcare reform to health transformation. The must-read aspect of this edition, however, is in its ability to translate complex principles of population health into a field manual that can serve as a guide for the difficult cultural transformation that will be necessary during this tumultuous time of both uncertainty and opportunity for all of us involved in providing health care.

As the president and CEO of an almost 200-year-old academic medical center (one that was smart enough to create the first school of population health), I recognize that what got us here won't get us there. The next few years will serve as a type of natural selection for those systems that begin the journey and create a road map for a culture of health. It's not what we were taught in medical school or business school, so for now the second edition of *Population Health: Creating a Culture of Wellness* will serve as a much-needed resource and reference on my desk and that of my trustees. I invite you to begin the journey with Dr. Nash and his colleagues of changing the DNA of health care—one population at a time.

Stephen K. Klasko, MD, MBA
President and CEO
Thomas Jefferson University and
Jefferson Health System

PREFACE

In July of 2008, the Board of Trustees of Thomas Jefferson University in Philadelphia, Pennsylvania, voted unanimously to approve the creation of the first College of Population Health in the United States, the Jefferson College of Population Health (JSPH). As part of a strategy to become a recognized national leader in health sciences education, the university has made an important public commitment to improving the health of its citizenry. As the first college of population health in the nation, we have a particular responsibility and burden. Our challenge is to train leaders for the future from across the healthcare spectrum who will go forward and improve the health of the population. This book provides a strong foundation for helping us meet that challenge.

A number of important questions needed to be answered as we began to develop a population health agenda, beginning with "What exactly is population health, and how does it differ from public health? Why create a multiauthored text on the subject? Who is the intended audience?" We tackled these issues in turn.

Population health is a term that has gained considerable traction in our everyday lexicon. Most thought leaders agree that population health refers to "the distribution of health outcomes within a population, the health determinants that influence distribution and the policies and interventions that impact the determinants."[1,2] Population health may also be viewed as "the aggregate health outcome of health adjusted life expectancy of a group of individuals, in an economic framework that balances the relative marginal returns from the multiple determinants of health. This definition proposes a specific unit of measure of population health and considers the relative cost-effectiveness of resource allocation to multiple determinants."[1] When applying the population health concept across the continuum, it is important to consider five essential goals: (1) keeping the well, well; (2) reducing health risks; (3) providing quick access to care for acute illness so that health does not deteriorate; (4) managing chronic illness to prevent complications; and (5) getting those with complex or catastrophic illnesses to centers of excellence or compassionate care settings. To accomplish these goals effectively, health informatics and organizational approaches to care must be leveraged and institutionalized, and progress must be regularly assessed across the spectrum of care.

As our school marks its sixth birthday, the leadership and faculty have coalesced around a deeper understanding of the differences between population health and public health (i.e., population health connects prevention, wellness, and behavioral health science with healthcare quality and safety, disease prevention, and management and economic issues of value and risk—all in the service of the specific population). Like public health, population health builds on epidemiology and biostatistics, but population health takes these disciplines in new directions by means of applied metrics and analytics.

Underlying the differentiation between population health and public health are some other critical aspects of our system. Historically, our healthcare system rewarded reactive care rather than proactive care and financially encouraged doctors to focus on treating acute episodes of illness and disease rather than managing those illness or diseases to avert future crises. In most cases, doctors were paid for "piecework" (i.e., they were paid more for providing higher volume and higher-intensity acute care services). At the same time, doctors were underpaid—or not paid—to coordinate effective preventive health care to keep their patients out of hospitals. This resulted in a "toxic payment system that undermines fiscal incentives for promoting wellness" and placed doctors in "the 'disease business' not the 'wellness business.'"[3]

Driven principally by the same payment system, hospitals have long been in the business of treating acute episodes that are the end result of preventable diseases. Although the mission statements of most hospitals read something like this, "Our mission is to improve the health of our community," the financial realities of the traditional payment system generated conflicts of interest. If hospitals were incentivized to succeed in their missions (e.g., payment for patient education, care coordination, and other efforts to reduce admissions for diabetes, smoking, asthma, and coronary disease), they and their patients would benefit. Population health represents the paradigm shift that has already begun to tackle the aforementioned challenges faced by doctors and hospitals.

Much has happened since the publication of the first edition of this book, principally, the continued implementation of the Patient Protection and Affordable Care Act (ACA), signed into law by President Obama on March 23, 2010. This book is not about red states or blue states. It is not about the troubled implementation of the insurance exchanges. It is not meant to be a treatise on healthcare reform. Rather this book is the lever with which we may begin to implement a new type of medicine—population health medicine—with a focus on changing the very nature of clinical practice so that it evolves into a "no outcome, no income" system, a system that is characterized by the following:

(1) practicing medicine based on the evidence and tying payments to those outcomes, (2) reducing unexplained clinical variation, (3) continually measuring and closing the feedback loop between physicians and the supply chain that supports them, (4) trading professional autonomy for clinical collaboration, and (5) engaging with patients across the continuum. The ACA makes this five-point plan a strategic imperative, and it offers a road map toward the creation of a more responsive and effective health system for the future.

Subsequent to the publication of the first edition, we've learned as a nation that our diet of unbridled access to high technology, a focus on illness, and an inequitable distribution of societal resources have led us to an unenviable spot (i.e., a nation that ranks 17th in the world with regard to the quality of life of our citizenry).[4] In a stunning Institute of Medicine report,[5] widely cited in the past several years, the United States ranks last, right behind Slovenia, of the world's wealthiest nations. This ranking is particularly disappointing in light of the fact that we spend more on health care than any other country. Certainly, if there ever was a time for us to embrace the concept of population health, it is now!

Population health is at the core of the Jefferson College of Population Health. Population health impels us to take a broader perspective to truly improve the health of the public. We must explicitly recognize the nature of care in our system. We must strive for better understanding of the evidentiary basis of what we do every day at the bedside and across every care setting—in ensuring wellness, preventing and treating illness, and supporting populations across the life-span. Finally, we must be responsible stewards of the vast public resources for which we are accountable to our citizens. Perhaps then our nation will become a world leader in providing a healthcare system characterized by the original Institute of Medicine's six domains of safety, effectiveness, efficiency, patient centeredness, timeliness, and equity.

WHY A SECOND EDITION OF THIS BOOK?

When we launched the Jefferson College of Population Health, there was no single unifying treatise that captured the philosophy and mission of our school. Although there were many contributors to the science of population health, no one had brought forth a single volume as an overview of the field. No one had previously articulated the scope of the field and the need for innovative approaches, strategies, and practices. This text continues to break new ground, and in so doing, it suggests new solutions and raises many vexing questions.

One lingering question remains unanswered: how will health systems deliver on the true mission of population health? There are promising reports of efforts that are already under way (e.g., some hospitals in the Midwest are growing crops to feed the poor in zip codes they serve, and others are interacting with local school systems and social institutions that help to determine the health of the population). As editors, we recognize that 85% of a society's well-being is driven by activities outside the four walls of any hospital or medical facility. The launch of our school, contiguous with one of the nation's oldest and largest private medical schools and health delivery systems, affords us a unique platform and a much-needed voice to meet the challenges at hand.

HOW IS THIS BOOK ORGANIZED?

This second edition brings the reader up to speed on the expanding role of population health and its importance in bringing about a nationwide culture of wellness. The entire text has been updated to incorporate considerable changes in the healthcare system and population health brought about by innovation as well as the implementation of the ACA. For example, a new opening chapter explains how the response of the healthcare system to the population health mandate has paved the way for the ultimate goal—a culture of health and wellness.

In this edition, chapters are regrouped under updated section headings to improve the flow and make the text more reader friendly. A number of chapters were added that recognize the new emphasis on emerging fields such as patient engagement, behavioral economics, and comparative effectiveness research. Several new and engaging case studies were added to the book as well (e.g., a case study focused on assessing the organizational readiness for population health in a national, not-for-profit hospital chain). The book is organized into five key sections:

- Section 1 provides an overview and a policy synthesis.
- Section 2 focuses on the consumer and his or her new role in a system characterized by population health.
- Section 3 recognizes the importance of the continuum of care, moving us beyond the hospital walls.
- Section 4 describes the connection between population health and the business case for achieving a "no outcome, no income" value-based delivery system.
- Section 5 discusses the key research questions for the future.

WHO SHOULD READ THIS BOOK?

The editors are grateful for the participation of a large number of nationally recognized experts from across the spectrum of population health practitioners. Principally organized for graduate work in population health, this edition could serve as the foundation for courses in schools of public health, health administration, medicine, nursing care, and pharmaceutical sciences. Every section contains important information for anyone who cares about how we might more effectively improve the health of our country. Practitioners in the field may benefit from the broad perspective and comprehensive approach of this book. Undergraduates in colleges and universities across the country may be moved to answer the call laid out by the Institute of Medicine to improve the public's understanding of these themes. We also hope that as they face the challenge of educating the physicians of tomorrow, many schools of medicine will adopt this book.

Many people played a role in the genesis of this edition. As the senior editor, I would particularly like to thank our new university president, Stephen Klasko, MD, MBA, for his visionary leadership and his ongoing support of the Jefferson College of Population Health. I also want to recognize other campus leaders, including Michael Vergare, MD, chairman of the Department of Psychiatry, who was a steadfast supporter of our school in his previous role as senior vice president for academic affairs, and the new provost, Mark Tykocinski, MD.

As the senior editor, I also am very appreciative of the hard work of Drs. Ray Fabius and Alexis Skoufalos, our coeditors, and Janice Clarke, a nurse and senior medical writer in our school. Finally, special thanks go to Melissa Horowitz as managing editor for all of her work in keeping the entire project on track and on time.

I am grateful to the faculty and the staff of the Jefferson College of Population Health who have traveled this unmarked path with us in the successful launch and early growth of our school. As authors, we would like to thank others who have built the foundation that has led to the development of this new discipline and our school. Without the pioneers in utilization management, case management, disease management, health informatics, public health, and health and productivity at the workplace, we would not be able to realize, measure, or improve the health status of the population. We also would like to mention our gratitude to friends and family who have supported us as we pursue our passion for improving the health and well-being of the population.

Of course, we are grateful to our current and future students, who challenge us with their complex questions and whose quest for solutions will bring about much-needed improvements in population health in the future. As dean, I am confident that our students will go forth and make a world of difference.

As editors, we take responsibility for any errors of omission or commission. Most importantly, we greatly value feedback from readers and fellow pioneers in population health. We are particularly interested in the value of the text as a pedagogic tool as well.

One of the hallmarks of good leadership is to help prepare those that will take the mantle tomorrow. I am confident that the content of *Population Health: Creating a Culture of Wellness* will provide the foundation for training the future healthcare leaders that our nation so desperately needs to help nurture a healthier, happier, and more productive nation.

David B. Nash, MD, MBA

REFERENCES

1. Kindig D, Stoddart G. What is population health? *Am J Public Health*. 2003;93(3):380-3.
2. Kindig DA. Understanding population health terminology. *Milbank Q*. 2007;85(1):139-61.
3. Kumar S, Nash DB. *Demand Better*! Bozeman, MT: Second River Healthcare Press; 2011.
4. Bayer R, Fairchild AL, Hopper K, et al. Confronting the sorry state of U.S. health. *Science* 2013;341:962-3.
5. U.S. Health in International Perspective: Shorter Lives, Poorer Health. Institute of Medicine Report Brief, January 2013. http://www.iom.edu/~/media/Files/Report%20Files/2013/US-Health-International-Perspective/USHealth_Intl_PerspectiveRB.pdf. Accessed November 7, 2014.

CONTRIBUTORS

Diane L. Bechel-Marriott, DrPH
Project Manager
Michigan Primary Care Transformation
    (MiPCT)
Belleville, MI
dbechel@umich.edu

Eric N. Berkowitz, PhD
Emeritus Professor of Marketing
Isenberg School of Management
University of Massachusetts, Amherst
Amherst, MA
eberkowitz@babson.edu

Bettina Berman, RN, MPH, CPHQ, CNOR
Project Director for Quality Improvement
Jefferson College of Population Health at
    Thomas Jefferson University
Philadelphia, PA
bettina.berman@jefferson.edu

Christy Calhoun, MPH
Vice President of Content
Healthwise
Boise, ID
ccalhoun@healthwise.org

Marna Canterbury, MS, RD
Director Community Heath
Lakeview Health Foundation
Stillwater, MN
marina.m.canterbury@lakeview.org

Ronda Christopher, MEd, OTR/L, LNHA
Executive Director
Healthspan Solutions
Cincinatti, OH
rchristopher@wellspan.org

John K. Cuddeback, MD, PhD
Chief Medical Informatics Officer
American Medical Group Association
Alexandria, VA
jcuddeback@amga.org

Suzanne Duda, MPP
Vice President
Government Strategy Healthways
Franklin, TN
Suzanne.Duda@healthways.com

Dee W. Edington, PhD
Founder and Chairman
Edington Associates
Ann Arbor, MI
dwe@edingtonassociates.com

Henry C. Fader, JD, MEd
Partner
Pepper Hamilton LLP
Philadlephia, PA
faderh@pepperlaw.com

Donald W. Fisher, PhD
President and CEO
American Medical Group Association
Alexandria, VA
dfisher@amga.org

Sharon Glave Frazee, PhD, MPH
Vice President of Research and Education
Pharmacy Benefit Management
Institutesfrazee@pbmi.com

Fredric S. Goldstein, MS
President
Accountable Health, LLC
Jacksonville, TN
fgoldstein@accountablehealthllc.com

Deborah M. Gorhan, MS, MCHES
Manager, Wellness & Health
    Promotion- Americas
Johnson & Johnson
Mansfield, MA
dgorhan@its.jnj.com

Leslie Kelly Hall
Senior Vice President
Policy Healthwise
Boise, ID
lkellyhall@healthwise.org

Gina Hemenway
Manager, Strategic Partnerships
Healthspan Solutions
Cincinatti, OH
rahemenway@healthspan.org

Fikry Isaac, MD, MPH, FACOEM
Vice President, Global Health Services
Johnson & Johnson
Flemington, NJ
fisaac1@its.jnj.com

Donald W. Kemper, MPH
Founder and CEO
Healthwise
Boise, ID
Dkemper@healthwise.org

Keith C. Kosel, PhD, MHSA, MBA
Executive Director, Center for
    Applide Healthcare Studies
VHA Inc.
Irving, TX
kkosel@vha.com

Thomas E. Kottke, MD, MSPH
Medical Director of Population Health
HealthPartners
Minneapolis, MN
Thomas.E.Kottke@HealthPartners.com

Jason S. Lee, PhD
Healthcare Forum Director
The Open Group
Burlington, MA
JasonLee.PhD@gmail.com

Jin Lee, DPhil
CEO
BabyNoggin Inc
San Francisco, CA
jinl16@gmail.com

Abbie Leibowitz, MD, FAAP
Executive Vice President and
Chief Medical Officer
Health Advocate
Plymouth Meeting, PA
aleibowitz@healthadvocate.com

C. Alan Lyles, ScD, MPH, RPh
Professor
University of Baltimore
Docent
University of Kelsinki
Bel Air, MD
alanlyles@comcast.net

Esther J. Nash, MD
Vice President and Medical Director
Comprehensive Care
Health Advocate
Plymouth Meeting, PA
enash@healthadvocate.com

Lynn Nishida, RPh
Assistant Vice President
Solid Benefit Guidance
Happy Valley, OR
mnishi@aol.com

Daniel A. Ollendorf, PhD
Chief Review Officer
Institute for Clinical and Economic Review
Boston, MA
dollendorf@icer-review.org

Steven D. Pearson, MD, MSc
President
Institute for Clinicial and Economic Review
Boston, MA
spearson@icer-review.org

Jennifer S. Pitts, PhD
Chief Science Officer
Edington Associates
Cambria, CA
jspitts@edingtonassociates.com

Ellen Plumb, MD
Department of Family and Community
Medicine
Sidney Kimmel Medical College at Thomas
Jefferson University
Philadelphia, PA
ellen.plumb@jefferson.edu

James D. Plumb, MD, MPH
Professor, Department of Family and
Community Medicine
Vice Chair, Community Medicine
Director, Center for Urban Health
Thomas Jefferson University
Philadelphia, PA
james.plumb@jefferson.edu

Valerie P. Pracilio, MPH, CPPS
Client Services Manager
Pascal Metrics
Philadelphia, PA
valerie.pracilio@pascalmetrics.com

James O. Prochaska, PhD
Professor and Director
Cancer Prevention Research Center
University of Rhode Island
Kingston, RI
jop@uri.edu

Janice Prochaska, PhD
President and CEO
Pro-Change Behavior Systems, Inc.
South Kingstown, RI
jmprochaska@prochange.com

Nico Pronk, PhD
Vice President and Chief Science Officer
HealthPartners
Minneapolis, MN
nico.pronk@healthpartners.com

Martha C. Romney, RN, MS, JD, MPH
Assistant Professor
Jefferson College of Population Health at
  Thomas Jefferson University
Philadelphia, PA
martha.romney@jefferson.edu

Vibin Roy, MD
Department of Family and Community
  Medicine
Sidney Kimmel Medical College at Thomas
  Jefferson University
Philadelphia, PA
vibin.roy@jefferson.edu

Brooke Salzman, MD
Department of Family and Community
  Medicine
Sidney Kimmel Medical College at
  Thomas Jefferson University
Philadelphia, PA
brooke.salzman@jefferson.edu

Alyssa B. Schultz, PhD
Assistant Research Scientist
University of Michigan Health
Management Research Center
Bellaire, MI
abelaireschultz@gmail.com

Vicki Shepard, ACSW, MPA
SVP Strategic & Government Relations
Healthways
Nashville, TN
vicki.shepard@healthways.com

Helen Sherman, PharmD
Vice President
Solid Benefit Guidance
Portland, OR
helen97225@yahoo.com

Jaan Sidorov, MD, MHSA
Principal
Sidorov Health Solutions
Harrisburg, PA
jaans@outlook.com

Matthew C. Stiefel, MPA, MS
Senior Director, Center for Population
Health / Care Management Institute
Kaiser Permanente
Oakland, CA
Matt.Stiefel@kp.org

R. Dixon Thayer
Chief Executive Officer
HealthNEXT
Unionville, PA
rdthayer@healthnext.com

Marianne Udow-Phillips, MHSA
Director
Center for Healthcare Research and
  Transformation
University of Michigan
Ann Arbor, MI
mudow@umich.edu

Bonnie L. Zell, MD, MPH
Principal
Zell Community Health Strategies
San Francisco, CA
bonnie@zellcommunityhealth.com

Donna Zimmerman, MPH
Vice President of Government and
  Community Relation
HealthPartners
Bloomington, MN
Donna.j.zimmerman@healthpartners.com

BUILDING CULTURES OF HEALTH AND WELLNESS

Raymond J. Fabius and Janice L. Clarke

Executive Summary

Creating a culture of wellness can sustain population health initiatives.

In many respects, population health is contingent upon the existence of a culture of health and wellness. Organizations and companies have demonstrated the ability to build a sustainable culture of health and wellness that produces improvements in **health status** and lowers healthcare costs for a target population. When legislators and politicians speak about bending the healthcare cost curve, those who have built cultures of health and wellness have done it. This chapter presents a clear picture of what it takes to achieve these best practices and informs readers who might one day embark on similar journeys within their organizations.

Learning Objectives

1. Define a culture of health and wellness.
2. Identify benchmark performance of a culture of health and wellness.
3. Explain how to create a road map for achieving a culture of health and wellness.
4. Analyze how a culture of health and wellness can contribute to solving the healthcare crisis in America.
5. Understand the connection between health and wealth.

Key Terms

alignment of constituencies	integrated data warehouse
behavioral economics	medically homeless
benchmark performance	risk reduction
best practice	road map
centers of excellence	value-based benefit design
culture of health	wellness champions
health status	workplace environment

INTRODUCTION

The population health movement has been gaining momentum over the past decade, particularly since the passage of the Patient Protection and Affordable Care Act (ACA) and the subsequent implementation of programs aimed at improving the health of the population. In terms of national statistics, population health remains a daunting challenge; however, some practical applications of its tenets by companies and organizations across the country show great promise. By enveloping population health in an environment that supports its delivery and sustainability, benchmark cultures of health and wellness are appearing throughout the country in large and small companies, in manufacturing and service-oriented organizations, in for-profit and not-for-profit entities, and even in governmental agencies. Since the previous edition of this text, the population health mandate has expanded to focus on building cultures of health and wellness.

WHAT IS A CULTURE OF HEALTH AND WELLNESS?

A **culture of health** and wellness is defined by its outcomes. Participants in a culture of health and wellness pursue and achieve higher levels of health and wellness than the general population does. The expected outcomes are comparatively better quality of life and reduced incidence of morbidity. Cultures of health and wellness surround participants with an environment, policies, and cues that lead regularly to healthy choices on both a conscious and unconscious basis.[1] To appreciate the all-encompassing nature of a culture of health and wellness, consider the following attributes:

A culture of health and wellness makes it easier and more rewarding to select lifestyles that foster health. Studies show that eating right, not smoking, exercising regularly, managing stress, and drinking alcohol only in moderation can markedly reduce chronic illness over time. In fact, the World Health Organization estimates that 80% of cardiovascular disease and type 2 diabetes and 40% of cancer could be eliminated by engaging in these activities.[2]

A culture of health and wellness cultivates the appropriate use of healthcare services. Studies by Barbara Starfield et al.[3] at Johns Hopkins University have demonstrated the importance of having a relationship with a trusted primary care provider within a medical home. Despite this, it is estimated that as many as half of all Americans have no satisfactory connection to primary care. Of perhaps even greater concern, most Americans access health care randomly. In retrospect, the Healthcare Maintenance Organization model that required members to declare an affiliation with a primary care provider was a good policy for cultivating health and wellness. Because a culture of health and wellness educates and helps its participants become better health consumers, there are fewer medical misadventures and a greater chance that critical medical concerns are treated within centers of excellence.

A culture of health and wellness leverages all population health strategies. The range of available options includes:

- Opportunities for physical activity (e.g., walking trails, intermural competitions, fitness centers, yoga, meditation, sponsored events)
- Policies forbidding the use of tobacco products
- Promoting and perhaps subsidizing healthy choices in cafeterias, restaurants, and vending machines or taxing unhealthy ones

The best marketing tactics—including a branded, coordinated campaign—must be deployed to effectively promote healthy choices. While I was the global medical leader of General Electric, we developed the "Health by Numbers 0 5 10 25" program. Offered in eight core languages, this program taught that one should always use 0 tobacco products, eat 5 fruits and vegetables daily, take 10 thousand steps a day (we distributed pedometers), and maintain a body mass index of 25. All efforts to promote the program were branded with a Health by Numbers logo.[4]

*A culture of health and wellness provides and tracks the progress of **risk reduction** programs.* All culture of health and wellness participants must know their health risks and develop action plans to mitigate them with the help of health coaches. Risks such as high cholesterol or high blood pressure are easily controlled by adherence to a regimen that includes a healthy diet, exercise, and medications. Obesity is a greater challenge, but participants are more likely to tackle it with social encouragement (e.g., Weight Watchers program), and they are more likely to maintain a lower weight in an environment that promotes healthy eating and exercise.

A culture of health and wellness assures that its participants have easy access to healthcare services. Access to prompt medical treatment for acute illnesses and to screening programs to identify chronic and potentially fatal conditions is essential to a culture of health and wellness program (e.g., breast and colon cancer deaths would be much rarer if mammographies and colonoscopies were conducted when recommended in all cases).

Vaccines are arguably man's greatest achievement. Within a culture of health and wellness, all participants receive age- and gender-appropriate immunizations. The availability of influenza and other vaccines at local pharmacies is a great step forward for population health and for promoting health and wellness.

A culture of health and wellness fosters the use of evidence-based clinical guidelines. Despite the availability of national guidelines for the treatment of many common chronic illnesses (e.g., heart disease, diabetes, asthma, chronic obstructive pulmonary disease, depression), only half of Americans with these conditions receive recommended care. A culture of health and wellness implements policies and programs that significantly improve the level of individual compliance.

A culture of health and wellness promotes health throughout the workplace environment. Social and environmental pressures influence behavior (e.g., a person placed in an environment where the majority of individuals are obese is more likely to become obese). In addition to leveraging **wellness champions** and leaders to promote healthy options, a culture of health and wellness has rituals and places symbols of health promotion throughout the environment (e.g., water bottles, T-shirts, wallet cards, pedometers, tracking bracelets, poster boards). The Internet and social media are utilized as well with messaging on dedicated websites, mobile devices applications, video screens, and telemedicine.

A culture of health and wellness assesses and improves its programs regularly. Things that are measured can be improved. Today, integrated warehouses of data track medical claims, laboratory values, pharmaceuticals, disability events, workers' compensation cases, durable medical equipment use, and even absence from work or work performance. A culture of health and wellness analyzes these data streams to identify healthcare trends and determine whether its population is experiencing better health, less illness, and in the case of a work environment, improved performance.

Many corporations, universities, and healthcare systems have been recognized as benchmark examples of cultures of health and wellness and much can be learned from studying them. One review of benchmark programs identified seven common elements:

1. Employ health and wellness program features and incentives that are consistent with the organization's core mission, goals, operations, and administrative structures
2. Operate at multiple levels, simultaneously addressing individual, environmental, policy, and cultural factors in the organization
3. Target the most important healthcare issues among the employee population
4. Tailor diverse components to the unique needs and concerns of individuals
5. Achieve high rates of engagement and participation, both in the short and long term
6. Achieve successful health outcomes, cost savings, and additional organizational objectives
7. Are evaluated based on clear definitions of success, as reflected in scorecards and metrics agreed upon by all relevant constituencies[5]

My research suggests that benchmark employers have deployed over 200 elements that are available to organizations seeking to build a culture of health and wellness and that a critical mass of these elements (approximately two-thirds) is required for success. It is now possible to measure any organization's pursuit of a culture of health and wellness against these elements and also to generate a score that can be tracked over time.

Experts suggest that both of the foregoing approaches to measuring a culture of health and wellness are helpful; the former quantifies a reduction of illness over time while the latter provides guidance on narrowing the gaps when compared with benchmark organizations.[6]

WHAT IS A CULTURE OF HEALTH AND WELLNESS BENCHMARK ORGANIZATION?

The literature is a good source of information on benchmark organizations (e.g., peer-reviewed articles, a book by Pitney Bowes about its journey).[7] Conferences are conducted throughout the year highlighting best practices (e.g., the National Business Group on Health, the National Business Coalition on Health, the Institute of Health and Productivity Management, the Population Health Alliance, and the Population Health Colloquium). Among the many award programs recognizing best efforts are the Wellness Council of America, the Health Education Resource Organization, the American College of Occupational and Environmental Medicine, and the National Business Group on Health.[8–12]

Because benchmark cultures of health and wellness demonstrate significant reductions in healthcare expenditures and trends, many employers are pursuing benchmark performance to address their escalating healthcare costs. A benchmark culture of health and wellness documents high screening rates, high compliance with nationally recommended guidelines for care and low levels of unhealthy lifestyles. For example, after targeting smoking cessation over many years, Johnson & Johnson has decreased the number of smokers in its workforce to 7%.[13] Compared to the national incidence of over 20%, this is a remarkable achievement. An IBM initiative encouraging the use of primary care and medical homes has markedly reduced the number of employees who are "**medically homeless.**"[14]

Research shows that benchmark culture of health and wellness organizations start with a strong commitment from leadership. The state of Delaware's DelaWELL program is supported by the governor's declaration.[15] The Dow Chemical Company's benchmark effort is led by its CEO.[16] All benchmark organizations have data warehouses, and many have developed scorecards, dashboards, and cockpits to drive improvement at the department, business, and organizational levels. Most have physician executives whose jobs are dedicated to promoting health and wellness within the population. Trained in medicine and population management, these professionals are given adequate resources to identify and address opportunities for improvement on a population basis. They monitor and integrate all of the health-related programs from a clinical perspective (e.g., health risk assessments, biometric screenings, disease management services, disability management, and worker's compensation).

As previously mentioned, many culture of health and wellness benchmark programs have sophisticated branding, marketing, and communication strategies. Most leverage the workplace to create an environment conducive to health and wellness. Some have built comprehensive primary care centers and pharmacies on their campuses.[17] Most of these organizations provide health benefits, at least for their workforce and dependents. They have leveraged the science of evidence-based benefit design[18] to foster the appropriate use of health services and healthy lifestyles. A few benchmark employers enable workers to earn higher levels of coverage by taking better care of themselves and family members. Increasingly, they are utilizing **behavioral economics**[19] and in some cases, reducing their contribution to healthcare coverage when recommendations are not met. All are involved in multiyear strategies and following detailed **road maps** to achieving or maintaining **benchmark performance**.

HOW DOES AN ORGANIZATION GET STARTED?

There are a number of resources from credible sources that can help to create an organizational road map (e.g., the Change Agent Workgroup,[20] the American Hospital Association,[21] the Centers for Disease Control and Prevention,[22] and the American College of Occupational and Environmental Medicine).[23] The Change Agent Workgroup (a diverse group of experts in this space) published the following seven-step process to achieve a culture of health and wellness:

1. Establish a vision for health
2. Engage senior leadership and align management
3. Develop supporting **workplace environment** changes and implement workplace policies
4. Construct a comprehensive **integrated data warehouse** to analyze what ails the employee population and their families
5. Determine the measurements and goals for success
6. Utilize **value-based benefit design** and behavioral economics
7. Implement broad population health activities[20]

ESTABLISH A VISION FOR HEALTH

Nearly every organization of significant size has developed vision and mission statements along with values and objectives. Benchmark culture of health and wellness companies embrace an organizational mission and vision that incorporates the value of a healthy workforce. Because these organizations strongly believe that a healthy workforce is a competitive advantage in the marketplace, they require employees to be responsible for maintaining their health as part of the job function. Employees may even be encouraged to assist coworkers in their quests for health and wellness. To begin building a culture of health and wellness, a company's vision, mission, and values statements may need to be amended to clearly state the individual and collective responsibility of all people in the organization to maintain their health and foster well-being among all members of the company.

ENGAGE SENIOR LEADERSHIP AND ALIGN MANAGEMENT

Once the vision for health has been established, it must be promoted by the leadership and the management of the organization. Under the best of circumstances, the CEO provides periodic messages to the workforce to reinforce the importance of maintaining health and well-being. One way to communicate this is by videotaping a senior leader "walking the talk" (e.g., exercising) with a tag line such as "If I can find time to do it, so should you." Many organizations do not actively support taking the time necessary to exercise; stating this as part of every job description goes a long way to building a culture of health and wellness.

A consequence of health benefits being paid through a corporate function is that management is removed from any oversight, understanding, or need to monitor the health of the workforce. Benchmark companies are changing this (e.g., some management compensation and bonuses are being calculated in part by the trend in medical costs and the health status of their employee bases).

DEVELOP SUPPORTING WORKPLACE ENVIRONMENTAL CHANGES AND IMPLEMENT WORKPLACE POLICIES

To establish a foundation for a culture of health and wellness, an organization must provide environmental cues. For instance, most companies have addressed smoking cessation through a series of incremental steps, from designated smoking areas, to no smoking in facilities, to no smoking on campus. This initiative is often accompanied by expanded health benefits to cover all treatments and services to support smoking cessation. Some cutting-edge organizations have gone further (i.e., testing new applicants for nicotine in their urine and not hiring smokers).

To promote exercise in the workplace, benchmark organizations ensure that the stairwells are safe and inviting (i.e., clean, carpeted, heated and air-conditioned, with paintings on the walls and music piped in to increase their use). Signage at elevators promotes stairwell use as well.

Cafeterias and vending machines in benchmark organizations offer healthy options that are marketed by means of prominent placement and labeling—unhealthy options are discouraged by making them more difficult to find or reach. Entrée choices are identified as being healthy or not. **Best practice** includes subsidizing the healthy choices and taxing the unhealthy ones. Progressive organizations work with nutritionists to eliminate unhealthy options from cafeterias, vending machines, and catering policies.

CONSTRUCT A COMPREHENSIVE INTEGRATED DATA WAREHOUSE TO ANALYZE THE EMPLOYEE POPULATION AND THEIR FAMILIES AND TO TRACK PROGRESS OVER TIME

Managing the health of a population requires understanding the key health risks, conditions, and diseases. Benchmark organizations integrate medical, pharmacy, disability, and workers' compensation claims along with laboratory values, biometrics, health risk appraisal survey results, and absence data. Highly enlightened companies include presenteeism data in their analyses and use validated tools such as the Work Limitations Questionnaire[24] or the Health and Work Performance Questionnaire.[25] With these integrated inputs, world-class culture of health and wellness organizations can determine the financial effect of specific health risks, conditions, and diseases and prioritize programs and approaches in the best interest of the organization and the employees.[26]

UTILIZE VALUE-BASED BENEFIT DESIGN AND BEHAVIORAL ECONOMICS

Companies and organizations whose employees receive compensation and benefits may take advantage of additional methods to promote a healthy culture (i.e., they can manipulate compensation and benefits to reward healthy choices and behaviors). State-of-the-art culture of health and wellness organizations offer different benefit packages that employees and dependents earn by taking better care of themselves and making healthy choices. Those that meet a full panel of required healthy activities can earn the highest level of coverage. These companies work closely with consultants and third-party administrators to deliver a health benefit package that is evidence based (i.e., covers proven treatments at a high level and either provides no coverage or charges a steep copayment for unproven or low-value therapies). Benchmark companies understand the nuances of behavioral economics (e.g., recognizing that loss avoidance has a three times greater influence on behavior than do rewards), and they utilize health savings and health spending accounts to adjust coverage and apply the most influential approaches to rewards and penalties.[27]

IMPLEMENT BROAD POPULATION HEALTH ACTIVITIES INCLUDING PATIENT-CENTERED MEDICAL HOMES AND CHRONIC CARE MANAGEMENT

Whether it be a single company or a national initiative, a benchmark culture of health and wellness must take a comprehensive approach that addresses five key population cohorts across the continuum:

1. Those who are well
2. Those who are at risk
3. The acutely ill
4. The chronically ill
5. Those with catastrophic conditions

Programs must be established to keep well people well using a holistic approach that includes support for social, physical, emotional, career, intellectual environmental, and spiritual wellness, or SPECIES.[28] People who are well have social connections, are physically fit and emotionally stable, have a purposeful stimulating occupation with potential for advancement, and live in a safe setting that supports physical activity and healthy eating. To keep its population well, a benchmark culture of health and wellness must employ a broad-based, systematic effort to help reduce risks for chronic illness (e.g., attacking obesity, smoking, drug and alcohol abuse, and sedentary lifestyles).[29]

Access to health services must be ensured so that acute illnesses are treated promptly and potentially serious medical issues are addressed early. People with chronic illnesses must be provided condition management support to mitigate potential complications (e.g., people with diabetes must receive an annual eye exam to reduce a leading cause of blindness in America).[30]

Lastly, a comprehensive population management platform must provide **centers of excellence**[31] and compassionate care for those with catastrophic illness.[32] This most seriously ill population segment benefits greatly from intensive and expensive medical management and coordinated social services. When properly managed, there is a significant return on the dollars spent and great value delivered to the patient and his or her loved ones. With advance directives in place, efforts to eliminate futile care will benefit families and society alike.

ALIGNING KEY CONSTITUENCIES

Organizations intent on building a culture of health and wellness should leverage constituency partners, with strong consideration given to collaborating with other like-minded organizations in the community through business coalitions and local chambers of commerce. Increasingly, payer organizations, health plans, insurance companies, and consolidated health delivery systems are positioning themselves to be allies in this pursuit. With better **alignment of constituencies** such as among employers, providers, payers, and the citizens, great progress can be made.[33]

COMPARISON TO BENCHMARKS

Today, there are many benchmark efforts worth studying. Johnson & Johnson and Dow Chemical have published their respective outcomes and presented their successful programs in many forums. The previous leadership at Pitney Bowes published a book on their approach. The state of Delaware's DelaWELL program[34] is an excellent governmental effort directed at state employees. The University of Michigan[35] publishes an annual report on its program. As mentioned earlier, several institutions confer awards on organizations that have built a culture of health and wellness (e.g., the National Business Group on Health, the Health Education Resource Organization, and the American College of Occupational and Environmental Medicine). By studying the scoring systems deployed by these organizations, any organization can determine where it stands in relation to a benchmark performance. To use benchmark program information effectively, an organization should first identify gaps between its efforts and the cultivated culture of health programs. Once identified, the gaps can be prioritized, and the organization can build a multiyear strategic plan to achieve benchmark organization outcomes (i.e., lower healthcare costs and engender greater employee engagement and higher performance).

A MARKET-BASED SOLUTION TO THE HEALTHCARE CRISIS

When a critical mass of organizations in a community or region achieves a culture of health and wellness, the problems of rising healthcare costs and the increasing prevalence of chronic illness are likely to be slowed. Social pressures are likely to shift from consumption to promoting wellness. The healthcare industry, especially providers and payers, will begin to direct their attention to economic models that support the elevation of health status rather than delivering more health services. Employers will recognize that focusing on the well-being of their workforces is more than a nice thing to do—it is good business.

JUSTIFICATION AND BUSINESS CASE: THE CONNECTION BETWEEN HEALTH AND WEALTH

For many years, the prevailing belief was that nations had to attain wealth before they could become healthy. The recent experience in Africa, where the AIDS epidemic has markedly affected the potential workforce, has reshaped our collective thinking on this. Without a healthy working-age population, a country faces insurmountable challenges with respect to productivity and growth in its gross national product (e.g., Japan has a stagnant economy largely due to an aging demographic). This situation will begin to burden the United States as baby boomers retire and are not replaced by a comparable number of healthy young workers to maintain and advance productivity. When life expectancy is used as a proxy for health, there is a correlation between it and income at the state and national levels. Hans Rosling demonstrated this phenomenon in a powerful short film that looks at 200 countries over a span of 200 years.[36]

The relationship between health and wealth plays out at an individual level. Recently, Fidelity Investments estimated that a couple retiring at 65 in average health will need over $220,000 to pay for their out-of-pocket medical costs. If the couple reaches retirement in poor health, the figure could easily double or triple.[37] Correlating income to health status, health informatics specialists Wendy Lynch and Hank Gardner[38] suggest that higher income earners are more engaged in health and wellness activities. Healthy individuals also are more likely to be higher performers as demonstrated by the Lamplighter Program at Unilever.[39]

Published articles also support the notion that companies emphasizing the pursuit of a culture of health and wellness experience less escalation in healthcare costs[40] and outperform in the marketplace.[40] Whether one examines the issue from an individual, company, state, national, or global basis, there is compelling evidence confirming the connection between health and wealth.

CONCLUSION

Studying the achievement of organizations and communities who have successfully built a culture of health and wellness can provide great insights for us as a nation. Replicating these best practices on a broader scale can improve the health status of large populations and enhance the quality of life and performance of individuals at work and at home. Healthier citizens are more productive. The positive outcomes may include more prosperous communities, more involved family members, and more willing civic contributors. As we gradually move toward a national culture of health and wellness, fewer financial resources will be consumed treating illness and more can be directed to keeping well people well.

STUDY AND DISCUSSION QUESTIONS

1. What is a culture of health and wellness?
2. How can you build a culture of health and wellness?
3. Why does it make sense to pursue a culture of health and wellness?
4. Is there a connection between health and wealth?
5. What does it mean to bend the healthcare cost curve?

SUGGESTED READINGS AND WEBSITES

READINGS

Allen J. *Wellness Leadership: Creating Supportive Environments for Heathier and More Productive Employees*. Burlington, VT: Human Resources Institute; 2011.

Barry R, Murcko AC, Brubaker C. *The Six Sigma Book for Healthcare: Improving Outcomes by Reducing Errors*. Chicago, IL: Health Administration Press; 2002.

Bray I., ed. *Healthy Employees, Healthy Business: Easy Affordable Ways to Promote Workplace Wellness*. Berkeley, CA: Nolo; 2009.

Cascio W, Boudreau J. *Investing in People: Financial Impact of Human Resource Initiatives*. Mahwah, NJ: Pearson Education, Inc; 2008.

Edington DW. *Zero Trends*. Ann Arbor: University of Michigan Health Management Research Center; 2009.

Frampton S, Gilpin L, Charmel P. *Putting Patients First: Designing and Practicing Patient-Centered Care*. San Francisco: Jossey-Bass; 2003.

Kaplan RS, Norton DP. *The Balanced Scorecard: Translating Strategy into Action*. Boston: Harvard Business School Press; 1996.

LaPenna M. *Workplace Clinics and Employer Managed Healthcare: A Catalyst for Cost Savings and Improved Productivity*. New York: Productivity Press; 2010.

Lynch W, Gardner H. *Who Survives? How Benefit Costs Are Killing Your Company*. Cheyenne, WY: Health as Human Capital Foundation; 2011.

Pronk NP, ed. *ACSM's Worksite Health Handbook: A Guide to Building Healthy and Productive Companies*. 2nd ed. Indianapolis, IN: American College of Sports Medicine; 2009.

Rath T, Harter J. *Well Being: The Five Essential Elements*. New York: Gallup Press; 2010.

Stephano RM, Edelheit J. *Engaging Wellness: Corporate Wellness Programs That Work*. Palm Beach Gardens, FL: Corporate Health and Wellness Association; 2012.

WEBSITES

National Business Group on Health: https://www.businessgrouphealth.org/
National Business Coalition on Health: http://www.nbch.org/
Health Enhancement Resource Organization: http://www.the-hero.org/
Institute for Health and Productivity Management: http://www.ihpm.org/
Centers for Disease Control and Prevention: http://www.cdc.gov/
Integrated Benefits Institute: http://www.ibiweb.org/

REFERENCES

1. Fabius R, Frazee S. The culture of health. *Health & Productivity Management*. Winter 2009; 7(2):13-15.
2. World Health Organization. Preventing Chronic Diseases: A Vital Investment. WHO Global Report; 2005:18. http://www.who.int/chp/chronic_disease_report/en/. Accessed November 7, 2014.
3. Starfield B, Shi L, Macinko J. Contribution of primary care to health systems and health. *Milbank Q.* 2005;83(3):457-502.
4. An Employer Case Study of General Electric Company: Improving Employee Health Through Prevention. Washington, DC: National Business Group on Health; April 2009. https://www.businessgrouphealth.org/pub/f3160d59-2354-d714-51e1-d2863f892f1c. Accessed November 7, 2014.
5. Goetzel RZ, Shechter D, Ozminkowski RJ, et al. Promising practices in employer health and productivity management efforts: findings from a benchmarking study. *J Occup Environ Med.* 2007;49(20)111-30.
6. C-Suite Reporting Tools and Strategies. WebEx Board Meeting of the Institute on Health, Productivity and Human Capital. National Business Group on Health; April 24, 2012.
7. Mahoney J, Hom D. *Total Value, Total Return*. Philadelphia: The GlaxoSmithKline Group of Companies; 2006.

Edington DW. *Zero Trends*. Ann Arbor: University of Michigan Health Management Research Center; 2009.

Frampton S, Gilpin L, Charmel P. *Putting Patients First: Designing and Practicing Patient-Centered Care*. San Francisco: Jossey-Bass; 2003.

Kaplan RS, Norton DP. *The Balanced Scorecard: Translating Strategy into Action*. Boston: Harvard Business School Press; 1996.

LaPenna M. *Workplace Clinics and Employer Managed Healthcare: A Catalyst for Cost Savings and Improved Productivity*. New York: Productivity Press; 2010.

Lynch W, Gardner H. *Who Survives? How Benefit Costs Are Killing Your Company*. Cheyenne, WY: Health as Human Capital Foundation; 2011.

Pronk NP, ed. *ACSM's Worksite Health Handbook: A Guide to Building Healthy and Productive Companies*. 2nd ed. Indianapolis, IN: American College of Sports Medicine; 2009.

Rath T, Harter J. *Well Being: The Five Essential Elements*. New York: Gallup Press; 2010.

Stephano RM, Edelheit J. *Engaging Wellness: Corporate Wellness Programs That Work*. Palm Beach Gardens, FL: Corporate Health and Wellness Association; 2012.

WEBSITES

National Business Group on Health: https://www.businessgrouphealth.org/

National Business Coalition on Health: http://www.nbch.org/

Health Enhancement Resource Organization: http://www.the-hero.org/

Institute for Health and Productivity Management: http://www.ihpm.org/

Centers for Disease Control and Prevention: http://www.cdc.gov/

Integrated Benefits Institute: http://www.ibiweb.org/

REFERENCES

1. Fabius R, Frazee S. The culture of health. *Health & Productivity Management*. Winter 2009; 7(2):13-15.

2. World Health Organization. Preventing Chronic Diseases: A Vital Investment. WHO Global Report; 2005:18. http://www.who.int/chp/chronic_disease_report/en/. Accessed November 7, 2014.

3. Starfield B, Shi L, Macinko J. Contribution of primary care to health systems and health. *Milbank Q.* 2005;83(3):457-502.

4. An Employer Case Study of General Electric Company: Improving Employee Health Through Prevention. Washington, DC: National Business Group on Health; April 2009. https://www.businessgrouphealth.org/pub/f3160d59-2354-d714-51e1-d2863f892f1c. Accessed November 7, 2014.

5. Goetzel RZ, Shechter D, Ozminkowski RJ, et al. Promising practices in employer health and productivity management efforts: findings from a benchmarking study. *J Occup Environ Med.* 2007;49(20)111-30.

6. C-Suite Reporting Tools and Strategies. WebEx Board Meeting of the Institute on Health, Productivity and Human Capital. National Business Group on Health; April 24, 2012.

7. Mahoney J, Hom D. *Total Value, Total Return*. Philadelphia: The GlaxoSmithKline Group of Companies; 2006.

individuals also are more likely to be higher performers as demonstrated by the Lamplighter Program at Unilever.[39]

Published articles also support the notion that companies emphasizing the pursuit of a culture of health and wellness experience less escalation in healthcare costs[40] and outperform in the marketplace.[40] Whether one examines the issue from an individual, company, state, national, or global basis, there is compelling evidence confirming the connection between health and wealth.

CONCLUSION

Studying the achievement of organizations and communities who have successfully built a culture of health and wellness can provide great insights for us as a nation. Replicating these best practices on a broader scale can improve the health status of large populations and enhance the quality of life and performance of individuals at work and at home. Healthier citizens are more productive. The positive outcomes may include more prosperous communities, more involved family members, and more willing civic contributors. As we gradually move toward a national culture of health and wellness, fewer financial resources will be consumed treating illness and more can be directed to keeping well people well.

STUDY AND DISCUSSION QUESTIONS

1. What is a culture of health and wellness?
2. How can you build a culture of health and wellness?
3. Why does it make sense to pursue a culture of health and wellness?
4. Is there a connection between health and wealth?
5. What does it mean to bend the healthcare cost curve?

SUGGESTED READINGS AND WEBSITES

READINGS

Allen J. *Wellness Leadership: Creating Supportive Environments for Heathier and More Productive Employees*. Burlington, VT: Human Resources Institute; 2011.

Barry R, Murcko AC, Brubaker C. *The Six Sigma Book for Healthcare: Improving Outcomes by Reducing Errors*. Chicago, IL: Health Administration Press; 2002.

Bray I., ed. *Healthy Employees, Healthy Business: Easy Affordable Ways to Promote Workplace Wellness*. Berkeley, CA: Nolo; 2009.

Cascio W, Boudreau J. *Investing in People: Financial Impact of Human Resource Initiatives*. Mahwah, NJ: Pearson Education, Inc; 2008.

8. Corporate Health Achievement Awards. Amercian College of Occupational and Environmental Medicine. http://www.chaa.org/. Accessed November 7, 2014.

9. C. Everett Koop National Health Awards. Health Enhancement Resource Organization. http://www.thehealthproject.com/awards/. Accessed November 7, 2014.

10. Best Employers for Healthy Lifestyles award program. National Business Group on Health. http://www.businessgrouphealth.org/bestemployers/. Accessed November 7, 2014.

11. Healthyroads. American Specialty Health. http://www.ashcompanies.com/News/Default.aspx?id=19-75159. Accessed November 7, 2014.

12. Well Workplace Awards Initiative. WELCOA. http://www.wellworkplaceawards.org/. Accessed November 7, 2014.

13. Henke RM, Goetzel RZ, McHugh J, et al. Recent experience in health promotion at Johnson & Johnson: lower health spending, strong return on investment. *Health Affs*. 2011;30(3):490-9.

14. IBM Institute for Business Value. Patient-Centered Medical Home: What, Why, and How? http://www-01.ibm.com/common/ssi/cgi-bin/ssialias?infotype=PM&subtype=XB&appname=GBSE_GB_TI_USEN&htmlfid=GBE03207USEN&attachment=GBE03207USEN.PDF. Accessed November 7, 2014.

15. State of Delaware. Governor's "Healthy State Workplace" Page. http://delawell.delaware.gov/healthy-workplace.shtml. Accessed November 7, 2014.

16. Partnership for Prevention. Andrew Liveris, CEO, Dow Chemical, on Leading by Example August 2010. http://www.prevent.org/MediaModule/video/183/Andrew-Liveris-CEO-Dow-Chemical-on-Leading-by-Example-.aspx. Accessed November 7, 2014.

17. The Disney Blog. Walt Disney World opens on-site health and wellness center for cast members and families. http://thedisneyblog.com/2008/10/15/walt-disney-world-opens-on-site-health-and-wellness-center-for-cast-members-and-families/. Accessed November 7, 2014.

18. Darling, H. Evidence-Based Benefit Design. Conversations on the Changing Face of Managed Care: Insights from the 2006–2007 Podcast Series. http://citeseerx.ist.psu.edu/viewdoc/download?doi=10.1.1.131.8838&rep=rep1&type=pdf#page=23. Accessed November 7, 2014.

19. Volpp K, Asch D, Galvin R, et al. Redesigning employee health incentives: lessons from behavioral economics. *N Engl J Med*. 2011;365:388-90.

20. Change Agent Work Group. Employer Health Asset Management: A Roadmap for Improving the Health of Your Employees and Your Organization; 2009. http://www.aon.com/attachments/improving_health.pdf. Accessed November 7, 2014.

21. American Hospital Association. A Call to Action: Creating a Culture of Health; January 2011. http://www.aha.org/research/cor/content/creating-a-culture-of-health.pdf. Accessed November 7, 2014.

22. Centers for Disease Control and Prevention. Workplace Health Model. http://www.cdc.gov/workplacehealthpromotion/model/index.html. Accessed November 7, 2014.

23. Hymel PA, Loeppke RR, Baase CM, et al. Workplace health protection and promotion: a new pathway for a healthier—and safer—workforce. *J Occup Environ Med*. 2011;53(6):695-702. http://www.acoem.org/uploadedFiles/Public_Affairs/Policies_And_Position_Statements/Guidelines/Guidelines/Workplace%20Health%20Protection%20and%20Promotion.pdf. Accessed November 7, 2014.

24. Burton WN, Pransky G, Conti DJ, et al. The association of medical conditions and presenteeism. *J Occup Environ Med*. 2004;46:538-45.

25. Kessler RC, Stang PE. *Health and Work Productivity: Making the Business Case for Quality Health Care*. Chicago: University of Chicago Press; 2006.

26. Goetzel RZ, Long SR, Ozminkowski RJ, et al. Health, absence, disability, and presenteeism: cost estimates of certain physical and mental health conditions affecting U.S. employers. *J Occup Environ Med*. 2004;46(4):399-412.

27. Houy M. Value-Based Benefit Design: A Purchaser's Guide. National Business Coalition on Health; January 2009. http://www.bailit-health.com/articles/valuebased_apg_bhp.pdf

28. Abbott Solutions Inc. SPECIES—7 Dimensions of Wellness: Survival of the Species. http://www

.7dimensionsofwellness.com/History-of-Wellness
.php. Accessed November 7, 2014.

29. Pronk N, Lowry M, Kottke T, et al. Association between optimal lifestyle adherence and short-term incidence of chronic conditions among employees. *Popul Health Manag.* 2010;13(6):289-95.

30. Schoenfeld ER, Greene MJ, Wu SY, et al. Patterns of adherence to diabetes vision care guidelines. *Opthalmology.* 2001;108(3):563-71.

31. Coulter CH, Fabius R, Hecksher V, et al. Assessing HMO centers of excellence programs: one employer's experience. *Manag Care Q.* 1998; 6(1):8-15.

32. Pawlecki JB. End of life: a workplace issue. *Health Aff.* 2010;29(1):141-6.

33. Environmental Scan: Role of Corporate America in Community Health and Wellness. Health Enhancement Resource Organization Research Project Submitted to the Institute of Medicine Roundtable on Population Health Improvement; January 2014. http://www.iom.edu/~/media/Files/Activity Files/ PublicHealth/PopulationHealthImprovementRT/ Background-Papers/PopHealthEnvScan.pdf. Accessed November 7, 2014.

34. Dela*WELL* Health Management Program 2013– 2014 Overview. http://delawell.delaware.gov/ documents/2013-2014-program-overview .pdf?ver=0905. Accessed November 7, 2014.

35. CY2012 Annual Report: Building a Model Community of Health at the University of Michigan. http://www.hr.umich.edu/mhealthy/news/ pdf/cy12-annual-report.pdf. Accessed November 7, 2014.

36. Hans Rosling's 200 Countries, 200 Years, 4 Minutes. www.youtube.com/watch?v=jbkSRLYSojo. Accessed November 7, 2014.

37. Fidelity Investments. Retiree Health Costs Hold Steady https://www.fidelity.com/viewpoints/retirement/ retirees-medical-expensesEAccessed December 30th 2014Lynch W, Gardner H. *Who Survives? How Benefit Costs Are Killing Your Company.* Cheyenne, WY: Health as Human Capital Foundation; 2011, Chapter 8.

38. Unilever Lamplighter Program. Report for John Cooper and Dean Patterson. Conference Presentations; 2013. http://www.world-heart-federation .org/fileadmin/user_upload/images/world-heart-day/2010/WHD_Employers_resource_guide/ case_studies/WHDCSUnileverLamplighter.pdf. Accessed January 9, 2015.

39. Goetzel RZ, Henke RM, Benevent R, et al. The predictive validity of the HERO scorecard in determining future health care cost and risk trends. *J Occup Environ Med.* 2014;56(2):136-44.

40. Fabius R, Thayer D. The link between workforce health and safety and the health of the bottom line. *J Occup Environ Med.* 2013;55(9):993-1000.

THE POPULATION HEALTH PROMISE

RAYMOND J. FABIUS, VALERIE P. PRACILIO,
DAVID B. NASH, AND JANICE L. CLARKE*

Executive Summary

The population health promise is to promote health and prevent disease; the strategy is to create an epidemic of health and wellness.

The Patient Protection and Affordable Care Act (ACA) of 2010 codified and set in motion an array of programs and initiatives aimed at improving the health of the U.S. population. Although considerable progress is being made on many fronts—from making health insurance accessible to more Americans to increasing accountability for and quality of healthcare delivery and services—the need for population health management continues to be urgent.[1]

Population health refers broadly to the distribution of health outcomes within a population, the health determinants that influence distribution, and the policies and interventions that affect those determinants.[2,3] Accordingly, population health is holistic in that it seeks to reveal *patterns and connections* within and among multiple systems and to develop approaches that respond to the needs of populations. Population health tactics include rigorous analysis of outcomes. Understanding population-based patterns of outcomes distribution is a critical antecedent to addressing population needs in communities (i.e., patterns inform the selection of effective population health management strategies to diminish problems and develop approaches to prevent reoccurrence in the future).

Convened by the National Quality Forum in 2008, the National Priorities Partnership addressed four major healthcare challenges that affect all Americans: eliminating harm, eradicating disparities, reducing disease burden, and removing waste.[4] One of the

---

*This chapter includes contributions made by JoAnne Reifsnyder, PhD, ACHPN, in the first edition.

six priorities identified to address these challenges is *improving the health of the population*. While ambitious, this goal is fundamental to healthcare reform. Improving the health of the population will require improved efforts to provide health insurance coverage, promote healthy behaviors, and prevent illness. The "silos" in healthcare delivery must be dismantled, and providers must work cooperatively to advance seamless, coordinated care that traverses settings, health conditions, and reimbursement mechanisms. Interdisciplinary teams of healthcare providers committed to diligent management of chronic conditions and providing safe, high-quality care will play a central role. Policy makers will be called upon to craft policies that support illness prevention, health promotion, and public health, and healthcare professionals must continue their efforts to enforce recommendations in communities. All of these efforts must align to promote health and wellness and to advance a new population health agenda. Population health is no longer a mere strategy—it is the solution that holds the greatest promise for creating *an epidemic of health and wellness*.

Learning Objectives

1. Explain the concept of population health.
2. Recognize the need for a population health approach to healthcare education, delivery, and policy.
3. Discuss the integration of the four pillars of population health.
4. Utilize this text as a resource for further population health study and practice.

Key Terms

chronic care management
health policy
healthcare quality
National Priorities Partnership

patient safety
population health
population health management
public health

INTRODUCTION

Although the term **population health** is not new, there is no clear consensus on a single definition. In the evolving U.S. healthcare environment, where the need for positive change is evident and ongoing, population health is viewed across constituencies as a promising solution for closing key gaps in healthcare delivery. In the context of this text, population health is defined as the distribution of health outcomes within a population, the health determinants that influence distribution, and the policies and interventions that affect the determinants.[2,3]

Population health embraces a comprehensive agenda—the healthy and unhealthy, the acutely ill and chronically ill, and the clinical and nonclinical as well as the public sector and private sector. While there are many determinants that affect the health of populations, the ultimate goal for healthcare providers, public health professionals, employers, payers, and policy makers is the same: healthy people comprising healthy populations that create productive workforces and thriving communities.

Population health is both a concept of health and a field of study.[2] Populations can be defined by geography or grouped according to some common element (e.g., employees, ethnicity, medical condition). As the name implies, population health is inclusive of every individual and group, comprising a heterogeneous population that wears many labels. For example, a man of Mexican descent who works for a carpenters union may be a member of three different populations: the Mexican community, an employer's organization, and the carpenters union. To address needs at the population level, all of these associations must be considered.

As a field of study, attention must be given to multiple determinants of health outcomes, including medical care, public health interventions, and the social environment, as well as the physical environment and individual behaviors, and the patterns among each of these domains.[5] The purpose of this chapter and those that follow is to promote an understanding of population health, to encourage discussions and engagement of key stakeholders (healthcare providers, public health professionals, payers/health plans, employers, and policy makers), and to foster the development and dissemination of strategies aimed at improving population health.

THE CURRENT STATE OF POPULATION HEALTH

Health care in the United States is complex, and many would argue that its healthcare "system" bears little resemblance to a true system. Considering the characteristics of systems (e.g., interactivity of independent elements to form a complex whole, harmonious or orderly interaction, and coordinated methods or procedures), U.S. health care may well represent the antithesis.

Despite devoting more than 17% of its gross domestic product (GDP) to health care (projected to approach 20% by 2020),[6] the United States performs lower on five dimensions of performance (quality, access, efficiency, equity, and healthy lives) compared to similar developed countries, including Australia, Canada, Germany, the Netherlands, New Zealand, and the United Kingdom. The common element among the aforementioned nations is a universal healthcare delivery system, and some argue that the absence of universal health care in the United States explains the access disparities, inequity, and poor outcomes in addition to the exorbitant and uncontrolled costs.[7]

Unfortunately, the health status of the U.S. population does not reflect the high level of spending on health care. For example:

- Of adults ages 18 to 64 years, 14% reported that they did not receive needed medical care in 2011, and 11% indicated they did not get needed prescription drugs in the past 12 months because of their cost.[8]

- Major disparities exist based on socioeconomic status. Roughly 40 million[9] Americans are still uninsured, and 112 million Americans (almost half of the U.S. population, 45%) suffer from at least one chronic condition.[10]
- **Healthcare quality** is suboptimal and **patient safety** is lagging.[8,11]
- The public health system continues to be egregiously underfunded.[12]

The passing of the ACA and the subsequent phased implementation of a broad range of regulations and initiatives aimed at improving the health of the U.S. population have brought about some positive change; however, it will take many years before the benefits are realized on a population scale,[1] and the need for population health management remains urgent.

Because important advances in science and technology have contributed to increases in life expectancy of more than 30 years in the 20th century,[13] unprecedented growth in the population of older adults has introduced new pressures on healthcare providers, payers, and communities. Roughly two-thirds of Medicare recipients contend with two or more chronic conditions, and 16% deal with six or more. In 2010, 58% of Medicare Fee-for-Service beneficiaries had hypertension, 31% had ischemic heart disease, and 28% were diabetic.[14] Chronic conditions require frequent monitoring and evaluation, which places a strain on the healthcare system and makes the need for care coordination imperative. Traditionally, the United States has supported a "sick care" system bolstered by payment policies that reward both consumers and providers for health care that is sought primarily when acute illness strikes or in an emergency. While caring for the sick will always be an integral part of health care, true population health can be achieved only by placing an equal emphasis on health promotion and disease prevention.

POPULATION HEALTH DEFINED

Population health is the distribution of health outcomes within a population, the determinants that influence distribution, and the policies and interventions that affect the determinants.[2,3] These three key components—health outcomes, health determinants, and policies—serve as the foundation for this chapter and those that follow.

Health determinants, the varied factors that affect the health of individuals, range from aspects of the social and economic environment to the physical environment and individual characteristics or behaviors.[15] Although some of these factors can be controlled by individuals, some are external to an individual's locus of control. For example, individuals may be coached to adopt healthier lifestyles, thereby reducing their risk for lifestyle-related diseases (e.g., hypertension, diabetes, and smoking-related illnesses). The same individuals may be genetically predisposed to cardiovascular disease or may reside in geographic locations where exercise outdoors is unsafe or air quality is extremely poor—these health determinants are outside of their control.

Health determinants are a core component of the ecological model used in **public health** to describe the interaction between behavior and health.[16] The model assumes that overall health and well-being are influenced by interaction among the determinants of health.[17] Relationships with peers, family, and friends influence behavior at the interpersonal level. At the community level, there are institutional factors (e.g., rules, regulations) that influence social networks. At the public level, policies and laws regulate certain behaviors.[13] These variables have a cumulative effect on health and the ability of individuals and populations to stay well in the communities where they live, work, and play.

Interaction among the determinants of health leads to outcomes, the second component of the population health definition. Population- and individual-level disparities and risk factors exert significant influence on health-related outcomes. General health outcomes could be improved by assuring access to quality health care for all populations, regardless of insurance status, with a primary focus on health maintenance and prevention to decrease health risks. Policy development is one mechanism used to support population health management and improvement. Support and guidance for these efforts is provided by policies at local, state, and federal levels.

Population health is not synonymous with public health. In fact, public health is a core element of population health that focuses on determinants of health in communities, preventive care, interventions and education, and individual and collective health advocacy and policies. The principal characteristic that differentiates population health from public health is its focus on a *broad set of concerns* rather than on just these specific activities.[2] Population health efforts generate information to inform public health strategies that can be deployed in communities. The combination of information gathered to define problems and build awareness and the strategies to address needs comprises **population health management**.

Consider Wendy McDonald, a hypothetical community member whose situation illustrates the importance of considering multiple factors when using a population health approach. Wendy is obese and lives in a lower-income community where healthy food is unavailable. Safe neighborhood parks and recreation centers are lacking, making physical activity a challenge. Inadequate health insurance restricts her ability to receive primary medical care or guidance from a healthcare provider on how to manage her weight, and she is unaware of the disease risk factors it presents. The population health conceptual model suggests effective approaches to care delivery in such situations. A primary care practice in communities such as Wendy's could be reengineered as a patient-centered medical home that applies a comprehensive, integrated approach to disease and **chronic care management** and supports health promotion and disease prevention, which would lead to better short- and long-term health outcomes. A community-based population health approach to address Wendy's challenges might include adding green space for recreation and supporting healthy food options through tax credits to food stores that offer them. Underlying both of these approaches are policies that support community improvements, make health a priority that leads to better health outcomes, and may be shared with public health initiatives.

Donald Berwick, MD, president and CEO of the Institute for Healthcare Improvement (IHI), once remarked health care has no inherent value, health does. The population health promise requires a broader focus—one that encompasses health promotion and disease prevention as well as caring for the sick. Under the traditional healthcare model, individuals seek care to restore health when it is compromised and seek prevention primarily when they are fearful about potential loss of health. Under an aspirational model of health and wellness promotion, individuals would value their health and seek preventive care as a means to optimize it. Ultimately, the intrinsic reward of feeling well should be a major driver of population health in a true "culture of wellness."

FOUNDATIONS OF POPULATION HEALTH

THE SCIENCE

Health is a state of well-being; population health provides a conceptual framework for the study of well-being and variability among populations.[5,13] In the United States, the delivery of healthcare services receives the lion's share of health-related resources and attention, and yet it is only one of many contributors to and drivers of a population's overall health (e.g., the business and political communities). There is substantial, yet unrealized, opportunity to advance the population health agenda and to improve health through efforts focusing on personal behavior and health promotion within each of these spheres.[18]

The expectation that healthcare providers must care for *their* own patients in *their* own practice settings is rapidly changing as new models for affecting outcomes at the population level are introduced. Treatment of populations aims to increase recommended prevention and screening practices and improve adherence to recommended treatment in accordance with evidence-based, nationally recognized guidelines. These aims can be achieved only with teams of healthcare providers cooperating within and across settings. While one-at-a-time treatment has been the traditional approach to patient care, population-level interventions that integrate a set of common aims and standards are needed to support significant and sustainable health improvements in the United States. This effort has been aided by the adoption of electronic medical records and the promotion of their meaningful use to improve accessibility of actionable health information.[19]

Management of chronic disease is a key priority in population health. The fact that nearly half of all Americans have one or more chronic diseases is only partly explained by population growth and increases in longevity. The present and predicted burden of chronic disease is the strongest signal that current strategies for helping people get well, and stay well, are ineffective. The burgeoning population, and the prevalence of chronic illness that accompanies it, drives both cost and utilization of healthcare services and threatens Americans' progress in life expectancy.

There is ample evidence to inform population health improvement strategies, but processes remain poorly defined and success is variable. Although numerous national goals for population health have been proposed and targeted outcomes have been defined, translating best practices into action is a daunting challenge. The Chronic Care Model is a well regarded conceptual model for guiding the development of effective programs to provide better chronic care to patients. The devil is, of course, in the details. Each of the six system components that comprise the Chronic Care Model (Patient Care and Practice Improvement Organization, Clinical Information Systems, Delivery System Design, Decision Support, Self-Management, and Community Resources) is covered in some detail in subsequent chapters of this text (Figure 1-1). The emerging understanding of what is required to build "cultures of health" will be of value, as will the recognition of complementary activities in support of an improved delivery process (e.g., social and environmental factors).[20]

The greatest contributor to premature death from preventable chronic illness is patient behavior. Of the six model components, the degree to which patients are informed and active is critical to improved patient outcomes. Informed, active patients are more likely to learn self-management strategies and to adopt healthy behaviors. Providers need an array of tools to effectively help patients manage their chronic conditions. Because they typically have neither the time nor the resources to consult the evidence base during a patient encounter, they need robust clinical decision support tools at the point of care. Further, providers need a reimbursement model that rewards appropriate interdisciplinary communication, collaboration, and follow-up, as well as access to interoperable

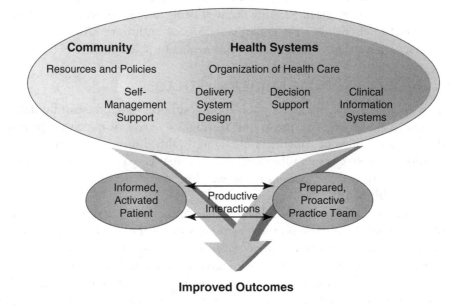

Improved Outcomes

Figure 1-1 The chronic care model.

technologies that permit data sharing in real time. All of these components must be supported by clinical information systems that track progress in the management of chronic conditions. These practice-based components, combined with community efforts (e.g., community-wide screenings, in-home support for elderly persons, nutritious school lunch programs) and active participation of patients who productively interact with healthcare providers, will support effective, quality chronic care management while reducing health risks and costs.[21]

One of the greatest challenges to improving the population's health is translating evidence into practice. Two state initiatives provide examples of successful population health strategies in action:

- Vermont: State legislation supports efforts to provide high-quality care and control costs. The Vermont Department of Health implemented a Blueprint for Health, which focuses on improving health and the healthcare system through prevention. Early assessment of these efforts shows reductions in health expenditure trends and hospitalization rates.[22]
- Wisconsin: David Kindig, a key thought leader in population health, is driving efforts to earn the designation of "healthiest state." The state earmarked 35% of monies realized from the sale of insurance stock to improve public health. Public health and **health policy** practitioners across the state are collaborating to assess population health status and to develop a plan to achieve health with less disparity.[23,24]

Both the Vermont and Wisconsin initiatives demonstrate that population health extends beyond health care. Achieving health and well-being at the individual, population, state, and national levels requires the collective efforts of healthcare providers, public health professionals, payers and health plans, employers, and policy makers.

THE EFFECT ON AND RESPONSE BY THE MARKETPLACE

There is a shared responsibility for population health. Although the cost burden of health care is shared among all constituents, the distribution of costs is not always proportionate. With more than 60% of Americans obtaining health insurance coverage through their employers, businesses have a substantial stake in their employees' health.[25] As healthcare costs continue to escalate, businesses are searching for strategies to decrease the cost of employee health benefits without compromising quality.

The health of its employees influences the economic health of a business—a healthy employee is more productive on the job and misses fewer days of work. The bottom line is that prevention generates a positive return on investment for employers. In 2009, an average of $3.27 in healthcare costs were saved for every dollar spent on employee wellness programs.[26] In this scenario everyone benefits—employees are healthier, businesses can operate more cost effectively through improved employee performance and reduced health benefits costs, and health plans reduce outlays for preventable morbidity. In some cases, the productivity gains exceed the healthcare cost savings for employers.[27] Moreover, there is evidence that companies focusing on the health and safety of their workforces produce greater returns for their shareholders.[28] Worksites are an ideal venue for promoting health and wellness because consumers spend the majority of their time at work.

While the business case for promoting wellness is clear, competing priorities present a challenge in many organizations. Corporate cultures, investment costs, incentives for participation in the initiative, and employee underlying health behaviors are potential barriers to implementing a successful workplace wellness program. However, workplace programs may be effective in three major domains of health: promoting behavior change to prevent illness, supporting employees to self-manage existing chronic conditions, and assisting in the navigation of a complex and fragmented healthcare system.

Forty percent of premature deaths can be attributed to behavior. In fact, behavior is a key contributor to two of the leading causes of preventable death: obesity and smoking.[26] Workplace smoking cessation programs have been effective in mitigating risk for health effects of smoking, which cost employers $3,391 per smoker per year.[29] Employer involvement in health plan–supported disease management efforts or health advocacy programs provides employees with access to education and tools to properly manage their conditions and seek the most appropriate care. The best available evidence concerning employer sponsorship of health and wellness programs supports the premise that employees who are well provide the greatest benefit to their organization.[30,31]

THE POLITICS

Prevention, health, and wellness efforts must be supported by policy and regulation to advance the population health agenda. Building awareness is the first step toward making lasting change, followed by identifying population health needs and recognizing the importance of data and measurements on which causal inferences are based and actions are taken. For example, current rates of obesity and smoking in the United States represent needs that must be addressed through population-based initiatives.[27] Policies that drive population health efforts must be created at the local, state, and national levels to serve as the foundation of the population health infrastructure. Because implementation of population health improvement policies often requires significant resources, stakeholders face difficult decisions about priorities. Federal monies made health improvement initiatives possible in Vermont and Wisconsin.[22,23,24]

The healthcare workforce that will provide high-quality, population-based health care in the future must be trained now, and education reform is under way to ensure the competency of future leaders and practitioners in health care, public health, business, and health policy. Finally, research is needed to inform strategies to address population health approaches. Similar to the potential benefits of disease management and wellness initiatives realized by employers, policies that support health and wellness will also contribute to the wealth of the nation.

FRAMEWORKS FOR INNOVATION

A few key initiatives provide a framework for innovation that aspires to make population health efforts the norm rather than the exception. As in all industries, common goals and objectives and guidelines and standards in health care provide an understanding of expectations and drive efforts to provide safe, quality care.

HEALTHY PEOPLE 2020

Since 1979, the U.S. Department of Health and Human Services (HHS) has been leading efforts to promote health and prevent disease through identification of threats and implementation of mechanisms to reduce threats. *Healthy People* sets national health objectives for a 10-year period based on broad consensus and founded on scientific evidence.[32] *Healthy People 2020* contains 38 focus areas and four overarching goals:

1. Attaining high-quality, longer lives free of preventable disease, disability, injury, and premature death
2. Achieving health equity, eliminating disparities, and improving the health of all groups
3. Creating social and physical environments that promote good health for all
4. Promoting quality of life, healthy development, and healthy behaviors across all life stages[33]

The *Healthy People* objectives are used by public health professionals to drive community efforts based on defined needs. Containing both clinical and nonclinical measures, *Healthy People* also serves as a guide for population health efforts and a road map for interdisciplinary collaboration that leads to shared responsibility for health and wellness. Also important, it introduces the concept of cultural transformation and the benefits of leveraging social and physical environmental influences to elevate the health status of populations.

TRIPLE AIM

In 2007, the IHI launched the Triple Aim, providing an agenda for optimizing performance on three dimensions of care: the health of a defined population, the experience of care for individuals in the population, and the cost per capita for providing care for this population.[34] "Population" is defined by enrollment or inclusion in a registry. Groups of individuals defined by geography, condition, or other attributes can be considered a population if data are available to track them over time. At the core of this initiative are efforts to optimize value. A number of integrators across the United States are working to implement strategies to achieve the Triple Aim. At the macro level, integrators pool resources and make sure the system structure and processes support the needs of the population. At the micro level, integrators ensure that the most appropriate care is provided to patients with respect to overuse, underuse, and misuse.[35] To successfully achieve the Triple Aim, healthcare institutions and delivery systems must reduce hospitalizations, apply resources to patient care that are commensurate with their needs, and build sustained relationships that are mindful of patient needs.[36] While a great deal of work remains to achieve optimal performance on the three objectives, the Triple Aim has built awareness and offers a framework for population health management.

NATIONAL PRIORITIES AND GOALS

Many groundbreaking reports have grabbed the public's attention and informed priorities for improvement, but few have set forth action plans to reach the goals. In this regard, the **National Priorities Partnership** (NPP) is unique. The NPP is a partnership of 52 major national organizations with a shared vision to achieve better health and a safe, equitable, and value-driven healthcare system.[36]

This collaborative was convened by the National Quality Forum and tasked with developing a set of national priorities and goals. Recognizing that "we must fundamentally change the ways in which we deliver care" to improve access to safe, effective, and affordable health care, the NPP envisioned a plan to achieve transformational change. The priorities were set with four key challenges in mind: eliminating harm, eradicating disparities, reducing disease burden, and removing waste. To address these challenges, six national priorities were established (in cooperation with the HHS) in September 2011:

1. Work with communities to promote wide use of best practices to enable healthy living and well-being
2. Promote the most effective prevention, treatment, and intervention practices for the leading causes of mortality, starting with cardiovascular disease
3. Ensure person- and family-centered care
4. Make care safer
5. Promote effective communication and care coordination
6. Make quality care more affordable for individuals, families, employers, and governments by developing and spreading new healthcare delivery models

To meet the first national priority and establish a population health framework, the NPP set forth the following questions that need to be addressed:

- How can individuals and multistakeholder groups come together to address community health improvement?
- Which individuals and organizations should be at the table?
- What processes and methods should communities use to assess their health?
- What data are available to assess, analyze, and address community health needs and to measure improvement?
- What incentives exist that can drive alignment and coordination to improve community health?
- How can communities advance more affordable care by achieving greater alignment, efficiency, and cost savings?

Achieving this national priority requires that health and wellness be fostered at the community level through a partnership between public health agencies, healthcare purchasers, and healthcare systems. The goal is to promote preventive services, healthy lifestyle behaviors, and measurement based on a national index to assess health status.[37] These priorities and projects will continue to spur action and innovation and serve as a model for population health improvement.

PREVENTIVE STRATEGIES AND PILLARS OF POPULATION HEALTH

To achieve the ambitious goal of improving the U.S. healthcare system, we must be prepared to broaden our current focus beyond acute, episodic health care. This implies a collective commitment to incorporating population-based primary and secondary prevention strategies—as citizens and as healthcare providers—as well as better coordinating care for those suffering from chronic illnesses to mitigate complications, also known as tertiary prevention.

PREVENTIVE STRATEGIES

National experts and policy analysts agree that focusing on primary prevention strategies (e.g., health promotion and wellness activities) will ultimately improve the overall health of citizens and decrease the costs associated with overmedicalization. Three lifestyle modifications—eliminating and reducing tobacco use, eating healthy foods with portion control, and increasing regular physical activity—are consistently identified in population-based epidemiologic research as most likely to reduce the prevalence of chronic conditions. Utilizing secondary preventive services (e.g., cancer screenings, blood pressure and cholesterol monitoring, health counseling) promotes early detection of disease. Secondary prevention strategies seek to reduce barriers to early treatment or completion of therapy, thereby improving treatment outcomes and reducing disease chronicity. Detecting an early stage breast cancer during mammography and initiating treatment is an example of secondary prevention.

Tertiary prevention focuses on minimizing disease complications and comorbidities through appropriate, evidence-based treatment and—critical to reducing healthcare costs—by coordinating and providing continuity of care for chronic conditions. This is best accomplished by incorporating the Chronic Care Model into healthcare systems and monitoring disease-specific indicators to ensure quality care and maximize quality of life for patients and their families.[30] Prevention and disease management are integral to maintaining population health and encouraging wellness. All healthcare professionals have a role to play.

THE FOUR PILLARS

Population health rests on four pillars (Figure 1-2):

- Care management
- Quality and safety

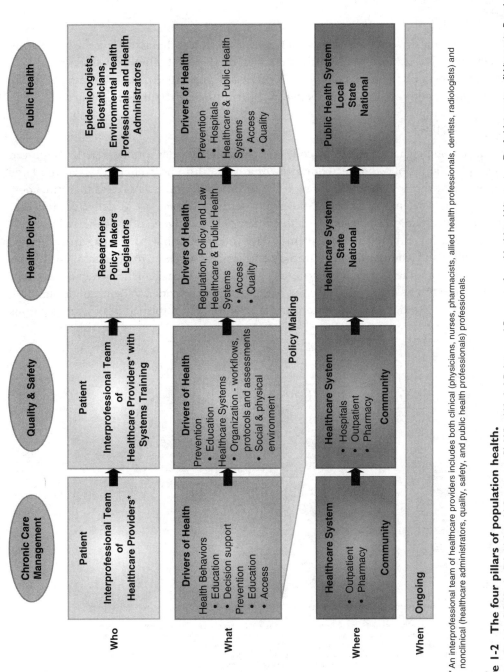

Figure 1-2 The four pillars of population health.
Data from Booske BC, Kindig DA, Nelson H, Remington PL. What Works? Policies and Programs for a Healthier Wisconsin—Draft. University of Wisconsin Population Health Institute; January 2009.

* An interprofessional team of healthcare providers includes both clinical (physicians, nurses, pharmacists, allied health professionals, dentists, radiologists) and nonclinical (healthcare administrators, quality, safety, and public health professionals) professionals.

- Public health
- Health policy

The interaction between each of these pillars in education and practice lays the foundation for achieving population health goals and strategies (Figure 1-3). National statistics show that only 55% of U.S. adults receive recommended preventive care, acute care, and care for chronic conditions, such as hypertension (high blood pressure) and diabetes.[11]

CARE MANAGEMENT

This fact alone signals a need for collective patient, provider, public health, employer, health plan, and policy maker efforts to improve health and wellness. Given the large proportion of the population suffering from chronic conditions, it is clear that care coordination must be improved across the many settings where care is delivered and that evidence-based clinical management and effective self-management must be actively promoted. Behavior and prevention play important roles in chronic care management. Access to screening and counseling for chronic conditions is integral to successful treatment. Education is another key component in chronic care management because treatment decisions need to be made jointly by the patient and the provider. Patients' understanding of their diseases and treatment options is essential for well informed healthcare decisions

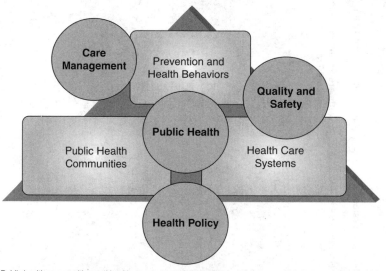

Public health communities and healthcare systems serve as the foundation on which the population health infrastructure rests. Healthcare providers, researchers, policy makers, legislators and public health professionals who work in the public health communities and healthcare systems partner with patients to focus on prevention and healthy behaviors. Professionals in chronic care management, quality and safety, public health, and health policy must work together to develop a framework to prevent conditions that burden the population both physically and economically. Interdisciplinary collaboration will strengthen the foundation of the population health infrastructure and lead to improved population health management.

Figure 1-3   An interdisciplinary model for population health.

and adherence to treatment. In combination, these efforts support quality of life and function, contribute to the health of populations, and reduce the use of costly acute care for preventable problems arising from poorly managed chronic illness.

QUALITY AND SAFETY

Quality and safety improvement rely on "activated" patients and provider teams that are motivated to examine the structure and organization of healthcare delivery and rectify the processes or workflows that lead to errors. Since the 1999 Institute of Medicine report, *To Err Is Human*, a number of national and professional organizations have identified best practices and made recommendations on how to design systems and processes to make healthcare safer.[38] Synergy between these groups will be integral to achieving gains in quality and safety. Local, state, and national public health efforts must support and complement the work being done in local healthcare institutions. The resulting public attention and awareness of quality and safety goals can serve to activate consumers.

PUBLIC HEALTH AND HEALTH POLICY

Through interaction with communities and healthcare institutions, public health professionals serve as educators and advocates. The third pillar, public health, provides a framework for identifying health determinants, health disparities, and disease burden and for implementing strategies to address community-wide health concerns. As the fourth pillar, policy efforts support population-focused care management, quality and safety, and public health (e.g., policy support in pay-for-performance initiatives that drive adoption of community-wide quality and safety standards). Taken a step further, making comparison data available for other healthcare constituents and consumers (i.e., transparency) creates a sense of accountability for performance and an impetus for improvement. Future policy changes supporting transparency and public accountability for health and wellness will be necessary to meet the population health promise. Taken together, the population health goals, strategies, and implementation tactics associated with the four pillars of care management, quality and safety, public health, and health policy will drive population health efforts to achieve health and wellness.

CONCLUSION

The United States is faced with many issues in health care, and the strategies used to address both existing and emerging challenges will determine the future health status of our nation. To improve the health of the nation, our focus must shift from health care that is reactive to health care that is proactive and promotes health and wellness.[30] Although population needs have been identified in current literature, a reproducible, population health action plan has yet to be established to address them. In the words of Goethe, "Knowing is not enough; we must apply. Willing is not enough; we must do."[39] It will require the collective efforts of many to truly create transformational change. This chapter is intended to prime readers for further exploration of population health efforts to promote health and wellness. In effect, it is a statement of population health's promise as well as a call to action.

STUDY AND DISCUSSION QUESTIONS

1. What is population health?
2. Why is a population health approach needed to promote health and wellness?
3. How do the four pillars of population health work together to improve population health?
4. What is your role in population health?

SUGGESTED READINGS AND WEBSITES

READINGS

Academic Medicine. 2008;83(4):319-421. Population health education theme issue.

Institute of Medicine. *Crossing the Quality Chasm: A New Health System for the 21st Century.* Washington, DC: National Academy Press; 2001.

Institute of Medicine. *To Err Is Human: Building a Safer Health System.* Washington, DC: National Academy Press; 2000.

Kindig D, Stoddart G. What is population health? *Am J Public Health.* 2003;93:380-83.

Kindig DA. Understanding population health terminology. *Milbank Q.* 2007;85:139-61.

National Priorities Partnership. *National priorities and goals: Aligning our efforts to transform America's healthcare.* Washington, DC: National Quality Forum; 2008. http://psnet.ahrq.gov/resource.aspx?resourceID=8745

WEBSITES

Dartmouth Atlas of Health Care: http://www.dartmouthatlas.org/

The Population Health Alliance: http://www.populationhealthalliance.org/

Institute for Healthcare Improvement: http://www.ihi.org/ihi

National Priorities Partnership: http://www.qualityforum.org/Setting_Priorities/NPP/National_Priorities_Partnership.aspx

Partnership to Fight Chronic Disease: http://www.fightchronicdisease.org/

Triple Aim: http://www.ihi.org/Engage/Initiatives/TripleAim/pages/default.aspx

Trust for America's Health: http://healthyamericans.org/report/61/shortchanging09

Understanding the U.S. Public Health System: http://www.cahpf.org/godocuserfiles/207.chi brief united states.pdf

REFERENCES

1. Chronic disease prevention and health promotion. Centers for Disease Control and Prevention. http://www.cdc.gov/chronicdisease/overview/. Accessed September 29, 2014.

2. Kindig D, Stoddart G. What is population health? *Am J Public Health*. 2003;93:380-83.

3. Kindig DA. Understanding population health terminology. *Milbank Q*. 2007;85:139-61.

4. Highlights: 2013 National Healthcare Quality & Disparities Reports. Rockville, MD: Agency for Healthcare Research and Quality; August 2014. AHRQ Pub. No. 14-0005-1. http://www.ahrq.gov/research/findings/nhqrdr/nhqr13/2013highlights.pdf. Accessed October 19, 2014.

5. Kindig DA, Asada Y, Booske B. A population health framework for setting national and state health goals. *JAMA*. 2008;299:2081-83.

6. US health spending projected to rise at an average annual rate of 5.8 percent over the next decade, reaching nearly $4.64 trillion by 2020. Health Affairs. http://www.healthaffairs.org/press/2011_07_28.php. Accessed September 30, 2014.

7. Davis K, Schoen C, Stremikis K. *Mirror, mirror on the wall: how the performance of the U.S. health care system compares internationally. 2010 update*. New York: The Commonwealth Fund; 2010. http://www.commonwealthfund.org/publications/fund-reports/2010/jun/mirror-mirror-update. Accessed October 29, 2014.

8. Health, United States, 2012: In Brief. http://www.cdc.gov/nchs/data/hus/hus12_InBrief.pdf. Accessed October 19, 2014.

9. Almanac of chronic disease. Partnership to Fight Chronic Disease. http://almanac.fightchronicdisease.org/. Accessed September 30, 2014.

10. Tavernise S. Number of Americans without health insurance falls, survey shows. New York Times, September 16, 2014. http://www.nytimes.com/2014/09/16/us/number-of-americans-without-health-insurance-falls-survey-shows.html?_r=0. Accessed October 29, 2014.

11. McGlynn EA, Asch SM, Adams J, et al. The quality of healthcare delivered to adults in the United States. *N Engl J Med*. 2003;348:2635-45.

12. Shortchanging America's health. Trust for America's Health. http://healthyamericans.org/assets/files/TFAH2010Shortchanging05.pdf. Accessed September 30, 2014.

13. Centers for Disease Control and Prevention. A framework for assessing the effectiveness of disease and injury prevention. *MMWR*. 1992;41:RR-3. http://www.cdc.gov/mmwr/preview/mmwrhtml/00016403.htm. Accessed September 30, 2014.

14. Chronic conditions among Medicare beneficiaries. Centers for Medicare and Medicaid Services. http://www.cms.gov/Research-Statistics-Data-and-Systems/Statistics-Trends-and-Reports/Chronic-Conditions/Downloads/2012Chartbook.pdf. Accessed September 30, 2014.

15. The determinants of health. World Health Organization. http://www.who.int/hia/evidence/doh/en/. Accessed September 30, 2014.

16. U.S. Department of Health and Human Services, National Cancer Institute. *Theory at a glance: A guide for health promotion practice*. U.S. Department of Health & Human Services National Institutes of Health; 2005. http://www.sneb.org/2014/Theory%20at%20a%20Glance.pdf. Accessed January 14, 2015.

17. Gebbie K, Rosenstock L, Hernandez LM, eds. *Who will keep the public healthy? Educating public health professionals for the 21st century*. Washington, DC: Institute of Medicine of the National Academies; 2003.

18. Schroeder SA. We can do better—improving the health of the American people. *N Engl J Med*. 2007;357:1221-8.

19. 2014 Definition stage 1 of meaningful use. Centers for Medicare and Medicaid Services. http://www.cms.gov/Regulations-and-Guidance/Legislation/EHRIncentivePrograms/Meaningful_Use.html. Accessed September 30, 2014.

20. Creating a culture of health. Cigna. http://healthiergov.com/docs/837897_CultureOfHealthWP_v5.pdf. Accessed September 30, 2014.

21. Changes. Institute for Healthcare Improvement. http://www.ihi.org/resources/Pages/Changes/ChangestoImproveChronicCare.aspx/. Accessed October 19, 2014.

22. Vermont blueprint for health. Vermont's Health Care Reform Agency of Administration. http://hcr.vermont.gov/blueprint. Accessed September 30, 2014.

23. University of Wisconsin Population Health Institute. http://uwphi.pophealth.wisc.edu/. Accessed November 3, 2014.

24. Health of Wisconsin: report card 2013. University of Wisconsin Population Health Institute. http://uwphi.pophealth.wisc.edu/programs/match/healthiest-state/report-card/2013/report-card-2013.pdf. Accessed September 30, 2014.

25. Baicker K, Cutler D, Song Z. Workplace wellness programs can generate savings. *Health Aff.* 2010;29(2):304-11.

26. Loeppke R, Hymel PA, Lofland JH. Health-related workplace productivity measurement: general and migraine-specific recommendations from the ACOEM expert panel. *J Occup Environ Med.* 2003;45:349-59.

27. Fabius R, Thayer RD, Konicki DL, et al. The link between workforce health and safety and the health of the bottom line: tracking market performance of companies that nurture a "culture of health." *J Occup Environ Med.* 2013;55(9):993-1000.

28. Smoking-attributable mortality, years of potential life lost, and productivity losses: United States, 2000-2004. Centers for Disease Control and Prevention. http://www.cdc.gov/mmwr/preview/mmwrhtml/mm5745a3.htm. Accessed September 30, 2014.

29. Why employee well-being matters to your bottom line. Society of Human Resource Management. http://www.shrm.org/hrdisciplines/benefits/Articles/Pages/EmployeeWellBeing.aspx. Accessed September 30, 2014.

30. Promoting employee well-being. Society of Human Resource Management. http://www.shrm.org/about/foundation/products/documents/6-11%20 promoting%20well%20being%20epg-%20final.pdf. Accessed November 3, 2014.

31. White M. The cost-benefit of well employees. *Harv Bus Rev.* December 2005. http://hbr.org/2005/12/the-cost-benefit-of-well-employees/ar/1. Accessed September 30, 2014.

32. History & development of healthy people. HealthyPeople.gov. http://healthypeople.gov/2020/about/history.aspx. Accessed September 30, 2014.

33. Leading health indicators development and framework. U.S. Department of Health and Human Services. https://www.healthypeople.gov/2020/leading-health-indicators/Leading-Health-Indicators-Development-and-Framework. Accessed September 30, 2014.

34. The IHI Triple Aim. Institute for Healthcare Improvement. http://www.ihi.org/Engage/Initiatives/TripleAim/pages/default.aspx. Accessed September 30, 2014.

35. Dentzer S. The 'Triple Aim' goes global, and not a minute too soon. *Health Aff.* 2013;32(4):638.

36. U.S. Department of Health and Human Services. Annual progress report to Congress. National Strategy for Quality Improvement in health care. (April 2012, corrected May 2014). Aligning federal and states efforts to the national quality strategy. http://www.ahrq.gov/workingforquality/nqs/nqs2012annlrpt.pdf. Accessed October 19, 2014.

37. Centers for Disease Control and Prevention. Framework for Evaluating Public Health Surveillance Systems for Early Detection of Outbreaks. *MMWR.* http://www.cdc.gov/mmwr/preview/mmwrhtml/rr5305a1.htm.

38. Institute of Medicine. *To Err Is Human: Building a Safer Health System.* Washington, DC: National Academy Press; 2000.

39. Johann Wolfgang von Goethe. Internet Encyclopedia of Philosophy. http://www.iep.utm.edu/goethe/. Accessed September 30, 2014.

Chapter 2

THE SPECTRUM OF CARE

JAAN SIDOROV AND MARTHA ROMNEY

Executive Summary

Population health—a strategy to address national health needs.

Population health provides unique opportunities to apply overlapping and synergistic interventions to care for populations, which can be defined by need, condition, or geography. Although this approach to care is rapidly evolving, there is a growing consensus that it will continue to be a key component in addressing the twin healthcare challenges of improving quality and cost.

An important feature of population health is the application of modern and culturally competent patient engagement and communication strategies that promote self-care. Such strategies include mutually agreed-upon goal setting and collaborative decision making to enable patients to identify opportunities to manage potential health risks or delay the onset of chronic conditions and their complications. The literature suggests that clinically and statistically significant increases in healthcare quality and corresponding decreases in unnecessary utilization are likely to result when populations have ready access to a medical home. A medical home issupported by a healthcare team that utilizes disease management approaches and health information technology (IT) that is integrated into the local community. This packaged care approach can be applied to both populations defined by the presence of a chronic illness (e.g., diabetes mellitus, coronary heart disease) and groups of people who would benefit from health-promotion and disease-prevention activities. Examples include employer- or insurer-based wellness, immunization, screening, and medication-compliance programs. Population health also has significant potential to reduce health disparities and serve as a building block in U.S. initiatives to address national health needs through many state-based programs and the **National Priorities Partnership**, as well as the *Healthy People* programs.

Learning Objectives

1. Define the concept and components of population health.
2. Identify determinants of health and their affect on health care.
3. Discuss the social and economic imperative of health promotion.
4. Define the concept of disease management and understand the business case.
5. Identify the need for and value of integrating healthcare services into the community, including worksites and healthcare institutions.

Key Terms

chronic care management

disease management

health determinants

health disparities

health promotion, prevention, and screening

National Priorities Partnership

patient-centered medical home

patient self-management

population health

INTRODUCTION

Population health is an organizing framework that seeks to align the components of the healthcare delivery system, which has been widely criticized as fragmented, ineffective, poorly managed, wasteful, and economically inequitable.[1] This chapter describes the population health paradigm and its promise of refocusing the system on achieving improved clinical and economic outcomes, reducing disparities of care, diminishing the prevalence of chronic illness, and realigning public and private healthcare financing. Ultimately, population health initiatives seek to improve health outcomes while "bending" or slowing the curve of the upward trajectory of healthcare spending.

WHAT IS POPULATION HEALTH AND WHY IS IT NECESSARY?

Population health can be defined as a "cohesive, integrated, and comprehensive approach to healthcare that considers the distribution of health outcomes within a population, the **health determinants** that influence distribution of care, and the policies and interventions that impact and are impacted by those determinants."[2] The Population Health Alliance, a trade organization representingmany for-profit population health service providers, describes the population health model as having seven components: population identification, comprehensive needs assessment, health promotion programs, self-management interventions, reporting, separate feedback loops that involve the healthcare consumer, and ongoing evaluation of outcomes.[3] In the context of a primary care practice, population health can be thought of as the use of clinical, demographic, and sociocultural information obtained from the patients served by the practice to improve care and clinical outcomes.[4]

Successful population health relies on the coordination of a variety of care interventions, which include **health promotion, prevention, and screening**; behavioral change; and consumer education with a special emphasis on self-management, **disease management**, and **chronic care management**. Simultaneously, population health seeks to eliminate healthcare disparities; increase safety; and promote effective, equitable, ethical, and accessible care.

Population health differs significantly from its predecessor, *disease management*.[5] One key difference is a greater reliance on data warehouses and *registries* to facilitate the collection and analysis of data regarding health outcomes. These types of data storage serve as the basis for efforts to improve those outcomes over time.[6] Once data are available, population health programs use a variety of mathematical or predictive models to *risk stratify* the population and identify patients with the greatest future vulnerabilities (e.g., declining health status, increased healthcare utilization).[7] Finally, by means of technology support tools, incentives, and tailored communications, population health seeks to engage at-risk patients and their healthcare providers in a collaborative approach to fostering high-value *self-care behaviors*.[8]

Supporters of population health believe that increasing the quality of care will eventually lead to decreasing costs. By promoting healthcare interventions where they are most needed, advocates are confident that enhanced quality will, in turn, support the achievement of improved economic and patient-centered outcomes[9] (e.g., enhanced quality of life; quality-adjusted life years; patient satisfaction; caregiver satisfaction; provider assessments; and reduced inpatient days, admissions, emergency department (ED) visits, and insurance claims expense).

From a clinical perspective, the population health paradigm requires that integrated care be focused on health promotion, illness prevention, and chronic condition management that rely on collaboration with active, engaged patient–consumers. In fact, improvements in **patient self-management** of chronic illness are the result of an increasingly sophisticated approach to behavior change and patient education that is based in *shared decision making*. Shared decision making is the term used to describe medical decisions involving interactions between patients and their providers that are informed by the best evidence and that reflect the individual patient's well considered goals and concerns.[10] By accommodating patients' preferences and values, traditional physician autonomy gives way to mutual agreement on the goals of treatment.[11,12] A growing body of evidence suggests that, in addition to greater satisfaction, shared decision making increases the rate of choosing more conservative treatment options over invasive surgery or certain types of elective testing.[13] This approach to care often relies on non-physician healthcare professionals who, when teamed with physicians in primary care settings, solicit input from patients and advance greater patient centeredness.[14]

Given the spectrum of cultural, linguistical, educational, and economic barriers to achieving equitable health care, behavior change management requires a tailored, multifaceted approach. Accordingly, population health seeks to integrate its personalized and culturally appropriate clinical care interventions with community health resources. Growing adoption of population health across multiple healthcare settings requires a high degree of patient care–team integration and alliances with local public health efforts that, in turn, promote well-being of populations in the surrounding community.

The prevalence and incidence rates, as well as the predicted trends of chronic illness and their associated economics, highlight the need for better prevention and chronic care management. The Centers for Disease Control and Prevention's (CDC's) summary of the burden of chronic illness in the United States documents a grim picture:

- Chronic diseases and conditions—such as heart disease, stroke, cancer, diabetes, obesity, and arthritis—are among the most common, costly, and preventable of all health problems.
- As of 2012, about half of all adults—117 million people—have one or more chronic health conditions. One of four adults has two or more chronic health conditions.
- Seven of the top 10 causes of death in 2010 were chronic diseases. Two of these chronic diseases—heart disease and cancer—together accounted for nearly 48% of all deaths.
- Obesity is a serious health concern. During 2009–2010, more than one-third of adults, or about 78 million people, were obese (defined as body mass index [BMI] ≥ 30 kg/m^2). Nearly one of five youths age 2–19 years was obese (BMI $\geq$ 95th percentile).
- Arthritis is the most common cause of disability. Of the 53 million adults with a doctor diagnosis of arthritis, more than 22 million say arthritis causes them to have trouble with their usual activities.
- Diabetes is the leading cause of kidney failure, lower limb amputations other than those caused by injury, and new cases of blindness among adults.[15]

With 80% of healthcare spending dedicated to the treatment of chronic care and an aging population experiencing one or more chronic diseases, substantial changes in our approach to healthcare delivery and financing will be necessary to reduce the year-after-rate increase in healthcare spending. A population health approach will realign the health focus, priorities, education, training, and incentives.

ATTRIBUTES OF THE POPULATION HEALTH PARADIGM

A healthcare delivery approach focused on individual care is limited by both the underuse and overuse of healthcare resources, and results in diminished clinical quality and increased expense. The population health paradigm integrates existing clinical delivery systems with public health–based models of care as the foundations for each of the components (see Box 2-1). The introduction of patient self-management distinguishes the population health approach from traditional approaches to healthcare education, training, servicing, and resourcing. Individual states and private healthcare entities are adopting population health models that differ only in the details of care delivery. Endorsement of this overall framework requires national support for the legislative, policy, and economic changes that will be necessary for its widespread adoption.

Investments will be required to build infrastructure to support the population health paradigm, address the bases for health inequities, integrate healthcare services, educate providers and consumers, and realign the financing of health care in the United States. As population-based care expands and the evidence accrues, many experts believe that the population health model will be proven effective in addressing the triple challenge of increasing quality of care, reducing costs, and improving the patient care experience.

BOX 2-1 BASIC ATTRIBUTES OF A POPULATION HEALTH PARADIGM

- Population identification
- Registry consisting of a searchable data warehouse
- Risk stratification modeling using patient surveys and health data inputs (e.g., insurance claims, electronic health record [EHR] information)
- Personalized, patient-centered care that includes self-management, shared decision making, health promotion, disease management, and case management
- An identified primary care provider (medical home)
- An interdisciplinary healthcare team to provide supportive services, including shared decision making
- Clinician knowledge about and recognition of determinants of health and their effect on population health and individual health
- Integration with public health and community systems
- Utilization of evidence-based guidelines to provide quality, cost-effective care
- Provision of culturally and linguistically appropriate care and health education
- Ongoing evaluation of outcomes with feedback loops
- Implementation of interoperable cross-sector health IT[16,17]

Data from the Population Health Alliance (formerly DMAA: The Care Continuum Alliance). DMAA definition of disease management, and Carney PA, Eiff MP, Saultz JW, et al. Aspects of the Patient-Centered Medical Home currently in place: initial findings from preparing the personal physician for practice. *Fam Med.* 2009;41(9):632–9.

COMPONENTS OF THE POPULATION HEALTH PARADIGM

The primary components of the population health paradigm are integrated health promotion and chronic disease management. Health promotion is the provision of clinical and public health services to collaboratively address the effect of health determinants on consumers for the purpose of improving and sustaining well-being. Disease management also relies on these integrated healthcare systems to apply evidence-based clinical guidelines for personalized, timely, high-quality, and cost-effective treatment that is based on level of risk. Health promotion and disease management can be offered both in healthcare and worksite settings, and both are ultimately intended to minimize the severity, length, and costs of care associated with chronic illness.[18]

Target populations can be identified on the basis of geography (e.g., the service area of a provider), insurance status (e.g., employer sponsorship), or the presence of a chronic condition (e.g., diabetes mellitus, hypertension). The identification process relies on a number of inputs, including health risk assessments (HRAs), assessments of willingness to change, insurance claims, EHR data, or public health statistics. Ideally, these data are stored in a registry, which is a searchable, secure data warehouse that facilitates the mathematical modeling used to assign a risk score to each individual in a population. Based on the level of risk and depending on individual preferences and goals, persons within the population are engaged in health promotion, disease management, or case management programs with links to public health and community-based health resources. Ongoing outcomes data collection may include quality of life assessments, satisfaction measures, specific clinical outcomes (e.g., blood pressure, diabetes testing and control, vaccination rates, referrals to community programs), and healthcare utilization as well as costs (e.g., hospitalization rates, ED visits, monthly insurance claims expense). These data can be used to compute summary statistics that assess the effect of the various health promotion and care management programs over time and inform program adjustments.[19]

These interlocking strategies leverage the determinants of health that affect an individual's well-being. Determinants include individual factors (e.g., gender, age, ethnicity, socioeconomic and educational status) and population-based factors[20] (e.g., geographic locale, environment and occupation exposures, physical safety, degree of psychological and physical stress in communities, economic stability, accessible and affordable quality preventive and disease management services, areas for adequate physical activity).[20] These determinants of health have an appreciable effect on inequities in prevention, screening, treatment, morbidity, and mortality.[20] As a result, disadvantaged populations bear a greater burden of disease and experience higher rates of infant mortality, cardiovascular disease, diabetes, cancer, and HIV/AIDS.[20]

HEALTH PROMOTION

The World Health Organization (WHO) defines health promotion as "the process of enabling people to increase control over their health and its determinants, and thereby improve their health."[21] Health promotion encompasses "activities . . . to maximize the development of resilience to . . . threats to health"[21] and involves an integrated, collaborative patient-centric approach to assessing, promoting, and managing health through prevention, screening, education, behavior change, and patient self-care.[22] As part of the national strategy to improve the health of all people through promotion of and increased access to care, Congress lowered the financial barriers to specific care and services. As of

January 1, 2014, the Patient Protection and Affordable Care Act (ACA) requires that all new health plans, both inside and outside of the Health Insurance Marketplace, cover a comprehensive package of items and services, known as essential health benefits.[23] Essential health benefits must include "ambulatory patient services; emergency services; hospitalization; maternity and newborn care; mental health and substance use disorder services, including behavioral health treatment; prescription drugs; rehabilitative and habilitative services and devices; laboratory services; preventive and wellness services and chronic disease management; and pediatric services, including oral and vision care."[24]

The ACA also established the first Prevention and Public Health Fund, with mandatory appropriations for "programs to improve health and help restrain the rate of growth in private and public health care costs."[25] For fiscal years (FYs) 2010 through 2022, $18.7 billion was mandated, with $2 billion annually thereafter. The initial allocation was $500 million in FY2010, with incremental increases up to $2 billion annually beginning in FY 2015.[25] Since that time, in response to both fiscal and political concerns, funding of many of the public health provisions of the ACA has been significantly modified.[26,27] How committed Congress and the administration remain to preserving the fund in the future remains an open question.

To set the national framework for prevention and health promotion, the ACA established the National Prevention, Health Promotion and Public Health Council (NPC).[28,29] Chaired by Surgeon General Regina Benjamin, with representation from 20 federal departments, agencies, and offices, the NPC created the first National Prevention Strategy and NPC Action Plan. Based on a vision and a goal, four strategic directions (i.e., Healthy and Safe Community Environments, Clinical and Community Preventive Services, Empowered People, and Elimination of Health Disparities), and priorities supported by evidence-based recommendations, the National Prevention Plan is the foundation for national, state, and local prevention efforts.[29,30]

Other prevention provisions support increased education, outreach, and access to clinical preventive services at the community level (e.g., school-based preventive services); additional health coverage for Medicaid[31] and Medicare[32] populations (e.g., annual wellness examination and designated preventive services); and encouraging value-based insurance design (VBID) to promote prevention and healthy lifestyles, to encourage adherence to recommended treatments, and to discourage use of low-value services.[33] For the past decade, employers across the country have been adopting VBID benefit plans to support healthier employees and dependents, and to reduce the costs associated with chronic illness from both health insurance and productivity perspectives.[34]

PREVENTION AND WELLNESS

Prevention consists of supportive strategies and interventions aimed at the deterrence, early detection, and minimization or cessation of disease and injury at a population level.[35] Preventive activities and care are critical to the health of the nation's population and economy. Although 70% of adult deaths are attributed to chronic diseases and an estimated 75% of U.S. healthcare expenditures are associated with treating chronic illness, a mere 3% is budgeted for health promotion and prevention.[36] Healthcare costs related to chronic illness include both direct medical expenditures and indirect costs (e.g., absenteeism, presenteeism, workers' compensation, and other associated labor costs).

Prevention activities are generally categorized as primary, secondary, and tertiary. Primary prevention involves interventions directed at preemptively preventing disease onset.[37] (e.g., immunizations, seat belt use, avoiding tobacco use).[38,39] Secondary prevention is the "early detection and swift treatment of disease . . . to cure disease, slow its progression, or reduce its impact on individuals or communities."[37] Screening is a form of secondary prevention and includes interventions for detecting diseases and high-risk behaviors associated with chronic illness (e.g., obesity, smoking, excessive alcohol consumption, illicit drug use).[37,40] Tertiary prevention is aimed at slowing the progression of confirmed disease[37] (e.g., routine foot and eye examinations for diabetic patients).[41,42] Numerous studies have demonstrated the efficacy of preventive measures in reducing the risks of chronic disease and mortality.[43] An excellent example of this approach is the U.S. childhood immunization initiative. While legislation, mandatory tracking, and incentives are not always necessary to ensure a cost-effective program, the collaboration and integration of health services, culturally and linguistically appropriate communication, education, care, tracking, reporting, and evaluation are all critical components of successful population health efforts.

General interventions in employer- and insurer-sponsored wellness programs include health risk assessments, health screenings, education and wellness coaching, and healthy behavior challenges.[38]

Although the health benefits are substantial, the short-term costs of preventive care are high,[44] and gaps in participation are common as a result of the traditional focus on sick care, diminished access to and availability of preventive services, lack of insurance coverage, health illiteracy, and minimal integration between public and clinical health.[44] Telling examples of these shortcomings include smoking cessation programs and increasing the appropriate use of aspirin among persons at high risk for blood clotting. Both initiatives are comparatively inexpensive and can reduce cardiovascular risks, yet concerns about the value and cost-efficacy of prevention programs have been raised.[36]

Over the past decades, different models of employee wellness and engagement have been incorporated into employer benefits packages. The benefits to employers are direct (i.e., expenses related to interventions such as medical treatment, medications, and hospitalizations) and indirect (i.e., manifested as increased employee productivity by decreasing presenteeism and absenteeism) cost savings.[38]

SCREENING

Screening is the "presumptive identification of unrecognized disease or health risks by the application of tests or other procedures that can be applied rapidly."[40] The efficacy of screening is based on two measures of validity: sensitivity and specificity. The four potential outcomes associated with screening are true positive (a positive test result in the presence of actual disease), true negative (a negative test result in the absence of disease), false positive (test is positive in the absence of disease), and false negative (negative test result in the presence of disease).[40] When assessing the appropriateness of screening, healthcare providers should consider the distribution of disease, the evidence supporting screening and validity of available tests, the benefits and risks associated with the screening, the availability and costs of treatment, and the determination of whether evidence-based and eligibility criteria exist.[40]

The benefits of screening include early detection of disease, with potential opportunities to institute preemptive treatment that results in better health outcomes and lower morbidity, mortality, and costs.[40] Screenings such as HRAs and measures of blood pressure, weight/BMI, vision, hearing, blood cholesterol/lipid profile, bone density, environment exposure (e.g., lead, asbestos, and toxic) measurement, and diagnostic examinations to rule out cancers have demonstrated benefits and lowered costs.[40]

Certain limitations and potential harms associated with screening (e.g., costs of unnecessary tests and unneeded care, risks linked to false-positive test results) warrant evidence-based assessment of the appropriateness of screening for individual patients.[40] Significant individual patient stress, harm, and death may result from test-associated complications or injuries, unnecessary interventions, and the failure to pursue further tests following a false-negative result.[40]

Under the ACA, insurance policies, both inside and outside of the Health Insurance Marketplace, must offer essential health benefits, including preventive health screenings for services that meet one of the following criteria:

1. Evidence-based items or services with an A or B rating in the current recommendations of the U.S. Preventive Services Task Force (USPSTF)
2. Immunizations recommended by the CDC's Advisory Committee on Immunization Practices with respect to the individual involved
3. Evidence-informed preventive care and screenings for infants, children, and adolescents as provided for in the comprehensive guidelines supported by the U.S. government's Health Resources and Services Administration (HRSA)
4. Additional preventive care and screenings for women not provided for in comprehensive guidelines supported by the HRSA[45]

States that opt to expand Medicaid must offer essential benefits to newly enrolled beneficiaries,[42] and the ACA provides Medicare coverage for annual wellness visits, including a personalized prevention plan.[46]

BEHAVIOR CHANGE (HEALTH MANAGEMENT)

An estimated 30% to 60% of patients are not compliant with their physician-directed treatment or medication regimens.[47] Because of the serious clinical and cost concerns this raises, behavior modification has become recognized as an integral part of the population health paradigm.[47] Behavior change encompasses a broad range of physical, emotional, habitual, and cultural factors that influence health status.

Population-based care is an interdisciplinary approach in which primary care providers collaborate with allied health staff to educate, engage, and support patients in behavior change through a process of shared decision making. A key strategy for accomplishing this is the assessment of *willingness to change*. A process of *motivational interviewing* leads to a better understanding of readiness, barriers, and effective strategies that lead to engagement.[48] When paired with usual clinical care, such participatory behavior change interventions have yielded positive patient outcomes in prevention and treatment of diabetes, hypertension, and lipid disorders; stress management; and tobacco cessation.[49]

PATIENT SELF-CARE

Population-based care acknowledges that consumers are essential partners in achieving good outcomes. Unlike traditional care models that view patients as passive recipients of treatment, a growing body of research has repeatedly demonstrated that health status is improved by means of behavior change and patient self-care. Through culturally and linguistically appropriate education, skills training, and integrated public and private healthcare delivery systems, healthcare consumers can readily learn to care for themselves and participate in goal setting and collaborative decision making.[47] Once patients engage with their providers to set goals of self-care, health service utilization is lowered as a result of improved compliance with health-promoting behaviors. Actively engaged patients also have an enhanced ability to identify potential health risks early, thereby enabling them to address the risks independently or via timely communication with their primary providers.[47]

PATIENT-CENTERED MEDICAL HOME

The **patient-centered medical home** (PCMH) concept is a professionally endorsed, integrated, and collaborative healthcare delivery model centered on primary care as a means to manage chronic illness, improve patient outcomes, and lower healthcare costs.[48] The Patient-Centered Primary Care Collaborative (PCPCC) defines the medical home as a team-based approach to care that is *patient centered* (involving a provider and patient and family partnership that respects patient preferences), *comprehensive* (maintaining a team that is accountable for the patient's care needs), *accessible* (offering ready in-person and remote communication access), *committed to quality and safety* (achieving continuous improvement), and *coordinated* (providing links across other elements of the broader care system, including community services).[49] The attribute of comprehensiveness has been expanded, with the growing recognition of the medical neighborhood concept (i.e., the constellation of supporting clinicians as well as community, social service organizations, and health agencies that serve the patients within a PCMH).[50] The PCMH model has been broadly implemented by government and private providers and is being adopted increasingly by health systems in response to healthcare reform.[36,51–53] A growing body of evidence indicates that the PCMH is associated with a reduction of medical errors, improved quality of care, and increased consumer satisfaction.[52,53]

The PCMH is rapidly emerging as a key component of the population health management model. As the consumer's primary point of contact, the primary care physician bears responsibility for team-based health coordination and disease management while ensuring that integrated clinical and community medical and psychosocial care are provided.[48] Services are based on evidence-based guidelines and enhanced through decision support, with an emphasis on patient self-care and behavior change.[48] Interoperable IT systems are necessary to integrate care across practices, sites, and the medical neighborhood, enabling appropriate access to medical records, e-prescribing capabilities, and disease registries.[48] IT systems make it possible to monitor, evaluate, report, and track improvement in the quality of care and patient outcomes, which is the basis for a majority of economic incentive programs (e.g., pay-for-performance).[54,55]

CHRONIC CARE MANAGEMENT AND DISEASE MANAGEMENT

Traditionally, disease management has been defined as a "system of targeted coordinated population-based healthcare interventions and communications for specific conditions in which patient self-care efforts are significant."[48,56] As population health has continued to evolve, healthcare delivery systems are placing greater emphasis on *chronic care management* (CCM) (i.e., the set of activities designed to assist patients and their support systems in managing medical conditions and related psychosocial problems more effectively, with the aims of improving patients' functional health status, enhancing the coordination of care, eliminating the duplication of services, and reducing the need for expensive medical services.[57] CCM builds on the integrated primary care health paradigm, which focuses on improving the quality of care and management of illness through "self-management, clinical information systems, evidence-based clinical decision support, redesigned integrated healthcare delivery clinical and community systems, and policies."[58,59] Both CCM and disease management seek to reverse the skyrocketing incidence and prevalence of serious, costly, chronic illness through improving patient outcomes with high-quality, cost-effective care that is optimally delivered by a PCMH.[48,60,61]

In response to the escalating prevalence of chronic illness and its associated economic burdens, many independent companies, self-insured employers, and health plans have implemented care management programs, often in partnership with vendors that provide these programs for a fee. Such programs utilize evidence-based, patient-focused strategies across populations to change patient behavior through collaborative healthcare, education, coaching, and financial incentives and to increase self-care and compliance.[25,48,62] Moreover, improvement initiatives must be accompanied by clearly defined outcome measures and evaluation processes to enable program modification.[25,48] Implementation of user-friendly, interoperable IT is integral to this health paradigm[25,48] Employers and health plans have demonstrated that these strategies increase productivity and decrease direct and indirect costs associated with chronic illness.[52] Many CCM strategies have been developed to combat obesity, coronary heart disease and heart failure, diabetes, chronic obstructive pulmonary disease, asthma, and cancer.[8,56,60]

Evaluation of care management programs yields mixed results. Some studies report improvements in congestive and coronary heart disease, diabetes, and depression.[56] Such programs are reported to increase productivity while decreasing absenteeism, presenteeism, and hospitalizations.[55] However, in many instances, the costs associated with implementing these programs are considerable and may not be offset by reductions in healthcare costs. As a result, the cost effectiveness of CCM programs remains an open question.[56,60,61] Proponents of CCM programs posit that increasing participation and measuring outcomes will improve cost effectiveness. To address the need for demonstrating and validating the cost effectiveness of CCM programs, public and private health and quality organizations (e.g., Agency for Healthcare Research and Quality, National Committee for Quality Assurance, The Joint Commission, the Population Health Alliance) are promoting clinical and financial outcome measurements to determine whether there is a financial return on investment.[39] Suggested outcome measures include healthcare utilization, clinical outcomes, and health care, including new comorbidity and pharmaceutical costs and productivity measures.[63]

CASE MANAGEMENT

Some individuals face unique or multiple care needs that cannot be adequately addressed through any single care management program. For this reason, *case management* is often used in population health. Case management is the collaborative process of assessment, planning, facilitation, and advocacy for options and services to meet an individual's health needs through communication and available resources to promote quality, cost-effective outcomes.[64]

Because case management focuses on the *individual*, it can provide high-intensity and personalized care planning. It is typically led by specially trained nurses and social workers. Once the individual's care needs are met, the corresponding reduction in risk can lead to a hand-off to a CCM program, ongoing physician follow-up, or a community-based resource.

HEALTH INFORMATION TECHNOLOGY

As described previously, health IT is a critical resource to support population health. In addition to data warehouse registries, risk stratification, and ongoing assessment of outcomes, health IT has important implications for the EHR and commercial and government insurance functions. Making risk assessments, program enrollment data, or case management care planning available electronically at the clinical point of care can greatly enhance care coordination. Theoretically, health insurers could use the same information that is available at the clinical point of care for actuarial modeling and traditional utilization management, and to advance the quality of care in their provider networks.

ELIMINATING HEALTH DISPARITIES

Health disparities can be defined as "differences in the incidence, prevalence, mortality, and burden of diseases, as well as other adverse health conditions or outcomes that exist among specific population groups," and have been well documented in subpopulations based on socioeconomic status, education, age, race and ethnicity, geography, disability, sexual orientation, or special needs.[65,66] These subpopulations experience disproportionate burdens of illness as a result of the barriers imposed by discrimination, as well as those from differences in culture, language, beliefs, and values, which lead to considerable social and economic burdens associated with poor quality of care and lack of access to affordable, quality primary care.[66–68]

Particularly for minority populations, disparities in health care are manifested in access to quality care, burdens of illness reflected in morbidity and mortality rates, life expectancy, and quality of life.[66–68] Racial and ethnic populations in the United States and residents of rural communities, children, the elderly, individuals with physical or psychological disabilities, and other disenfranchised populations tend to live in lower socioeconomic communities with higher rates of violence and environmental exposures, work in jobs with greater occupational hazards, have less access to affordable nutritious foods, and have higher rates of being uninsured.[66–68] These populations have less access to preventive and diagnostic care and treatment, resulting in higher rates of morbidities, emergency department utilization, hospitalizations, and mortalities.[67–69] The Institute of Medicine's report, *Unequal Treatment: Confronting Racial/Ethnic Disparities in Health Care*, cited more than 175 studies documenting diagnostic and treatment disparities of various conditions among racial/ethnic populations, even when confounding factors (e.g., insurance and socioeconomic status, comorbidities, age, healthcare venue, stage of diseases) were controlled for in analyses.[67,68]

Since the mid 1990s, many strategies, initiatives, and programs have been implemented to reduce healthcare disparities at the federal, state, and local levels with public and private funding.[70] However, according to the CDC "Health Disparities and Inequalities Report—United States, 2013," disparities persist in the prevalence and outcomes of chronic disease, suicide, and infant mortality among racial and ethnic populations.[71] African American adults have the highest prevalence of hypertension and obesity and are at least 50% more likely to die prematurely from stroke or heart disease than Caucasians.[71]

Barriers to health care have been conceptualized as organizational, structural, and clinical, including lack of diversity in the healthcare workforce, lack of cultural and linguistic competency, lack of health literacy, and inadequate access to and coordination of care.[72] In practical terms, health disparities include a spectrum of factors that affect access, diagnostics, treatment, follow-up, and continuity of care. These barriers result in the day-to-day inability to obtain prescription medications, prevent illness, and avoid hospitalizations or ED use, all of which lead to poorer clinical outcomes and higher costs.[72]

The population health approach integrates clinical and public healthcare approaches to explicitly address these cultural determinants of health through the targeted provision of appropriate services that seek to reduce the myriad barriers to care.

CULTURAL COMPETENCY

Cultural competency involves "acknowledg[ing] and incorporat[ing] [and] . . . understanding the importance of social and cross-cultural influences of different populations' values, health beliefs and behaviors, disease prevalence and incidence and treatment outcome; considering how these factors interact with and impact multiple levels of healthcare delivery systems; and implementing interventions to assure quality care to diverse patient populations."[73] This requires the assessment of cross-cultural relations and barriers, expansion of cultural knowledge, and awareness of integration of health beliefs and behaviors.[72] Organizational, structural, and clinical barriers include the following:[72]

- Inadequate diversity in institutional leadership, healthcare providers, and workforce; limited clinic hours; and extended waiting for appointments and care.[81] Studies have demonstrated correlations between consumer satisfaction and racial concordance with providers.[72]
- Healthcare providers' lack of knowledge of and/or sensitivity to differences in ethnic, religious, or health beliefs; values; and culturally endorsed treatments.[72]
- Language differences without availability of interpreters (i.e., monolingual or unilingual education and patient information resources that are available only in English) create important structural barriers that significantly impede provider and consumer understanding of assessments, diagnosis, and care recommendations; the necessity of specialty referrals; and mutually agreed-upon compliance with treatments.[72]

Access to and the provision of culturally and linguistically appropriate/competent care are necessary to reduce disparities in healthcare access, delivery, costs, and outcomes. Recognition of the need for and value of culturally and linguistically appropriate services across the healthcare continuum is reflected in governmental, quasi-regulatory, professional, and educational policies. Although the federal mandate to make accommodations for individuals with low English proficiency has been codified since the Civil Rights Act of 1964,[74] more recent legislation, regulations, and guidelines[75–78] reinforce the imperative of effective provider–patient communications. Additionally, organizations such as The

Joint Commission,[79] the National Committee for Quality Assurance,[80] and the National Quality Forum (NQF)[81] have developed and implemented cultural and linguistic competency accreditation standards and quality measures, guidelines, and tools. At the state level, six states have required or are in the process of requiring cultural competency training for physician state licensure. Thirty-five states have enacted legislation requiring provisions for language access.[73]

In 2001, the U.S. Department of Health and Human Services Office of Minority Health published *National Standards for Culturally and Linguistically Appropriate Services in Health and Health Care*[82] (the National CLAS Standards) to assist healthcare organizations in developing a framework to respond to diverse patient populations, to support the elimination of ethnic and racial disparities, and to improve the health of all consumers.[58,61]

In recognition of current and projected demographic changes; persistent racial, ethnic, and cultural health disparities; the expansion of knowledge about cultural and linguistic competency; and national initiatives to improve access, quality, and costs of care, the Office of Minority Health issued revised standards following a 2-year comprehensive, multifaceted stakeholder assessment and consultation initiative.[82] The enhanced National CLAS Standards, published in September 2013, broaden the definition of culture to "include religion and spirituality; lesbian, gay, bisexual, and transgender community individuals; deaf and hearing impaired individuals; and blind and vision impaired individuals; include health literacy issues, patient safety and satisfaction principles; establish congruency with other standards in the field and reflect concurrent changes in the healthcare environment and continuum of delivery of care and services."[82] Because each of the now 15 standards are considered to have equal importance, healthcare organizations are pursuing adoption of all of the provisions to more effectively achieve improved health outcomes.[82]

CHALLENGES AND OPPORTUNITIES IN IMPLEMENTING A POPULATION HEALTH APPROACH

Population health is no longer a theoretical construct; it is the new healthcare paradigm that must be implemented to improve the health and health outcomes of our population; to reduce risk, harm, waste, and costs; to eliminate health disparities; and to sustain future generations. The challenges and opportunities of implementing a population health approach amidst the restructuring of our national healthcare delivery and payment system are tremendous. The scope, volume, and complexity of the ACA affect our entire healthcare structure and infrastructure, workforce, financing, delivery, and accountability. A number of the challenges and opportunities have been identified in this chapter, but many more exist and are yet to be defined.

Many of the most pressing challenges related to implementing a population health paradigm fall into three broad areas: clinical, business, and policy.

CLINICAL: CAPACITY CHALLENGES

One key determinant of the success of healthcare reform is the capacity of the healthcare workforce to provide care to the increased number of consumers. The Congressional Budget Office estimates that by 2023, tens of millions of additional individuals will be seeking health care.[83] Capacity encompasses the volume, competencies, distribution, and composition of health care disciplines. But increasing capacity alone is not enough; realignment of the healthcare workforce is essential. Our traditional system of health workforce education and training is siloed and uncoordinated. Disparate state licensing and practice acts, insurance coverage, and institutional policies have contributed to discordant, fragmented, and perilous delivery of care.[84] Transitioning to new models and venues of care in which systems and providers are held accountable for the quality, costs, and patient experience of care necessitates the restructuring and realigning of the healthcare workforce. The roles and responsibilities of healthcare professionals must be reassessed and redefined to accommodate transitions of care across a person's lifespan. An interdisciplinary population health model of care must be integrated into the education, training, and development of healthcare professionals.[84] There are many untapped opportunities to eliminate professional silos to address the need for competent, quality, evidence-based, patient-centered care; to promote health and wellness; to manage and reduce chronic illness; to engage patients, families, and communities; and to collaboratively address complex health issues and treatment.

In 2013, the Institute of Medicine's Global Forum on Innovation in Health Professional Education convened a workshop to create a transdisciplinary code of ethics for health professionals—a social contract that would reflect an integrated approach among diverse disciplines working with shared values and purpose to address the populations' health needs, standards, and expectations.[85]

BUSINESS: NAVIGATING THE QUALITY MEASUREMENT LABYRINTH

Since the release of the Institute of Medicine's seminal report, *Crossing the Quality Chasm*, in 2001, the scope and imperative of identifying, measuring, and reporting quality metrics have expanded and become a prominent component of our health delivery and reimbursement system.[86]

The NQF, the Centers for Medicare & Medicaid Services, and other federal and state authorities as well as professional, business, and consumer groups have implemented diverse mandatory and voluntary measurements at the health system, provider, and insurer-provider levels.[87] Recently, the ACA codified the importance of quality measurement through the mandate for the creation and implementation of a National Quality Strategy.[88] The ensuing plethora of measures has caused confusion, redundancies, inconsistencies, and logistical challenges.[87] Panzer and colleagues recommend the following changes to improve the structure and value of quality measurement:

- Setting higher quality standards and measurement
- Harmonizing measures and reporting

- Continuing support and reliance on NQF endorsements
- Replacing claims-based measures with measures reflecting true clinical relevance
- Developing and expanding data-rich registries in key domains
- Paying less attention to proprietary report cards
- Transiting carefully to "eMeasures"
- Allocating adequate resources to support data capture and reporting[87]

CONCLUSION

Population health is a dynamic approach to health care that consists of a variety of inter-related approaches; it ultimately seeks to simultaneously improve healthcare quality and optimize healthcare spending. At its core, population health advances patient self-care so that recipients are better able to work with the healthcare system to improve their health status, intervene early in any exacerbations of chronic illness, reduce the incidence of complications, and rely on efficient and effective healthcare options.

The ACA advances population health by increasing access to healthcare services through expanded insurance coverage and by establishing national strategies (e.g., prevention, health promotion, public health, quality) to guide improved healthcare quality and delivery, thereby reducing disparities and improving consumer outcomes through government-funded initiatives and new reimbursement models. The opportunity exists to implement a health promotion and prevention infrastructure that incorporates increased consumer engagement, use of interoperable health IT (e.g., EHRs), interdisciplinary healthcare teamwork, coordinated transitions of care across the life spectrum, and primary care reform with the patient-centered medical home and innovative payment reform models (e.g., accountable care organizations).

While other health reform efforts are underway, population health promises to be a key component of the United States'—and possibly the rest of the world's—efforts to reduce chronic illness. Given the twin challenges of increasing quality and reducing cost, population health remains the best strategy for meeting our national healthcare goals.

STUDY AND DISCUSSION QUESTIONS

1. What is the definition of population health and what are its key attributes?
2. What are the determinants of a population's health status and what are the roles of health promotion and disease management?
3. What are the roles of behavior change and self-care in achieving population health outcomes?
4. How can population health address healthcare disparities?
5. How can population health assist in achieving goals of the national and state initiatives that address population health needs?

SUGGESTED READINGS AND WEBSITES

READINGS

Adler NE, Rehkopf DH. U.S. disparities in health: descriptions, causes, and mechanisms. *Annu Rev Public Health*. 2008;29:235-52.

Barr VJ, Robinson S, Marin-Link B, et al. The expanded Chronic Care Model: an integration of concepts and strategies from population health promotion and the Chronic Care Model. *Hosp Q*. 2003;7(1):73-82.

Betancourt JR, Green AR, Carillo JE, et al. Defining cultural competence: a practical framework for addressing racial/ethnic disparities in health and health care. *Public Health Rep*. 2003;118:293-302.

Bodenheimer T. Helping patients improve their health-related behaviors: what system changes do we need? *Dis Manag*. 2005;8(5):319-30.

Bodenheimer T, Chen E, Bennett HD. Confronting the growing burden of chronic disease: can the U.S. health care workforce do the job? *Health Aff*. 2009;28(1):64-74.

Braveman P, Gruskin S. Defining equity in health. *J Epidemiol Community Health*. 2003;57(4):254-58.

Carney PA, Eiff MP, Saultz JW, et al. Aspects of the Patient-Centered Medical Home currently in place: initial findings from preparing the personal physician for practice. *Fam Med*. 2009;41(9):632-39.

Frazee SG, Sherman B, Fabius R, et al. Leveraging the trusted clinician: increasing retention in disease management through integrated program delivery. *Popul Health Manag*. 2008;11(5):247-54.

Goetzel RZ, Ozminkowski RJ, Villagra VG, et al. Return on investment in disease management: a review. *Health Care Financing Rev*. 2005;26(4):1-19.

Grandes G, Sanchez A, Cortada JM, et al. Is integration of healthy lifestyle promotion into primary care feasible? Discussion and consensus sessions between clinicians and researchers. *BMC Health Serv Res*. 2008;8:213.

Musich SA, Schultz AB, Burton WN, Edington DW. Overview of disease management approaches: implications for corporate-sponsored programs. *Dis Manage Health Outcomes*. 2004;12(5):299-326.

Rosenthal TC. The medical home: growing evidence to support a new approach to primary care. *J Am Board Fam Med*. 2008;21(5):427-40.

Sisko A, Truffer C, Smith S, et al. Health spending projections through 2018: recession effects add uncertainty to the outlook. *Health Aff*. 2009;28(2):w346-57.

WEBSITES

Centers for Disease Control and Prevention: http://www.cdc.gov/

Health Policy and Reform of the *New England Journal of Medicine*: http://healthcarereform.nejm.org/?query=rthome

Healthy People 2020: http://www.healthypeople.gov/

Kaiser Family Foundation: http://www.kff.org/

National Business Coalition on Health: http://www.nbch.org/

National Coalition on Health Care: http://nchc.org/

National Prevention Strategy: http://www.surgeongeneral.gov/initiatives/prevention/strategy/

National Priorities Partnership: http://www.qualityforum.org/Setting_Priorities/NPP/National_Priorities_Partnership.aspx

National Quality Forum: http://www.qualityforum.org/

Patient-Centered Primary Care Collaborative: http://www.pcpcc.net

Population Health Alliance (formerly DMAA: The Care Continuum Alliance): http://www.populationhealthalliance.org

U.S. Preventive Services Task Force: http://www.uspreventiveservicestaskforce.org/

World Health Organization: http://www.who.int/en/

REFERENCES

1. National Coalition on Health Care. High health spending and rapid growth in that spending are the result of a variety of causes and http://www.nchc.org/wp-content/uploads/2012/09/NCHC_Report_Card_on_113th_Congress.pdf. Accessed January 16, 2014.

2. Kindig D, Stoddart G. What is population health? *Am J Public Health*. 2003;93(3):380-3.

3. Population Health Alliance. About PHA. http://www.populationhealthalliance.org/pha.html. Accessed January 13, 2015.

4. Cusack CM, Knudson AD, Kronstadt JL, et al. Practice-based population health: information technology to support transformation to proactive primary care. http://pcmh.ahrq.gov/sites/default/files/attachments/Information Technology to Support Transformation to Proactive Primary Care.pdf. Accessed September 29, 2014.

5. Mattke S, Seid M, Ma S. Evidence for the effect of disease management: is $1 billion a year a good investment? *Am J Man Care*. 2007;13:670-6.

6. Larsson S, Lawyer P, Garellick G, et al. Use of 13 disease registries in 5 countries demonstrates the potential to use outcome data to improve health care's value. *Health Aff.* 2012;31:220-7.

7. Wennberg DE, Marr A, Lang L, et al. A randomized trial of a telephone care-management strategy. *New Engl J Med* 2010;363:1245-55.

8. Population health guide for primary care models. Care Continuum Alliance. http://selfmanagementalliance.org/wp-content/uploads/2013/11/A-Population-Health-Guide-for-Primary-Care-Models-CareContinAlliance.pdf. Accessed September 29, 2014.

9. Stiefel M, Nolan K. A guide to measuring the triple aim: population health, experience of care, and per capita cost. Institute for Healthcare Improvement. IHI Innovation Series white paper. Cambridge, MA: Institute for Healthcare Improvement; 2012.

10. Fowler FJ, Levin CA, Sepucha KR. Information and involving patients to improve the quality of medical decisions. *Health Aff.* 2011;30(4):699-706.

11. Kon AA. The shared decision-making continuum. *JAMA*. 2010;304(8):903-4.

12. Barry MJ, Edgman-Levitan S. Shared decision making: the pinnacle of patient-centered care. *N Engl J Med* 2012;366:780-1.

13. Stacey D, Bennett CL, Barry MJ, et al. Decision aids for people facing health treatment or screening decisions. *Cochrane Database Syst Rev*. doi:10.1002/14651858.CD001431.pub3

14. Rittenhouse DR, Shortell SM. The patient-centered medical home. Will it stand the test of health reform? *JAMA*. 2009;301(19):2038-40.

15. National diabetes fact sheet, 2011. Centers for Disease Control and Prevention. http://www.cdc.gov/diabetes/pubs/pdf/ndfs_2011.pdf. Accessed September 29, 2014.

16. PHA definition of population health management. The Population Health Alliance. http://www.populationhealthalliance.org/research/phm-glossary/d.html. Accessed October 29, 2014.

17. Carney PA, Eiff MP, Saultz JW, et al. Aspects of the Patient-Centered Medical Home currently in place: initial findings from preparing the personal physician for practice. *Fam Med*. 2009;41(9):632-9.

18. Starfield B. Basic concepts in population health and health care. *J Epidemiol Community Health*. 2001;55(7):452-4.

19. A population health guide for primary care models. Care Continuum Alliance. http://www.populationhealthalliance.org/publications/program-measurement-evaluation-guide-core-metrics-for-employee-health-management-executive-summary.html. Accessed November10, 2014.

20. Gehlert S, Sohmer D, Sacks T, et al. Targeting health disparities: a model linking upstream determinants to downstream interventions. *Health Aff*. 2008;27(2):339-49.

21. World Health Organization. The Bangkok charter for health promotion in a globalized world (11 August 2005). http://www.who.int/healthpromotion/conferences/6gchp/bangkok_charter/en/. Accessed September 29, 2014.

22. Shenson D. Putting prevention in its place: the shift from clinic to community. *Health Aff*. 2006;25(4):1012-5.

23. U.S. Government Printing Office. Patient Protection and Affordable Care Act (P.L. 111-148 §1001(5)), 2010.

24. U.S. Government Printing Office. Patient Protection and Affordable Care Act (P.L. 111-148 §1302), 2010.

25. U.S. Government Printing Office. Patient Protection and Affordable Care Act (P.L. 111-148§4002), 2010.

26. Prevention and public health fund resources. American Public Health Association. https://www.apha.org/topics-and-issues/aca-basics/prevention-and-public-health-fund-resources. Accessed September 29, 2014.

27. U.S. Government Printing Office. Consolidated Appropriations Act, 2014 (H.R. 3527). Passed January 17, 2014 (Pub. L. 113-76). http://www.gpo.gov/fdsys/pkg/PLAW-113publ76/html/PLAW-113publ76.htm. Accessed September 29, 2014.

28. U.S. Government Printing Office. Patient Protection and Affordable Care Act(P.L. 111-148§4001), 2010.

29. U.S. Government Printing Office. Patient Protection and Affordable Care Act (P.L. 111-148 §4002), 2010.

30. U.S. Government Printing Office. Patient Protection and Affordable Care Act (P.L. 111-148 §4003), 2010.

31. U.S. Government Printing Office. Patient Protection and Affordable Care Act (P.L. 111-148 §4108), 2010.

32. U.S. Government Printing Office. Patient Protection and Affordable Care Act. (P.L. 111-148 §4103), 2010.

33. U.S. Government Printing Office. Patient Protection and Affordable Care Act (P.L. 111-148 §4103), 2010.

34. Wagner RB. The search for value: Value-based insurance design in both public and private sectors. *Compensation and Benefits Review*. http://www.sph.umich.edu/vbidarchive/registry/pdfs/CompensationBenefitsReviewApril2011.pdf. Accessed September 29, 2014.

35. Starfield B. Basic concepts in population health and health care. *J Epidemiol Community Health*. 2001;55(7):452-4.

36. Chatterjee A, Kubendran S, King J, et al. Checkup time: chronic disease and wellness in America. http://assets1c.milkeninstitute.org/assets/Publication/ResearchReport/PDF/Checkup-Time-Chronic-Disease-and-Wellness-in-America.pdf. Accessed September 29, 2014.

37. Oleckno WA. Selected disease concepts in epidemiology. In: Oleckno WA. *Essential Epidemiology: Principles and Applications*. Long Grove, IL: Waveland Press; 2002:30-1.

38. Goetzel RZ, Ozminkowski RJ. The health and cost benefits of work site health-promotion programs. *Ann Rev Public Health*. 2008;29:303-23.

39. Chapman LS, Pelletier KR. Population health management as a strategy for creation of optimal healing environments in worksite and corporate settings. *J Altern Complement Med.* 2004;10(Suppl 1):S-127-40.

40. Durojaiye OC. Health screening: is it always worth doing? *Internet J Epidemiol.* 2009;7(1). http://ispub.com/IJE/7/1/3995. Accessed September 29, 2014.

41. National diabetes fact sheet, 2011. Centers for Disease Control and Prevention. http://www.cdc.gov/diabetes/pubs/pdf/ndfs_2011.pdf. Accessed September 29, 2014.

42. USPSTF A and B recommendations. U.S. Preventive Services Task Force. http://www.uspreventiveservicestaskforce.org/uspstf/uspsabrecs.htm. AccessedSeptember 29, 2014.

43. Kahn R, Robertson RM, Smith R, et al. The impact of prevention on reducing the burden of cardiovascular disease. *Diabetes Care.* 2008;31(8):1686-96.

44. U.S. Government Printing Office. Patient Protection and Affordable Care Act (P.L. 111-148 §1302), 2010.

45. U.S. Government Printing Office. Patient Protection and Affordable Care Act (P.L. 111-148 §2713), 2010.

46. U.S. Government Printing Office. Patient Protection and Affordable Care Act (P.L. 111-148 §4103), 2010.

47. Bodenheimer T. Helping patients improve their health-related behaviors: what system changes do we need? *Dis Manage.* 2005;8(5):319-30.

48. Söderlund LL, Madson MB, Rubak S, et al. A systematic review of motivational interviewing training for general health care practitioners. *Patient EducCouns.* 2011;84(1):16-26.

49. Defining the medical home: a patient-centered philosophy that drives primary care excellence. Patient-Centered Primary Care Collaborative. http://www.pcpcc.org/about/medical-home. Accessed September 29, 2014.

50. Taylor EF, Lake T, Nysenbaum J, et al. Coordinating care in the medical neighborhood: critical components and available mechanisms. Agency for Healthcare Research and Quality. http://pcmh.ahrq.gov/sites/default/files/attachments/Coordinating Care in the Medical Neighborhood.pdf. Accessed September 29, 2014.

51. Rittenhouse DR, Shortell SM, Fisher ES. Primary care and accountable care—two essential elements of delivery-system reform. *N Engl J Med.* 2009;361:2301-3.

52. Rosenthal TC. The medical home: growing evidence to support a new approach to primary care. *J Am Board Fam Med.* 2008;21(5):427-40.

53. National health expenditure data. Centers for Medicare and Medicaid Services. http://www.cms.gov/Research-Statistics-Data-and-Systems/Statistics-Trends-and-Reports/NationalHealthExpendData/Downloads/tables.pdf. Accessed September 29, 2014.

54. For the public's health: investing in a healthier future. Institute of Medicine. http://www.iom.edu/Reports/2012/For-the-Publics-Health-Investing-in-a-Healthier-Future.aspx. Accessed September 29, 2014.

55. Musich SA, Schultz AB, Burton WN, et al. Overview of disease management approaches: implications for corporate-sponsored programs. *Dis Manage Health Outcomes.* 2004;12(5):299-326.

56. Mattke S, Seid M, Ma S. Evidence for the effect of disease management: is $1 billion a year a good investment? *Am J Managed Care.* 2007;12(12):670-6. http://www.allhealth.org/briefingmaterials/Soeren_Mattke_AJMC-1230.pdf. Accessed September 29, 2014.

57. Bodenheimer T, Berry-Millett RL. Follow the money—controlling expenditures by improving care for patients needing costly services. *New Engl J Med.* 2009;361:1521-3.

58. Bodenheimer T, Wagner EH, Grumbach K. Improving primary care for patients with chronic illness. *JAMA.* 2002;288(14):1775-9.

59. Wagner EH, Austin BT, Davis C, et al. Improving chronic illness care: translating evidence into action. *Health Aff.* 2001;20(6):64-78.

60. Lewis A. How to measure the outcomes of chronic disease management. *Popul Health Manag.* 2009;12(1):47-54.

61. An analysis of the literature on disease management programs. Congressional Budget Office. http://www.cbo.gov/sites/default/files/10-13-diseasemngmnt.pdf. Accessed September 29, 2014.

62. Barr VJ, Robinson S, Marin-Link B, et al. The expanded Chronic Care Model: an integration of concepts and strategies from population health promotion and the Chronic Care Model. *Hosp Q.* 2003;7(1):73-82.

63. Goetzel R, Ozminkowski RJ, Villagra VG, et al. Return on investment in disease management: a review. *Health Care Financing Rev.* 2005;26(4):1-19.

64. What is a case manager? Case Management Society of America. http://www.cmsa.org/Home/CMSA/WhatisaCaseManager/tabid/224/Default.aspx. Accessed September 29, 2014.

65. Carter-Pokras O, Baquet C: What is a "health disparity"? *Public Health Reports* 2002;117(5):426-34. http://www.ncbi.nlm.nih.gov/pmc/articles/PMC1497467/pdf/12500958.pdf. Accessed November 10, 2014.

66. Betancourt JR, Corbett J, Bondaryk, MR. Addressing disparities and achieving equity: cultural competence, ethics and health-care transformation. *Chest.* 2014;145(1):143-8.

67. Adler NE, Rehkopf DH. U.S. disparities in health: descriptions, causes, and mechanisms. *Annu Rev Public Health.* 2008;29:235-52.

68. Gillespie CD, Hurvitz KA. Prevalence of hypertension and controlled hypertension—United States, 2007-2010. *MMWR.* 2013;62(3):144-48. http://www.cdc.gov/mmwr/preview/mmwrhtml/su6203a24.htm. Accessed September 29, 2014.

69. Bodenheimer T, Chen E, Bennett HD. Confronting the growing burden of chronic disease: can the U.S. health care workforce do the job? *Health Aff.* 2009;28(1):64-74.

70. Chin MW, Clarke AR, Nocon RS et al: A roadmap and best practices for organizations to reduce racial and ethnic disparities in health care. *JGIM.* 2012;27(8):992-1000.

71. Centers for Disease Control and Prevention. CDC Health Disparities and Inequalities Report—United States, 2013. *MMWR Supplement.* 2013;62(Suppl 3):1-187. http://www.cdc.gov/mmwr/preview/ind2013_su.html. Accessed September 29, 2014.

72. Betancourt JR, Corbett J, Bondaryk, MR. Addressing disparities and achieving equity: cultural competence, ethics and health-care transformation. *Chest.* 2014;145(1):143-8.

73. State licensing requirements for cultural competency. Quality Interactions. http://www.qualityinteractions.org/cultural_competence/cc_statelicreqs.html. Accessed September 29, 2014.

74. U.S. Government Printing Office. Civil Rights Act of 1964 (P.L. 88-352), 1964.

75. U.S. Government Printing Office. Emergency Medical Treatment & Labor Act (42 USC §1395-100), 1986.

76. U.S. Government Printing Office. Plain Writing Act of 2010 (P.L. 111-274), 2010.

77. U.S. Government Printing Office. Patient Protection and Affordable Care Act. (P.L. 111-148), 2010.

78. National action plan to improve health literacy. U.S. Department of Health & Human Services. http://www.health.gov/communication/hlactionplan/. Accessed September 29, 2014.

79. Advancing effective communication, cultural competence, and patient- and family-centered care: a roadmap for hospitals. The Joint Commission. http://www.jointcommission.org/assets/1/6/ARoadmapforHospitalsfinalversion727.pdf. Accessed September 29, 2014.

80. Multicultural health care: a quality improvement guide. National Committee for Quality Assurance. http://www.ncqa.org/portals/0/hedisqm/CLAS/CLAS_toolkit.pdf. Accessed September 29, 2014.

81. Cultural competency measurement and implementation strategies: summary report. The National Quality Forum. http://www.qualityforum.org/Projects/c-d/Cultural_Competency_2010/Cultural_Competency_2010.aspx. Accessed September 29, 2014.

82. National standards for culturally and linguistically appropriate services in health care: final report. U.S. Department of Health and Human Services. Office of Minority Health. http://minorityhealth.hhs.gov/assets/pdf/checked/finalreport.pdf. Accessed September 29, 2014.

83. Banthin J, Masi S. CBOs' estimate of the net budgetary impact of the affordable care act's health insurance coverage provisions has not changed much

over time. http://www.cbo.gov/publication/44176. Accessed September 29, 2014.

84. Ricketts TC, Fraher EP. Reconfiguring health workforce policy so that education, training, and actual delivery of care are closely connected. *Health Aff.* 2013;32(11):1874-80.

85. Wynia MK, Kishore SP. A unified code of ethics for health professionals: insights from an IOM workshop. *JAMA.* 2014;311(8):799-800.

86. Institute of Medicine. *Crossing the Quality Chasm: A New Health System for the 21st Century.* Washington, DC: National Academies Press; 2001.

87. Panzer RJ, Gitomer RS, Greene WH, et al. Increasing demands for quality measurement. *JAMA.* 2013;310(18):1971-80.

88. U.S. Government Printing Office. Patient Protection and Affordable Care Act. (P.L. 111-148 §3011), 2010.

| Chapter 3 | POLICY IMPLICATIONS FOR POPULATION HEALTH: HEALTH PROMOTION AND WELLNESS |

POLICY IMPLICATIONS FOR POPULATION HEALTH: HEALTH PROMOTION AND WELLNESS

FREDERIC S. GOLDSTEIN,
VICKI SHEPARD, AND SUZANNE DUDA*

Executive Summary

Population health management is a systematic approach to enable all people in a defined population to maintain and improve their health. This is accomplished by providing individually customized programs, information, and support designed to promote healthy lifestyles and improve adherence to evidence-based care.

Critical to the success of population health management is understanding the population through data analytics, facilitating scalable and standardized delivery through enabling technology, promoting participant and support system engagement, and securing the active participation of healthcare providers and community resources.

Rising costs and increasing prevalence of chronic conditions among various segments of the U.S. population have caused policy makers to seek alternative models of care to address the needs of at-risk and chronically ill populations. In 2009, the new Obama administration, congressional leaders, interest groups, and others declared healthcare delivery system reform a top priority for the 110th Congress. Congress passed the Patient Protection and **Affordable Care Act** (ACA), which is widely acknowledged as the most comprehensive healthcare reform legislation in decades. In addition to expanding health insurance coverage, the ACA includes many provisions that reform the healthcare delivery system to encourage providers to better manage the health of the populations they serve. This chapter provides an overview of the key players in federal policy making (both enactment and implementation), experiences from early disease management demonstrations

*This chapter was based on contributions made by Tracey Moorhead; Jeanette C. May, PhD; and Kip MacArthur in the first edition.

and pilot programs enacted at the federal level, specific provisions of the ACA, and key components for consideration in developing policy to advance population health.

Learning Objectives

1. Describe the factors that play a role in the shift to population health management.
2. Identify the key players and their roles in federal policy making for population health.
3. Appreciate the components of population health under the Medicare program and how Medicare policy has shaped commercial insurance.
4. Understand the design and use of incentives and their potential for discrimination.
5. Understand the key components of the ACA and how it influences the adoption of disease prevention services and initiatives in the system.

Key Terms

accountable care organization	fee-for-service
Affordable Care Act	health information technology
discretionary spending	mandatory spending

INTRODUCTION

Population health management programs are continually evolving to better address the needs and resources of the populations and providers they serve. Population health management has become a catch phrase for those seeking to improve the healthcare system. Population health approaches have evolved from programs focused on single chronic disease management, to comprehensive programs and interventions that address all of the individuals within a given population regardless of their health status. Many of the population health management "innovations" were previously introduced and delivered by health plans and later industry vendors, like case or disease management, and are now being delivered by newly formed provider arrangements such as **accountable care organizations** (ACOs) and patient-centered medical homes. Many experts believe that this is an improvement. Embedding state-of-the-art population health management approaches closer to the doctor–patient relationship increases the likelihood of engagement and adherence.

Population health also recognizes that many of the factors that influence a person's health are outside of the care system (e.g., community-based issues, access to sidewalks and nutritious foods). Given the broad range of services and structures required to improve the health of populations, the most effective approaches are dependent on (or rely on) collaboration and support. As the ACA drives more providers to move into the population health space, new reimbursement methodologies and organizational structures are taking effect (e.g., integrated delivery systems [IDSs] and ACOs). Recognizing that they have a vital interest in the health of their constituents, communities are beginning to form broader partnerships and engage in collaborative efforts to address the range of services necessary to maintain and improve population health and well-being.

The ACA established many new legislative initiatives targeting population health to improve care and outcomes and reduce costs. These include delivery system and payment reforms that reward efforts that add value rather than volume (i.e., moving away from a fee-for-service methodology), such as quality measures, specific prevention and wellness activities, incentives for outcomes-based programs, and implementation of **health information technology (HIT)**. There was and continues to be considerable congressional debate regarding the components of population health management and their efficacy and use. In any event, the ACA will have a profound effect for years to come on the development, implementation, and use of population health management tools, strategies, and systems.

KEY PLAYERS IN FEDERAL POLICY MAKING

There are many stakeholders that affect healthcare policy at both the federal and state levels. At the federal level, these players include the U.S. Congress, congressionally mandated independent organizations, and cabinet-level agencies and offices.

The federal government influences policy and population health directly as one of the largest purchasers of health care and indirectly as an influencer of private sector healthcare purchasing and delivery. As the largest employer and purchaser of healthcare services, the federal government finances and provides coverage to nearly 130 million government employees; the poor, disabled, and elderly; active duty and former military personnel and their dependents; and Native Americans and other populations.[1] Given this role, federal government purchasing and healthcare delivery policies can often significantly influence other purchaser and provider populations. For example, independent health plans and providers who participate in federal programs (e.g., Medicare **fee-for-service plans**, military-focused TRICARE program) may impose payment and rate policies on nongovernment clients similar to those imposed by large government-managed programs. Private sector purchasers, especially those seeking coverage options for thousands of employees, dependents, or retirees, may seek to negotiate contract rates similar to those paid by government programs, or they may follow the government's lead in directly contracting with newly formed ACOs. Clearly, government coverage, payment policies, and ideas regarding system structure extend beyond government-managed programs and can directly affect coverage, rate policies, and contracting for other purchasers, as well as coverage and payment policies for healthcare practitioners.

U.S. CONGRESS AND CONGRESSIONAL ADVISORY AGENCIES AND COMMISSIONS

The U.S. Congress plays a key role in establishing healthcare policy and directly influences population health management in the context of broader health policy and healthcare reform. Several congressional committees, in both the U.S. House of Representatives and the U.S. Senate, share jurisdiction over portions of the healthcare delivery and payment systems at the federal level. In the House, several committees have jurisdiction over healthcare delivery and payment systems for the private sector as well as for government programs:

- The Education and the Workforce Committee considers legislation relating to employer-sponsored health benefits.
- The Energy and Commerce Committee addresses public health, Medicaid, pharmaceutical, and other national health insurance issues.
- The Committee on Ways and Means has authority over bills and matters pertaining to health programs under the Social Security Act and many public health programs.

There are two Senate committees with jurisdiction over healthcare policy:

- The Committee on Finance considers healthcare programs under the Social Security Act, including Medicare, Medicaid, and other health programs financed by certain taxes or trust funds.
- The Health, Education, Labor and Pensions Committee (HELP) considers legislation that affects primary health and aging, including issues related to the Health Resources and Services Act and the Older Americans Act.

Congressional legislative efforts to enact policy changes are informed by numerous sources, including a variety of congressionally mandated, independent organizations. Among these organizations, the Medicare Payment Advisory Commission (MedPAC) and the Congressional Budget Office (CBO) are integral to advancing the population health agenda.

MedPAC was created by the Balanced Budget Act of 1997 as an independent congressional agency. The 17-member commission, comprising health policy experts, healthcare providers, and academicians, provides the U.S. Congress with analyses, recommendations, and reports on issues affecting the Medicare program (e.g., payment, access, and quality). MedPAC convenes publicly several times a year to review staff research and to seek comment and input from healthcare researchers, providers, and beneficiary advocates on financing and delivery and other trends affecting the Medicare program. Congressional leaders and the Centers for Medicare and Medicaid Services (CMS) rely heavily on MedPAC analyses for critical examination of existing policy and case studies to understand the effect of potential policy or payment changes.

MedPAC has studied models of care coordination in treating those with chronic disease and the feasibility of applying these models to a broader Medicare population. CMS has implemented many of the models as demonstration programs and other initiatives to improve care coordination. These care coordination efforts are expected to foster better patient understanding and adherence to various treatment regimens, and to drive patients toward more appropriate and less costly care settings (e.g., primary care providers and urgent care centers rather than emergency departments). Care coordination and appropriate utilization are key components of any successful population health management program.

In several recent reports to Congress, MedPAC reiterated concerns that poor care coordination, combined with a growing prevalence of beneficiaries with chronic disease, will continue to put a strain on Medicare resources. A 2003 MedPAC analysis of Medicare fee-for-service beneficiaries found that a Medicare beneficiary saw, on average, five different physicians each year. For those who were diagnosed with at least three common chronic conditions, the number increased to 10 or more per year.[2] When viewed from a population health perspective, such fragmented care is inefficient and ineffective.

The report goes on to review several Medicare pilot programs and demonstration projects that address chronic conditions and associated costs in the fee-for-service Medicare population.[2] These pilots and demonstrations are discussed later in the chapter. In addition, MedPAC analyzed the feasibility of developing a Medicare Chronic Care Practice Research Network to continue testing models of care coordination for the Medicare population. These findings can help move population health forward through the testing and validation of various models designed to address whole-person, whole-population needs.

The CBO was established in 1974 as an objective, nonpartisan entity to provide data, estimates, and analyses on the fiscal implications of congressional proposals and federal spending on the economy. For legislative proposals reported out of a congressional committee or upon request, the CBO is required to produce estimates on the effect of both **discretionary spending** (i.e., budget authority that is provided and controlled by appropriation acts and the outlays that result from that budget authority) and **mandatory spending** (i.e., budget authority provided and controlled by laws other than appropriation acts and the outlays that result from that budget authority).[3] Increasing healthcare costs and expanding public sector program populations have caused great emphasis to be placed on the CBO's scoring reports for healthcare reform and policy proposals.

Current CBO analytic models have not attributed financial savings to proposed prevention and wellness programs, and this presents a challenge for the population health management industry in terms of demonstrating cost savings associated with disease prevention. In its December 2008 analysis of key issues in health insurance proposals, the CBO stated that although initiatives to improve people's health (e.g., adopting healthy lifestyles, obtaining preventive screenings, implementing programs to better manage chronic disease) lead to better quality of life, they do not necessarily reduce healthcare spending. Although the programs may be worthwhile, the CBO has questioned whether certain types of initiatives save enough to cover their cost. As of 2010, the CBO has concluded that the clinical and economic effect of prevention services is not sufficiently well understood to precisely estimate costs and benefits.

Several reports dispute the CBO's assertion that prevention will not reduce healthcare spending. In a white paper commissioned by the Partnership to Fight Chronic Disease, economists Michael O'Grady and James Capretta suggest that there are limitations to the

CBO's cost-estimating practices.[4] Because the CBO does not forecast beyond a 10-year budget window, it is unable to capture the long-term cost savings associated with preventing chronic disease. A recent study titled "Potential Medicare Savings Through Prevention and Health Risk Reduction" aimed to identify the relationship between cost and risk.[5] Researchers developed models to better understand how cost would be affected if the population were able to shift to a lower risk category and/or maintain a low-risk status longer. The models suggest that the Medicare program could save $65 billion annually, approximately $650 billion over 10 years, by increasing the number of low-risk individuals who are 65 years of age and reducing the health risk progression by 10%.

Another barrier to the CBO's demonstrating savings is that it must include all costs to the government made by the proposed change, including those that are outside of the healthcare system (e.g., the legislation's effect on life expectancy and the increase in Social Security and other costs that are associated with increased life span).

U.S. DEPARTMENT OF HEALTH AND HUMAN SERVICES

Cabinet-level agencies and other offices are also key players in policy making, with primary responsibility for implementing legislative policy on healthcare issues. Most prominent is CMS, formerly known as the Health Care Financing Administration, which is an office of the U.S. Department of Health and Human Services (HHS). Established as the regulatory agency for federal healthcare programs, CMS administers the Medicare program (including covered healthcare services, benefits, eligibility, enrollment, and provider participation), Medicaid, and the Children's Health Insurance Program (CHIP) (the latter two of which are jointly administered by CMS and individual states). As of 2012, there were nearly 110 million people covered under the Medicare, Medicaid, and CHIP programs.[1] As discussed earlier, the federal government has a significant role in the financing and delivery of health care, developing health policy, and managing population health as one of the largest administrators and purchasers of healthcare services.

The role of HHS in promoting population health management extends beyond the public programs it administers. For example, HHS plays a role in administering regulations related to the use of financial incentives to promote wellness. The Health Insurance Portability and Accountability Act (HIPAA) prohibits health plans from charging higher premiums or cost sharing for individuals with preexisting conditions, with limited exceptions. The population health management industry has pioneered the use of innovative incentive programs to encourage sustained behavior change. After the ACA expanded the allowable use of wellness-related financial incentives, HHS, the Department of Treasury, and the Department of Labor collaborated to issue new regulations to enhance and clarify requirements related to the use of nondiscriminatory wellness incentives. The Equal Employment Opportunity Commission (EEOC) also plays a role in regulating the use of wellness incentives and is expected to issue clarifying regulations in the near future.

The establishment of the Center for Medicare & Medicaid Innovation within CMS has created opportunities for further development of models that support population health.

The CMS Innovation Center funds a broad range of demonstration programs, including alternative payment and delivery models, intended to promote care coordination.

The Office of the National Coordinator for Health Information Technology (ONC) is the principal federal agency charged with the coordination of national efforts to implement the use of HIT and the electronic exchange of health information. The ONC is engaged in promoting the development of a nationwide HIT infrastructure that will lead to the interoperability of health information. This has been largely supported by funds allotted within the stimulus package prior to the passage of the ACA.

HIT plays an important role in population health management and is a key strategy for achieving population health improvement. HIT is an essential element in improving patient safety and the overall quality of care.[6] Patients, particularly those with chronic conditions, often see multiple healthcare providers. Like electronic health records (EHRs), HIT allows each provider access to the same information, thereby increasing access to vital information and improving transparency among healthcare providers. HIT provides actionable data and analytic systems, such as embedded clinical decision support and clinical alerts, that facilitate improved delivery of healthcare services and population health management.

The federal government has placed a major emphasis on moving providers away from paper records to an electronic format with the passage of the Health Information Technology for Economic and Clinical Health (HITECH) Act, under section XIII of the American Recovery and Reinvestment Act of 2009. Under the HITECH Act, HHS has spent billions of dollars to promote and expand provider use of EHRs. Many of the "meaningful use" criteria set by HITECH are related to population health approaches, including the following:

- Improve care coordination
- Reduce healthcare disparities
- Engage patients and their families
- Improve population and public health
- Ensure adequate privacy and security

Recent federal government efforts in HIT include a broad approach to create linkages for patients through the federal Blue Button initiative, a U.S. Department of Veterans Affairs program expanded on by the ONC. The Blue Button is a tool that promotes care coordination by making medical records easily available for patients to share with their healthcare providers.

OVERVIEW OF DEMONSTRATION PROJECTS AND PILOTS

The expected growth of the Medicare population, coupled with the prevalence and costs associated with the treatment of chronic illness, has caused policy makers to seek alternative models of care to address the needs of chronically ill beneficiaries. Passage of the

Medicare Modernization Act (2003) gave CMS the authority to explore other care delivery models for the fee-for-service Medicare population through demonstration projects and pilot programs.

Demonstrations and pilots are requested by Congress and carried out by CMS for the purpose of testing the viability and feasibility of new healthcare delivery systems and services. Results from previous demonstrations and pilots are used to shape new models for testing and application to more broadly affect population health. This exercise is integral to population health (i.e., building on previous successes to achieve further improvements and advancing the agenda to achieve high-quality, affordable, coordinated care).

In terms of disease state control and quality of life, population health management has shown mixed results in commercial and other government programs, and further research is needed to determine whether these programs can be adapted successfully and implemented in the Medicare environment. Pilot tests of these strategies on Medicare-managed populations include Medicare Advantage plans and special needs plans for chronically ill populations.[7] Both of these plans offer population health approaches, including assessments, care coordination, unique exercise programs, and other services that are not available in the fee-for-service Medicare program and that may provide some insight and experience that lead to better care coordination within the Medicare population. Preliminary results suggest that a population health management strategy that includes wellness, disease management, case management, and care coordination may improve outcomes, reduce costs, and improve the patient experience, which are all consistent with the Triple Aim[8] (improve the patients' experience of care and the health of populations, and reduce the per capita cost of health care).

In contrast to the commercial and public sector managed care markets, identifying ideal health management models for Medicare fee-for-service beneficiaries is in the early stages of development. Although promotion of wellness and reduction of health risks are crucial components of population health, prevention and wellness solutions have not yet been tested in fee-for-service Medicare populations. Roughly three-quarters of Medicare beneficiaries receive care through original fee-for-service Medicare (i.e., the provider of services is paid for each unit of service). Original Medicare consists of Part A (inpatient hospital, skilled nursing facility, and hospice) and Part B (doctor's visits, outpatient care, and some preventive services).

Permanently authorized as part of the Balanced Budget Act of 1997, Medicare Advantage, or Medicare Part C (formerly known as Medicare+Choice), is a form of managed care run by private health plans and approved by CMS. Varying by plan, Part C provides coverage granted through Parts A and B, often including additional benefits not covered by Medicare fee-for-service (e.g., vision, hearing aids). Medicare Advantage is an alternative for Medicare-eligible individuals wherein enrollees are encouraged to seek care with participating providers. In many cases, Medicare Advantage plans charge premiums (in addition to the Part B premium) to offset benefits that are beyond those of traditional Medicare coverage.

Medicare currently provides healthcare benefits and coverage to nearly 50 million Americans; the vast majority of these beneficiaries are older than 65 years of age. A growing number of Medicare beneficiaries with multiple chronic conditions are responsible for the greatest percentage of healthcare expenses. These beneficiaries are likely to have more provider visits, see multiple clinicians, fill more prescriptions, and have far more hospitalizations. Care coordination and wellness and disease management programs offer these populations crucial support services to assist with the management and mitigation of diseases and risk factors. Care coordination and disease management are among the approaches now being tested for Medicare fee-for-service beneficiaries.

STATE CASE STUDIES IN DISEASE MANAGEMENT

Early on, states recognized the value of disease management programs as a strategy to improve quality and control the increasing costs of healthcare delivery, especially to those with chronic illnesses. In the late 1990s, states began to implement disease management programs for chronically ill Medicaid patients in an effort to address the rising costs associated with treatment. By the early 2000s, nearly all 50 states had implemented disease management or care coordination programs for some segment of the Medicaid population. Because federal policy allowed many states to develop and implement various approaches to care management, case studies were reported demonstrating the potential for care management in public populations. In effect, states were permitted exceptional flexibility in the design and implementation of such programs, going far beyond interventions tested in the Medicare populations.

The state of Missouri transformed its Medicaid program from a provider-centered model to an individual-centered, outcomes-focused model by combining primary care case management, care coordination, and disease management services offered through targeted disease state and risk assessment.[9] The expectation was that the newly designed program would improve adherence, increase appropriate service utilization, increase provider use of electronic tools, and improve both participant and provider satisfaction. In fact, it led to improvements in outcomes (e.g., adherence, service utilization, cost for participants with a variety of chronic conditions). For participants with diabetes, adherence to recommended diabetic testing and screening improved. Other improved outcomes included lipid panel compliance for populations with diabetes and coronary artery disease (CAD), and improved medication adherence for populations with asthma and chronic obstructive pulmonary disease. Lastly, emergency department (ED) visits and costs decreased substantially for the population enrolled in the program.

In Pennsylvania, a pay-for-participation (P4P) program was instituted with selected providers in 2003 in an effort to reduce inpatient admissions and ED visits by Medicaid beneficiaries. Incentives were paid to providers who practiced guideline-based care and who ensured that patients receiving certain interventions experienced improved health outcomes. Results demonstrated that Medicaid beneficiaries associated with a provider receiving P4P incentives had fewer inpatient admissions and ED visits than beneficiaries receiving care from a provider not receiving additional payments.

These two state efforts are examples of successful population health approaches that have informed practitioners and policy makers alike.

THE PATIENT PROTECTION AND AFFORDABLE CARE ACT OF 2010

Although much of the effect of the ACA will take years if not decades to realize, there has been considerable debate as to its merits and its implementation to date.

The ACA addresses population health in four ways: expands insurance coverage, seeks to improve quality, enhances prevention and health promotion, and promotes community and population health activity.[10] Some of the specific changes addressed in the Act include the following:

- The establishment of a National Prevention, Health Promotion, and Public Health Council, involving more than a dozen federal agencies, which will develop a prevention and health promotion strategy for the country.[11]
- A new Prevention and Public Health Fund, with an annual appropriation that begins at $500 million fiscal year 2010 and increases to $2 billion in fiscal year 2015 and beyond, which will invest in a range of prevention and wellness.
- Coverage of a range of recommended preventive services with no cost sharing by the beneficiary. These service include those rated as A (strongly recommended) or B (recommended) by the U.S. Preventive Services Task Force (USPSTF), vaccinations recommended by the Advisory Committee on Immunization Practices (ACIP), and preventive care and screening included both in existing health guidelines for children and adolescents and in future guidelines to be developed for women through the U.S. Health Resources and Services Administration (HRSA). Coverage has also been extended for obesity treatment programs.
- Coverage of an annual Medicare wellness visit to establish a personalized prevention plan.
- Payments to providers for care coordination.
- Expanded incentives for wellness programs.
- Medicare shared savings methodology with ACOs.
- Health Insurance Marketplace (public exchange).

KEY CONSIDERATIONS IN POLICY DEVELOPMENT

Policy makers acknowledge the effects of chronic illness on the Medicare population and are seeking solutions to improve health outcomes and prevent avoidable healthcare costs. There is widespread acknowledgment of the need to better manage and prevent chronic illness through whole-person, whole-population management. Organizing care, information, and services around the health needs and desires of individuals is a concept that all healthcare stakeholders have embraced. For policy makers, redesigning care delivery models to meet these goals requires understanding existing barriers to management and prevention, recognizing innovative delivery models, and identifying key components that contribute to the success of delivery models. Further complicating the challenge of care delivery redesign is the need to align financing and payment models with new delivery approaches.

Population health management continues to move toward collaborative models of care delivery, and it has become clear that no single model is appropriate for all settings or populations. Rather, flexible models, developed and aligned with the needs of the target population and existing services, have demonstrated considerable success. Many models seek to transform provider practice design, integrate HIT, and develop partnerships among interdisciplinary healthcare teams. As these new models and collaborations evolve, population health management strategies can provide significant support and expertise based on experiences in service delivery and outcomes improvement.

Population health management strategies and their components are essential solutions for policy makers to consider at both the federal and state levels. Population health management places the patient at the center of the model and aims to improve the health status of the entire population through prevention, wellness, chronic condition support, and advanced care management services. Key components of population health management are identification of the population; determination of the individual's risks; stratification based on identified risk; implementation of a person-centered model of intervention that recognizes and coordinates community resources; organization and tailored approaches based on the risk level; and measurement of the outcomes in the areas of psychosocial behavior change, clinical and health status, quality of life, and financial realms.[12]

A review of successful commercial and public sector programs offers key design principles for consideration in the implementation of future population health management programs in Medicare fee-for-service. These principles include the following:

- Appropriate use of data and analytic capabilities to target populations most appropriate for intervention
- Availability of care coordination and coaching resources for targeted populations
- Widespread adoption of interoperable health information technologies
- Clearly defined metrics for outcomes measurement

These principles are common to a variety of delivery system models and are readily transparent in traditional managed care and physician-led care delivery models, cooperative healthcare models, and newly designed ACOs.

The use of timely clinical and self-reported data and analyses, using predictive modeling methods, is essential to identifying individuals and population cohorts that might benefit from a broad variety of population health management services. Timely data ensure that individuals have not progressed in their conditions beyond the scope of the services to be delivered, a key consideration in elderly populations served by fee-for-service Medicare. Predictive modeling applications are rapidly improving in their ability to identify appropriate individuals and population cohorts for intervention.

Enhanced care coordination and coaching support services are key to effectively teaching patients or their caregivers to manage their conditions and to navigate the healthcare system. Models of care coordination may range from a physician group that provides care coordination services to its patients, to an external care management or health advocacy organization that offers these services, to automated responses that use technology and mobile health tools.[12] There is evidence that programs aimed at improving coordination of care for the chronically ill have resulted in positive health outcomes (e.g., reduction in hospital readmissions among patients who are provided assistance with care transition between settings). Care coordination also has proven beneficial in assisting patients to manage their own conditions.[13] Population health management has played a vital role in successfully managing transitions from acute care to home for many patients. Working with hospitals, providers, and ancillary care organizations, population health management can reduce avoidable morbidity associated with transitions across different sites and levels of care by leveraging experience and employing the most advanced technology.

The explosion in mobile technologies (e.g., smartphone technology and usage, consumer demand for monitoring and tracking devices and applications) has been moving into the population health space. This technological explosion has resulted in initial efforts by the Food and Drug Administration (FDA) to better understand the use and potential of mobile devices and apps, and to regulate them as appropriate.

Widespread adoption and integration of HIT is another key strategy for improving population health management. Paired with skilled and coordinated interdisciplinary healthcare teams and activated patients and families, this technology provides access to relevant data and supports improved outcomes. Systematic improvements in management of information are crucial to improving the quality of health care for patients with chronic diseases and decreasing costs of their care. Specifically, tools available to individuals for health support in the home setting are proliferating. Devices such as biometric monitors and diagnostic devices can populate data fields in providers' and care managers' EHRs. Further, EHRs and personal health records hold great promise for enhancing care coordination, eliminating waste and duplication, and providing individuals with greater resources for improving their own health. Because issues such as integration, usability, and relevance are still being defined, the goal of a seamless, smart system of devices, data, analytics, and interventions is yet to be attained.

Population health management leaders continue the process of defining guidelines and best practices for evaluating program outcomes. Just as a single-care delivery model is not appropriate for all settings or populations, policy makers must recognize that no single measure or method of value assessment is appropriate to all programs. Examining specific program components, strategies, and goals is essential to ensuring the appropriate evaluation of outcomes for all metrics.

CONCLUSION

Significant new opportunities for the population health management industry have been brought about by the HITECH Act and the ACA. The ACA places a greater emphasis on prevention and population health while moving the implementation of many of these programs to provider-based care models. The new focus on population health is intended to improve access to care coordination and support programs to targeted beneficiaries; expand use of prevention and wellness services; and further encourage widespread adoption of HIT to collect, share, and analyze health-related data. Many of the approaches designed to test and implement these models present new opportunities and challenges for the population health management industry.

Proponents of a medical home or other physician-led care models underscore the benefits of a designated primary care physician or healthcare team leader. In addition, many providers recognize the benefits of practice transformation, workflow enhancement, capacity-expanding health information technologies, and expanded provider partnerships to better meet the ever-diversifying needs of various patient populations. This recognition has led to innovative collaborations among healthcare providers who recognize that although physicians must lead these efforts, they can benefit from additional staff and capabilities, both within their practice walls and beyond, to provide comprehensive support to patients. Healthcare delivery system reform debates have centered on these practice model changes and collaborative delivery approaches. Expanded pilot programs and payment mechanisms are likely to provide new opportunities for population health management to offer services and resources to physicians implementing these models.

Transitions of care for vulnerable populations have been another key focus of healthcare reform debates. Healthcare reform advocates have recognized the importance of managing transitions for vulnerable populations between acute care settings and the home, especially for those with Medicare. Population health management providers that have incorporated strategies such as use of advanced technologies and collaboration with hospitals, providers, and ancillary care organizations have demonstrated the ability to eliminate avoidable morbidity associated with transitions across different sites and levels of care. Healthcare reform efforts will undoubtedly provide opportunities to test these programs in Medicare populations with the likelihood of expansion in the coming years.

Federal government efforts in recent years have focused on the expansion and use of health information technologies, including EHRs. Clearly, EHRs and personal health records hold greater promise than ever before for enhancing care coordination, eliminating waste and duplication, and providing individuals with greater resources for improving their health. Healthcare reform's goal of improved quality and more cost-efficient care makes the expanded adoption and use of HIT resources significant and timely. Population health management strategies have greatly expanded service delivery and improved outcomes through the utilization of varied HIT applications.

The ACA has placed prevention and population health management front and center. With the myriad changes accompanying the ACA, it will be years before its implications are understood and the full impact is recognized. But it has created a profound shift in the way patients, providers, and payers work together to implement population health approaches.

STUDY AND DISCUSSION QUESTIONS

1. What factors have influenced the need for a population health focus?
2. Who are the key players for federal policy making and what role do they play?
3. Why was the Medicare Payment Advisory Commission created and what role does it play?
4. What is the Congressional Budget Office? What is its role? What has been its assessment of population health?
5. What role does health information technology play in population health?
6. How does Medicare shape the commercial side of population health?
7. Describe and discuss the key design principles of population health for Medicare.
8. Is care coordination important to population health? Why or why not?
9. What are some of the key concepts and proposals shaping the population health strategy debate?

SUGGESTED READINGS AND WEBSITES

READINGS

Baicker K, Cutler D, Song Z. Workplace wellness programs can generate savings. *Health Aff.* 2010;29(2):304-11.

Caloyeras J, Hangsheng L, Exum E, et al. Managing manifest diseases, but not health risks, saved PepsiCo money over seven years. *Health Aff.* 2014;(33)1:124-31.

Congress of the United States, Congressional Budget Office. *Budget Options.* Washington, DC: *Health Care.* 2008;(1) Pub No. 3185. http://www.cbo.gov/sites/default/files/12-18-healthoptions.pdf. Accessed October 20, 2014.

Congress of the United States, Congressional Budget Office. *Key Issues in Analyzing Major Health Insurance Proposals.* Washington, DC: 2008. Pub No. 3102. http://www.cbo.gov/sites/default/files/12-18-keyissues.pdf. Accessed October 20, 2014.

Congress of the United States H.R.3590—Patient Protection and Affordable Care Act. 111th Congress (2009-2010). http://beta.congress.gov/bill/111th-congress/house-bill/3590?q=%7B"search"%3A%5B"Affordable+care+act"%5D%7D. Accessed September 30, 2014.

Fisher ES, McClellan MB, Bertko J, et al. Fostering accountable health care: moving forward in Medicare. *Health Aff (Millwood)*. 2009;28(2):w219-31.

Mattke S, Hangsheng L, Caloyeras JP, et al. Workplace wellness program study final report report. http://www.rand.org/content/dam/rand/pubs/research_reports/RR200/RR254/RAND_RR254.pdf. Accessed September 30, 2014.

WEBSITES

Agency for Healthcare Research and Quality: http://www.ahrq.gov

Centers for Medicare and Medicaid Services: http://www.cms.gov

Committee on Finance: http://www.finance.senate.gov

Committee on Health, Education, Labor and Pensions: http://help.senate.gov

Committee on Ways and Means: http://waysandmeans.house.gov

The Commonwealth Fund: http://www.commonwealthfund.org

Congressional Budget Office: http://www.cbo.gov

Education and the Workforce Committee: http://edworkforce.house.gov/

Energy and Commerce Committee: http://www.energycommerce.house.gov

Health Affairs: http://www.healthaffairs.org

Health information technology: http://www.healthit.gov

Institute of Medicine: http://www.iom.edu

Kaiser Family Foundation: http://www.kff.org

Medicare Overview: http://www.medicare.gov/sign-up-change-plans/decide-how-to-get-medicare/your-medicare-coverage-choices.html

Medicare Payment Advisory Commission: http://www.medpac.gov

The New England Journal of Medicine: http://www.nejm.org

Partnership to Fight Chronic Disease: http://www.fightchronicdisease.org

Patient Protection and Affordable Care Act: http://www.hhs.gov/healthcare/rights/law/

Population Health Alliance: http://www.populationhealthalliance.org/

U.S. House of Representatives: http://www.house.gov

U.S. Senate: http://www.senate.gov

REFERENCES

1. Jaffe S. Health policy brief: key issues in health reform. *Health Aff*. August 20, 2009. http://www.healthaffairs.org/healthpolicybriefs/brief.php?brief_id=10. Accessed October 20, 2014.

2. Report to the Congress: improving incentives in the Medicare program. Medicare Payment Advisory Commission. June 2009. http://www.ehidc.org/resource-center/reports/view_document/158-reports-report-to-congress-improving-incentives-in-the-medicare-program-accountable-care. Accessed October 2, 2014.

3. Congressional Budget Office. Frequently asked questions about CBO cost estimates. https://www.cbo.gov/about/products/ce-faq. Accessed October 20, 2014.

4. O'Grady MJ, Capretta JC. Health-care cost projections for diabetes and other chronic diseases: the current context and potential enhancements. http://www.fightchronicdisease.org/sites/fightchronicdisease.org/files/docs/PFCD_whitepaper5.21.09.pdf. Accessed December 15, 2014.

5. Rula E, Pope J, Hoffman JC. Potential Medicare savings through prevention & health risk reduction: a report from the Center for Health Research. http://www.healthways.com/trillions/download/medicaresavings.pdf. Accessed September 30, 2014.

6. Hillestad R, Bigelow J, Bower A, et al. Can electronic medical record systems transform health care? Potential health benefits, savings, and costs. *Health Aff.* 2005;24(5):1103-17.

7. Caloyeras JP, Liu H, Exum E, et al. Managing manifest diseases, but not health risks, saved PepsiCo money over seven years. *Health Aff.* 2014;33(1):124-31.

8. Carmona RH. Evaluating care coordination among Medicare beneficiaries. *JAMA.* 2009;301(24):2547-8.

9. Oestreich G, Rogers D. Engaging providers in achieving chronic care improvement in a Medicaid population. Paper presented at 10th Annual Meeting of DMAA: The Care Continuum Alliance; November 2008; Hollywood, FL.

10. Stoto MA. Population health in the Affordable Care Act era. *Academy Health.* February 21, 2013. https://www.academyhealth.org/files/AH2013pophealth.pdf. Accessed September 30, 2014.

11. Koh HK, Sebelius KG. Promoting prevention through the Affordable Care Act. *N Engl J Med.* 2010;363(14):1296-9.

12. Population Health Alliance. Outcomes guidelines report, volume 5. Washington, DC. Population Health Alliance. 2010.

13. Wennberg D, Doyle M. *From Hospital to Home: A New Approach for Reducing Readmissions and Easing Transitions in Care for the Medicare Population.* Boston, MA: Health Dialog; 2009.

POPULATION HEALTH EDUCATION

JAMES D. PLUMB, ELLEN PLUMB, VIBIN ROY, AND BROOKE SALZMAN

Executive Summary

Since 2004, several reports exposed serious flaws in education for health professions that contributed to many of the recognized failures in the American healthcare delivery system. The Institute of Medicine (IOM) provided compelling evidence that our current approach to educating health professionals falls woefully short of adequately preparing the healthcare workforce.[1] In 2004, the Healthy People Curriculum Task Force emphasized that "an essential element of any effort to change a healthcare system must be the education of future clinicians who will practice new approaches in new contexts."[2] Failure to fundamentally alter health professions education can be a serious obstacle to realizing actual transformation of healthcare delivery and improving the health of populations.

Traditional education for clinicians focuses narrowly on acute medical conditions and neglects the principles of population health and prevention that are necessary to achieve a greater positive impact on our nation's health. Health professional education reform requires fundamental redesign to integrate new skills and approaches that support the health of populations. In this way, education reform will play a key role in "transforming the nation's health care delivery system from one that historically has focused on care for acute illness . . . to one that values patient-centered care, quality improvement, and resource conservation."[3]

In responding to the challenge, many academic and professional organizations have made recommendations regarding healthcare education reform, and developed and piloted educational alternative designs utilizing a population health approach. The aim is to create and reflect positive changes in the larger healthcare system while preparing and supporting healthcare providers and leaders in the new healthcare delivery models.

The Patient Protection and Affordable Care Act (ACA) moves these efforts forward with several provisions and policy initiatives that relate to population health education. The majority of the ACA provisions deal with health insurance reform and regulations to afford millions of uninsured and underinsured Americans the opportunity to obtain health insurance coverage. However, the ACA also includes policy elements that address the composition and training of the healthcare workforce; innovation in care delivery; health disparities; data mining; and renewed investments in primary care, public health, and prevention.[4]

Learning Objectives

1. Explain the vital role of educating health professionals and preparing the health professions workforce to both create and reflect transformed models of care.
2. Identify essential knowledge and skills required by health professionals in a transformed healthcare delivery system.
3. Discuss key concepts and methods of population health to frame education reform for health professions.

Key Terms

core competencies   interdisciplinary teams

INTRODUCTION

The need for healthcare reform in the United States remains compelling. Despite the good intentions and best efforts of healthcare professionals and other stakeholders, the U.S. healthcare system remains fragmented, inefficient, and ineffective in promoting population health and in providing full value for the resources invested.[5] Compared to other health systems, the World Health Organization (WHO) ranks the U.S. healthcare system 37th for its ability to provide health care.[6] Although the United States spends $8,467 in per capita total expenditure on health, it ranks 34th in the world in life expectancy and 39th in infant mortality.[6]

Substantial disparities in health outcomes and access to care are known to exist in the United States. Former Surgeon General David Satcher estimated that the "black–white mortality gap" results in more than 80,000 excess preventable deaths each year among African Americans.[7] Furthermore, the IOM estimates that as many as 24,000 people die each year in the United States because they lack health insurance.[8]

While the need for healthcare reform remains uncontested, debate continues regarding the scope and specific elements of reform. In general, efforts address two major aspects of health care: reforming the insurance system with the goal of broadening coverage and transforming the delivery system. The call for healthcare delivery reform derives from the recognition that current approaches fail to ensure safety and quality, and contribute to health disparities and excessive costs. Most proposals for healthcare delivery reform call for realigning payment incentives to promote quality, leveraging skill sets of healthcare professionals, adopting and relying on evidence-based systems of care, and ensuring that care is provided by **interdisciplinary teams** of prepared professionals.

In *Health Professions Education: A Bridge to Quality*, the IOM provided compelling evidence that the traditional approach to educating health professionals does not address the central needs of a workforce development in a transformed delivery system.[1] Failure to fundamentally alter health professions education remains an obstacle to transformation of healthcare delivery and improving the health of populations.

In 2004, the Healthy People Curriculum Task Force emphasized that "an essential element of any effort to change a health care system must be the education of future clinicians who will practice new approaches in new contexts."[2] Traditional education for clinicians in all disciplines focuses on acute medical conditions and fails to incorporate the principles of population health and prevention that are necessary to achieve a broader positive impact on the nation's health. To meet the challenge of system transformation, health professions education must be fundamentally redesigned to integrate new skills and approaches that support population health. In this way, education reform will play a key role in transforming the nation's healthcare delivery system.[3]

Although a majority of the 2010 ACA's provisions deal with health insurance reform and regulations, several provisions relate to population health education (e.g., the composition and training of the healthcare workforce; innovation in care delivery; health disparities; data mining; and renewed investments in primary care, public health, and prevention).[10]

A population health approach to educating health professionals will create and reflect positive changes in the broader healthcare system and will better prepare and support healthcare providers and leaders. This chapter will describe existing shortcomings in current health professions education and review recommendations for educational reforms that are rooted in the principles of population health. Using examples, this chapter demonstrates how such reforms create and reflect positive changes in the larger healthcare system while preparing health professionals to deliver care and provide leadership in new and emerging healthcare delivery models.

THE NEED FOR HEALTH PROFESSIONAL EDUCATION REFORM

The inadequacy of traditional health professions education to adapt to a changing healthcare environment has been well established.[1,4,9–17] Multiple reports have described deficiencies in the preparation of future health professionals to deal with major contemporary realities, which include suboptimal and inconsistent healthcare quality and safety, unsustainable rising healthcare costs, rapidly expanding science and technology, increasing public accountability, escalating burden of chronic disease, and widening disparities in health and health care.[16] The IOM reported in 2001 that "clinical education [for health professionals] simply has not kept pace with or been responsive enough to shifting patient demographics and desires, changing health system expectations, evolving practice requirements and staffing arrangements, new information, a focus on improving quality, or new technologies."[9]

Several leading organizations have identified key sets of knowledge and skills that must be integrated into education curricula to better prepare the health professions workforce and enable transformation of the healthcare delivery system. The IOM proposes a core set of competencies that *all* health clinicians should possess to meet the needs of the 21st century healthcare system. This set of **core competencies** includes the ability to provide patient-centered care, work in interdisciplinary teams, employ evidence-based practice, apply quality improvement, and utilize informatics.[1] The report describes the rationale supporting each selected competency and notes the current lack of knowledge and skills in these key domains (Table 4-1).

Table 4-1 Proposed Set of Core Competencies and Examples of Deficiencies in Health Professions Education

Definition	Examples of Deficiencies
Provide patient-centered care	
• Identify, respect, and care about patients' differences, values, preferences, and expressed needs; relieve pain and suffering; coordinate continuous care; listen to, clearly inform, communicate with, and educate patients; share decision making and management; and continuously advocate disease prevention, wellness, and promotion of healthy lifestyles, including a focus on population health.[1]	• Dominance of the biomedical model of practice whereby patients are viewed in terms of signs and symptoms.[18] • Belief in physician-only decision making.[19] • Training in communication for pharmacists can be irregular and not well developed.[20] • Limited training in pain assessment and management.[21.] • Inconsistent training for nurses regarding end-of-life care.[22] • Limited training in cross-cultural communication.[23]
Work in interdisciplinary teams	
• Cooperate, collaborate, communicate, and integrate care in teams to ensure that the care of populations and communities is continuous and reliable.[1]	• Social isolation of health professionals and isolated decision making.[24] • Separate schedules prevent interprofessional curriculum design.[25] • Fewer than 15% of U.S. nursing and medical schools had any interdisciplinary programs.[26] • Attitudes among students may present a barrier to interprofessional teamwork.[24]

Table 4-1 **Proposed Set of Core Competencies and Examples of Deficiencies in Health Professions Education (*Continued*)**

Definition	Examples of Deficiencies
Employ evidence-based practice	
• Integrate best research with clinical expertise and patient values for optimum care, and participate in learning and research activities to the extent feasible.[1]	• More than 25% of medical school graduates from schools teaching skills related to evidence-based medicine feel unprepared to interpret clinical data, research, literature reviews, and critiques.[27] • Limited diffusion of evidence-based practice into nursing curriculum.[28]
Apply quality improvement	
• Identify errors and hazards in care; understand and implement basic safety design principles, such as standardization and simplification; continually understand and measure quality of care in terms of structure, process, and outcomes in relation to patient populations and community needs; design and test interventions to change processes and systems of care, with the objective of improving quality.[1]	• Little available information on the extent to which students are educated about error reduction, process measurement and redesign, and monitoring of patient data.[29–31] • Limited education for nurses on quality improvement strategies in clinical areas.[32]
Utilize informatics	
• Communicate, manage knowledge, mitigate error, and support decision making using information technology to study the care delivered to populations and communities.[1]	• Fewer than one-third of nursing schools addressed informatics.[33]

Data from Institute of Medicine. *Health Professions Education: A Bridge to Quality*. Washington, DC: National Academies Press; 2003.

In response to the IOM report, the Association of American Medical Colleges (AAMC), the Accreditation Council for Graduate Medical Education (ACGME), the National League for Nursing (NLN), and the Federation of Associations of Schools of the Health Professions (FASHP) published their respective positions on the need for health professions education reform. The AAMC set forth learning objectives as part of the Medical School Objectives Project (MSOP) to assist medical schools in developing curricula to better align educational content and goals with "evolving societal needs, practice patterns, and scientific developments."[10]

The MSOP is an ongoing process of examining the state of clinical education at U.S. medical schools and specifying necessary reforms. Several reports have come out of the MSOP that propose education reform relating to improving quality and safety of care, population health, medical informatics, communication and coordination of care, and interdisciplinary teamwork.[10–12]

The ACGME Outcome Project generated six general competencies and outlined the skills considered essential for all practicing physicians: patient care, medical knowledge, professionalism, systems-based practice, practice-based learning and improvement, and interpersonal and communication skills.[15] Competency in practice-based learning and improvement requires that physician residents "systematically analyze practice using quality improvement methods, and implement changes with the goal of practice improvement."[15]

Competency in systems-based practice entails that physician residents "demonstrate an awareness of and responsiveness to the larger context and system of health care" and work in interdisciplinary teams, incorporate considerations of cost awareness, advocate for quality patient care, and participate in identifying system errors and implementing solutions.[15]

In 2012, the ACGME introduced the Next Accreditation System (NAS), which bases graduate medical program accreditation on measurable educational outcomes related to the six clinical competencies. The restructuring of the accreditation system is accompanied by an increased educational emphasis on patient safety, quality improvement, and health disparity reduction.[34,35] Leading organizations from multiple health professions other than medicine are calling for innovations in education to create and shape the future of healthcare delivery. In its position statement on transforming nursing education (2005), the NLN recommended that education programs be redesigned to address significant changes arising from healthcare reform and embrace principles of accountability and evidence-based practice.[33] The FASHP, a forum for representatives from organizations of health professions education, asserts the need to reshape and invest in health professions education to provide high-quality, team-based, and patient-centered care.[36]

Other key organizations have weighed in on the discussion. The Medicare Payment Advisory Commission (MedPAC), an independent congressional agency established to advise the U.S. Congress on issues affecting the Medicare program, expressed concern that "health professionals are not gaining certain skills they need to provide the kinds of care that will best serve the public's needs."[3] MedPAC contracted with RAND Corporation researchers to evaluate the content of curricula for medical graduates in internal medicine and found that curricula fell far short of the instruction recommended by the IOM and others. In particular, the study identified a lack of formal instruction and experience in interdisciplinary teamwork, cost awareness in clinical decision making, comprehensive health information technology, and patient care in ambulatory settings.[3]

The Institute for Healthcare Improvement (IHI) recommends that new health system designs be developed to simultaneously accomplish three critical objectives, or the Triple Aim: improve the health of the population, enhance the patient's experience of care (including quality, access, and reliability), and reduce, or at least control, the per capita cost of care.[5] Recognizing that achieving such objectives requires new approaches to health professions education, the IHI identified eight essential quality improvement knowledge domains as part of the core content. These domains focus on understanding the organization of healthcare systems; the processes involved in healthcare delivery; and the utilization of outcomes measurement to allow increased accountability, collaboration, and quality improvement.[5]

Finally, the IOM report titled *Who Will Keep the Public Healthy: Educating Public Health Professionals for the 21st Century* emphasized the central role of health professionals from diverse disciplines in contributing to the health of the public and the critical need to strengthen public health education for all health professionals to improve health on a population level.[16] The report offers a framework and recommendations for advancing public health education and integrating eight vital new areas: informatics, genomics, communication, cultural competence, community-based participatory research, policy and law, global health, and ethics.[16]

Failure to adequately prepare the healthcare workforce will impede our ability to transform healthcare delivery and improve health on a population level. Although various organizations have identified slightly different knowledge and skills as core content areas, there is general agreement that new approaches to education must impart competence to deliver patient-centered care (including effective communication and cultural competence), perform practice-based quality improvement, work in interdisciplinary teams, navigate growing bodies of information and new technology to employ evidence-based practices, utilize information technology in clinical practice, demonstrate cost awareness, and apply population-based approaches to improve health on a population level.

THE NEED FOR A POPULATION HEALTH APPROACH TO HEALTH PROFESSIONS EDUCATION

Despite the well documented need for fundamental change in health professions education and multiple efforts by leading organizations to revise and expand curricula, widespread transformation has been slow to materialize. The NLN position statement proposes that "more must be done than merely updating or rearranging content."[33] However, there is limited room to incorporate all the aforementioned content into already overcrowded curricula. Most leading organizations in health professions education agree that health professions education reform requires a systems-based approach to prepare clinicians for making meaningful and lasting contributions to the delivery of health care and to the emerging field of population health.

A systems approach to improving health education requires consideration of fundamental features of educational systems, including the composition of the population of learners, characteristics of the learning environment, organizational structures, and sources of support (institutional and financial). Although defining major competencies and learning objectives is an essential aspect of curriculum redesign, a pedagogical shift is required to truly reform current health professions education and provide an understanding of the treatment of populations as well as that of individual patients.

A population health perspective is essential for reshaping the way in which health and health care are understood and approached and, more to the point, the way in which the education of health professionals can be redesigned. It follows that a useful, dynamic framework for formulating a broadly supported new approach to health professions education is one that utilizes the concepts and methods of population health. The AAMC Population Health Perspective Panel (part of the Medical School Objectives Project) defines a population health perspective as one that "encompasses the ability to assess the health needs of a specific population; implement and evaluate interventions to improve the health of that population; and provide care for individual patients in the context of culture, health status, and health needs of the populations of which that patient is a member."[10] Major concepts and methods employed in a population-based approach to health (e.g., measurement, system change, accountability) provide a structure for organizing and integrating key approaches into education.[35]

A fundamental principle of population health, developing an understanding of the determinants of health and health disparities, goes beyond providing individual medical care.[35,37] This broader view enables health professions students to consider influences on health that exist both inside and outside the healthcare system and to link the medical care provided to individuals to the larger contexts of family, community, and society. In this context, population health becomes a vital strategy for integrating clinical care with community and public health. Although the call for building bridges between medical care and public health is hardly new, the urgent need for healthcare delivery reform has created the opportunity for the two fields to unite in a population-based approach that facilitates their synergy.[38–41]

In 1997, the New York Academy of Medicine called for medicine and public health to reevaluate their relationship and better coordinate their efforts.[42] The Academy presented multiple examples of improving health on both individual and population levels that are achievable through collaboration between medical care and public health. Examples include the following:

- Improve health care by coordinating services for individuals
- Improve access to care by establishing frameworks to provide care for the uninsured and underinsured
- Improve the quality and cost-effectiveness of care by applying a population health perspective to medical practice
- Use clinical practice to identify and address community health problems
- Strengthen health promotion and health protection by mobilizing community campaigns
- Shape the future direction of the health system by collaborating about policy, training, and research[42]

To facilitate an alliance between medical care and public health, health professionals need to understand and value their role as public health professionals.[36,43] The IOM report titled *Training Physicians for Public Health Careers* (2007) states that "effective public health actions rely upon a well-trained public health workforce," which is "composed of individuals from many disciplines, including physicians, nurses, environmental health specialists, epidemiologists, and health educators, among others."[43] To advance health on a population level, public health education and training must be embedded into the education of all health professionals. Moreover, education reform utilizing a population-based approach that is aimed at overcoming the deficiencies and disparities in our current healthcare system may produce health professionals that become "agents of change, committed to designing a system of care that is equitable, cost-effective, prevention-oriented, universal, and thus moral."[45]

ESTABLISHING A FRAMEWORK IN POPULATION HEALTH EDUCATION

UNDERGRADUATE PUBLIC HEALTH EDUCATION

As part of its report titled *Who Will Keep the Public Healthy?* (2003), the IOM concluded that a healthy public requires both an educated public health workforce and an educated citizenry and recommended that "all undergraduates should have access to education in public health."[46] This recommendation stimulated a movement connecting undergraduate public health education to the Liberal Education and America's Promise (LEAP), an effort on the part of the Association of American Colleges and Universities to produce a more educated citizenry.[47]

The 2006 Consensus Conference on Undergraduate Public Health brought together educators in the fields of public health, arts and sciences, and clinical health professions to develop a core undergraduate public health curriculum and implementation recommendations. According to consensus guidelines, an educated citizen "should be prepared to understand emerging public health issues, analyse options for addressing these issues, and provide the necessary political and financial support needed to address these issues."[48,49] General principles and recommendations that emerged from the conference toward developing a more educated citizenry included making a core public health curriculum (composed of course work in Public Health 101, Epidemiology 101, and Global Health 101) available to students at all undergraduate institutions with fulfillment of general education requirements. Additional implementation recommendations included provision of the following:

- Websites to provide information on undergraduate public health and shared curriculum
- Faculty development measures to assist colleges and universities in developing new introductory public health courses
- Encouragement of applicants by health professions education and graduate public health degree programs to enroll in introductory public health courses

- Continued discussion of approaches for developing minors in public health and global health in institutions with and without schools or programs in public health
- Participation by public health practitioners in experiential or service learning[48,49]

POPULATION HEALTH AND MEDICAL EDUCATION

There has been a large shift in the healthcare needs of the U.S. population ranging from acute episodic care to care for chronic conditions. With this shift, there is a commensurate realization that the predominant drivers of health involve social and environmental factors.[50,51] To improve health outcomes and reduce healthcare costs, medical education requires a greater emphasis on public health.[12] Although medical education and public health education utilize different approaches, they are actually complementary. The primary difference is that medicine is typically focused on an individual patient's diagnosis and treatment, whereas public health is focused on the health of populations, prevention, and health promotion.[52] For practical reasons, public health and medical education have operated as distinct and parallel entities rather than working cooperatively. Because of increasing calls from various medical organizations, population health is gradually being incorporated into medical education. The AAMC Population Health Perspective Panel developed education objectives related to population health and strategies for designing and implementing population health education.[11] The panel formulated a foundation of knowledge, skills, and attitudes involved in a population health curriculum (Table 4-2).

The panel also identified three education principles to guide effective implementation of a population health curriculum: teaching students the practical fundamentals of the core disciplines that underpin the effective application of population health, giving students valuable experiences in studying real populations, and integrating teaching and learning into all parts of the medical curriculum rather than relying solely on a stand-alone population health course.[11]

Additionally, the panel recommended strategies to facilitate the widespread development of a curriculum to teach population health:

- Develop an explicit list of mechanisms by which population health objectives are to be met by each school and conduct periodic evaluations to track their success
- Identify faculty to serve as teachers and mentors; support their development
- Form liaisons with others to help, such as the American Board of Preventive Medicine and Association for Prevention Teaching and Research
- Ensure that the Liaison Committee on Medical Education (LCME) requires that schools show evidence that they have developed objectives, designed and delivered a curriculum, and tested students for these competencies
- Ensure that national board examinations test population health competencies[11]

Table 4-2 Population Health Perspective Panel's Population Health Curriculum: Knowledge, Skills, and Attitudes

Knowledge	Skills	Attitudes
Evidence-based medicine	Mechanisms to gather information from diverse sources	Cultural responsiveness
Social and behavioral determinants of health, at an individual and population level	Use of nonquantitative descriptors	Constructive attitudes and ability to work with other disciplines
Ethics:	Measuring performance in populations:	Influence of doctors on the health system
Distribution of resources	Patient satisfaction	Field experience with economically disadvantaged populations
Barriers to access	Functional status	
Distributive justice—use of scarce resources for individuals vs. populations	Costs and cost effectiveness	Identification and collaboration with external organizations
	Clinical outcome measurement	
Organization and financing of U.S. health care	Performance scorecards	
The principles, practice, and financing of preventive care	Severity adjustment approaches	
	Skills to cause change (leadership skills, advocacy, change strategies, communication)	
Cost-analysis approaches and information in prioritizing the use of resources	Use of test characteristics in routine decisions of day-to-day practice	
Describe population demographics	Application of quality improvement methods to improve the systems and individual care	

Reproduced from Association of American Medical Colleges. *Report II—Contemporary Issues in Medicine: Medical Informatics and Population Health.* Washington, DC: Association of American Medical Colleges; 1998.

Of interest, the panel also identified three important barriers to change that must be addressed to advance the teaching of population health: the lack of ownership of population health by any one department in the medical school organization, the absence of dedicated funding to support new initiatives in teaching population health, and the misconception within the academic community that population health is simply a response to concerns expressed by the managed care industry.[11] The panel underscored the need for accountability among leading national organizations, including the AAMC, to clearly articulate the priority of ensuring instruction and support of a population health curriculum.

In a collaborative effort to improve population health/public health education for medical students and residents, the AAMC and the Centers for Disease Control and Prevention (CDC) established Regional Medicine-Public Health Education Centers (RMPHECs) and Regional Medicine-Public Health Education Centers-Graduate Medical Education (RMPHEC-GMEs).[53,54] RMPHEC and RMPHEC-GME sites were required to partner with at least one state or local public health agency to help integrate population health/public health content into their curricula. Grantees developed their own education approaches and materials that were consistent with their institutions' curricular structures and themes.

The RMPHECs provided a list of competencies that all medical students should possess as demonstrated by the ability to do the following:

- Assess the health status of populations using available data (e.g., public health surveillance data, vital statistics, registries, surveys, electronic health records, and health plan claims data)
- Discuss the role of socioeconomic, environmental, cultural, and other population-level determinants of health on the health status and health care of individuals and populations
- Integrate emerging information on individuals' biologic and genetic risk with population-level factors when deciding upon prevention and treatment options
- Appraise the quality of the evidence of peer-reviewed medical and public health literature and its implications at patient and population levels
- Apply primary and secondary prevention strategies that improve the health of individuals and populations
- Identify community assets and resources to improve the health of individuals and populations
- Explain how community engagement strategies may be used to improve the health of communities and to contribute to the reduction of health disparities
- Participate in population health improvement strategies (e.g., systems and policy advocacy, program or policy development, or other community-based interventions)
- Discuss the functions of public health systems including those that require or benefit from the contribution of clinicians, such as public health surveillance, preparedness, and prevention of chronic conditions
- Describe the organization and financing of the U.S. healthcare system, and their effects on access, utilization, and quality of care for individuals and populations
- Discuss the ethical implications of healthcare resource allocation and emerging technologies on population health
- Identify quality improvement methods to improve medical care and population health

The April 2008 edition of *Academic Medicine*, which had a theme of population health education, profiled 6 of the 16 schools that participated in the RMPHEC program, describing the strategies employed at their schools to integrate population health across their curricula.[55-58] In 2010, the AAMC and CDC hosted the "Patients and Populations: Public Health in Medical Education" conference to discuss the lessons learned from the RMPHEC and RMPHEC-GME initiatives. A supplement to the *American Journal of Preventive Medicine* (October 2011) highlighted several of the new curricular models for population health in graduate medical education in the fields of pediatrics, family medicine, internal medicine, emergency medicine, and surgery.

In part because of the growing recognition of the importance of public health education in medical education, the LCME revised two of its educational standards to explicitly include public health sciences and preventive medicine in student curriculum in 2010. Data from the LCME and AAMC's graduation questionnaire have shown that beginning in 2004, more schools are including a broader range of public health topics in their curricula, students are more satisfied with the public health education they are receiving, and more schools are offering MD-MPH opportunities to meet the interests of their students.[59]

PATIENT SAFETY AND QUALITY IMPROVEMENT

The decade following 2004 has seen remarkable shifts in healthcare delivery, largely influenced by reports on the need for quality improvement and patient safety (QI/PS), changes in the healthcare system itself, and new regulations and accreditation requirements. These shifts have resulted in innovations in QI/PS education among U.S. medical schools and teaching hospitals, fostered in part by Integrating Quality (a 2008 initiative of the AAMC) and Best Practices for Better Care (a joint initiative of the AAMC and University Health System Consortium).[60]

To augment these initiatives and to support faculty development in QI/PS, the expert panel report titled "Teaching for Quality" articulates a broad vision for healthcare delivery, offers a strategy to increase faculty capacity, and makes three core recommendations.[60] The report defines "teaching" as a broad concept that includes curriculum design, competency assessment, experiential learning, and aspects of the hidden curriculum, such as role-modeling. The report outlines three important recommendations:

- Recommendation 1: To achieve QI/PS goals for education and practice, the medical schools, teaching hospitals, accreditation bodies, examination organizations, and specialty bodies should ensure the integration of QI/PS concepts into meaningful learning experiences across the educational continuum.
- Recommendation 2: To improve the processes and outcomes of care, medical schools and teaching hospitals should expect all clinical faculty to be proficient in QI/PS competencies and be able to identify, develop, and support a critical mass of faculty as expert educators to create, implement, and evaluate training and education in QI/PS for students, residents, and colleagues.

- Recommendation 3: Academic and clinical leadership should share a common commitment to QI/PS and demonstrate a concrete alignment of the academic and clinical enterprises in a manner that produces excellent health outcomes valued by healthcare professionals and the public.[60]

POPULATION HEALTH AND INTERPROFESSIONAL EDUCATION

In 2004, the Healthy People Curriculum Task Force (convened by the Association of Prevention Teaching and Research [APTR]) introduced the Clinical Prevention and Population Health Curriculum Framework, with the intent of increasing health promotion and disease prevention content in health professions education.[2,53] The task force included representatives from eight health professions education associations on behalf of allopathic and osteopathic medicine, dentistry, nursing, nurse practitioners, pharmacy, allied health, and physician assistants. The updated framework (released in 2009) consists of four components: evidence-based practice, clinical preventive services and health promotion, health systems and health policy, and population health and community aspects of practice.[53] The full Curriculum Framework comprises 19 domains organized under the four components (Table 4-3). In addition, a variety of methods are recommended for teaching the materials and integrating them into existing curricula (e.g., the use of service learning and problem-based learning) as well as innovative approaches to interdisciplinary education.[59]

Formed in 2010, the Interprofessional Education Collaborative (IPEC) comprises health profession education associations from the disciplines of nursing, medicine, pharmacy, dentistry, and public health. An expert panel from IPEC produced a report in an effort to define a common language for interprofessional education and collaborative practice. The report identified 38 behavioral expectations across four competency domains: Values and Ethics for Interprofessional Practice, Roles and Responsibilities, Interprofessional Communication, and Teams and Teamwork. The rationale for the formation of the IPEC captures the essence of the changing educational landscape:

> Offering students the opportunity to address population health issues as members of teams will equip them with an understanding of what each health professional brings to the care of patients and health of communities. Connecting the Core Competencies with the Curriculum Framework can guide educational programs as they build a robust curriculum that will prepare students for future service to populations.[61]

Released in May 2011, the Core Competencies for Interprofessional Collaborative Practice are aimed at preparing health profession students for integrated, team-based, high-quality healthcare delivery in evolving healthcare systems.[60]

The Healthy People Curriculum Task Force prepared a guide to inform curriculum development focused on students' abilities to participate effectively as members of

Table 4-3 The Clinical Prevention and Population Health Curriculum Framework

Evidence-based practice	• Problem description—descriptive epidemiology • Etiology, benefits, and harms—evaluating health research • Evidence-based recommendations • Implementation and evaluation
Clinical prevention services and health promotion	• Screening • Counseling for behavioral change • Immunization • Preventive medication • Other preventive interventions
Health systems	• Organization of clinical and public health systems • Health services financing • Health workforce • Health policy process
Population health and community aspects of practice	• Communicating and sharing health information with the public • Environmental health • Occupational health • Global health issues • Cultural dimensions of practice • Community services

Data from Association for Prevention Teaching and Research. *Clinical Prevention and Population Health Curriculum Framework.* Washington, DC: Association for Prevention Teaching and Research; 2009. https://www.aacom.org/docs/default-source/med-ed-presentations/revised_cpph_framework_2009.pdf?sfvrsn=0. Accessed February 4, 2015.

interprofessional healthcare teams in delivering clinical prevention and population health services. Users are encouraged to adapt this guide and customize activities to an institution's specific learning environments and health professions education programs.[60] The Healthy People Curriculum Task Force provides several examples of integrative interprofessional learning activities that address selected *Core Competencies* and content elements within the *Curriculum Framework* (Table 4-4).

Interprofessional teams can also support "community health teams," a concept that is established and supported by grant funding under the ACA, for the establishment of community-based interdisciplinary, interprofessional (health) teams, which support primary care providers and receive capitated payments for their services. The model is based on prior work by healthcare experts who have focused on the task of strengthening the capacity of the primary healthcare system to address the highest cost patients.[61–63] Going well beyond upgrading practice, this strengthening of capacity is envisioned as embedding practice in a broader public health model. Entities eligible for grants are state or tribal entities that can demonstrate a plan for long-term financial sustainability and a plan for incorporating prevention initiatives, patient education, and care management

Table 4-4 Learning Activity 3—Responding to Sentinel Events in Health Care

Case study that requires the student team to analyze a sentinel event in a healthcare institution and make quality improvement recommendations

IPEC core competencies	Clinical prevention and population health curriculum framework elements
VE1. Place the interests of patients and populations at the center of interprofessional health delivery.	**Evidence-Based Practice** 3. Evidence-Based Recommendations • Assessing the quality of the evidence (e.g., types and quality of studies and relevance to target populations)
VE8. Manage ethical dilemmas specific to interprofessional patient-/population-centered care situations.	• Assessing the magnitude of the effect • Grading of the recommendations

RR5. Use the full scope of knowledge, skills, and abilities of available health professionals and healthcare workers to provide care that is safe, timely, efficient, effective, and equitable.	4. Implementation and Evaluation
	  • At whom to direct intervention
	  • How to intervene
	  • Evaluation

CC2. Organize and communicate information with patients, families, and healthcare team members in a form that is understandable, avoiding discipline-specific terminology when possible.	**Health Systems and Health Policy**
	2. Health Services Financing
	  • Methods for financing healthcare institutions
	  • Ethical frameworks for healthcare financing

CC6. Use respectful language appropriate for a given difficult situation, crucial conversation, or interprofessional conflict.	3. Health Workforce • Methods of regulation of health professionals and healthcare institutions
CC7. Recognize how one's own uniqueness, including experience level, expertise, culture, power, and hierarchy within the healthcare team, contributes toeffective communication, conflict resolution, and positive interprofessional working relationships.	• Legal and ethical responsibilities of healthcare professionals (e.g., malpractice, HIPAA, confidentiality) 4. Health Policy Process • Process of health policy making
CC8. Communicate consistently the importance of teamwork in patient-centered and community-focused care.	• Methods for participation in the policy process
TT5. Apply leadership practices that support collaborative practice and team effectiveness.	• Impact of policies on health care and health outcomes including impacts on vulnerable populations and eliminating health disparities
TT7. Share accountability with other professions, patients, and communities for outcomes relevant to prevention and health care.	
TT9. Use process improvement strategies to increase the effectiveness of interprofessional teamwork and team-based care.	
TT10. Use available evidence to inform effective teamwork and team-based practices.	

Data from Interprofessional Education Collaborative Expert Panel. (2011). *Core competencies for interprofessional collaborative practice: Report of an expert panel.* Washington, DC: Interprofessional Education Collaborative.

resources into the delivery of health care in a highly integrated fashion.[4] Teams must be interdisciplinary; the statute contains references to the full range of medical, nursing, nutritional, social work, and mental health professionals.[4]

COMMUNITY HEALTH WORKERS AND EDUCATION

The use of community health workers (CHWs) to reduce disparities in health care and health outcomes represents a growing trend and adds another dimension to interdisciplinary teams that are working with patient-centered medical homes and accountable care organizations. CHWs represent a systematized approach to providing self-management support for care of chronic conditions and navigation through a complex, fragmented healthcare system. In addition to providing linkages with community services and resources, CHWs (e.g., doulas, outreach advisers, patient navigators, peer counselors/educators and promoters) help patients to access primary care and preventive services, maintain healthy behaviors, and manage chronic conditions in culturally and linguistically relevant ways.[63]

The Community Health Worker National Education Collaborative, representing 22 college-based educational institutions and other stakeholders, has developed educational resources, curricula, and promising delivery strategies for the CHW field. The CDC has developed Promoting a training course, Policy and Systems Change to Expand Employment of Community Health Workers, designed to provide state programs and other stakeholders with basic knowledge about CHWs. The course includes information and examples of how states can become engaged in policy and systems change efforts to establish sustainability for the work of CHWs.[64] The six-session online modules cover CHWs' roles and functions, current status of the CHW occupation, areas of public policy affecting CHWs, credentialing CHWs, sustainable funding for CHW positions, and examples of states that have been successful in moving policy and systems change forward. In addition, the Health Resources and Services Administration's (HRSA) Office of Rural Health Policy has developed a Community Health Workers Evidence-Based Models Toolbox.[65,66] Despite these efforts, there is no standardized training curriculum for CHWs; because each community's needs are different, training content differs from program to program. CHWs often participate in on-the-job training programs to develop competencies directly related to their activities. Such trainings are administered by the coordinator of the CHW program or informally through mentoring by an experienced CHW or healthcare provider. Some CHWs pursue formal training at an educational institution.

Many rural CHW programs have created their own educational and training curricula from existing resources and best practices. Curricula may include training on accessing health care and social services systems; translating, interpreting, and facilitating client–provider communications; gathering information for medical providers;

delivering services as part of a medical home team; educating social services providers on community/population needs; teaching the concepts of disease prevention and health promotion to lay populations; managing chronic conditions; home visiting; understanding community prejudices; and other topics.

Many programs have developed resources for on-the-job training. By adapting existing materials from the CDC, other federal and state agencies, and academic institutions, these programs have created their own training materials and curricula to ensure that CHWs acquire the skills necessary to serve the target population. Common components of on-the-job CHW training materials are cultural competency, patient intake and assessment, protocol delivery, screening recommendations, risk factors, insurance eligibility and enrollment, communication skills, health promotion, and disease prevention and management. Some states require training on the legal and ethical dimensions of CHW activities.

Dumbald and associates describe a unique method of community engagement that utilizes an interactive course on research fundamentals as a component of a Clinical and Translational Science Award (CTSA) program for CHWs.[65] The course was designed and implemented jointly by a community agency that serves a primarily Latino rural population and an academic health center. A focus group of community members and input from community leaders comprised a community-based participatory research model to create three 3-hour interactive training sessions. The resulting curriculum successfully stimulated dialogue between trainees and academic researchers. By choosing course activities that elicited community-specific responses into each session's discussion, researchers learned as much about the community as CHW trainees learned about research. The approach is readily adaptable, making it useful to other communities where CHWs are part of the health system.[66,67]

COMMUNITY-BASED LEARNING AND POPULATION HEALTH

Community-Campus Partnerships for Health (CCPH) has long championed the idea that community-based education and organized service-learning activities are essential in preparing health professionals to effectively understand and practice in a new healthcare system.[68] In an effort to equip health professions educators with the necessary knowledge and skills to expand prevention and population health curricula and promote *Healthy People 2010* objectives in partnership with the community, the CCPH developed a guide titled "Advancing the Healthy People 2010 Objectives Through Community-Based Education: A Curriculum Planning Guide."[68]

The CCPH guide emphasizes the central value of incorporating the perspectives of community partners and students into the development of the curriculum. Of note, the guide was designed for multidisciplinary health professions faculty and for community leaders interested in establishing partnerships with leaders of health professions schools. The partnerships driving the inclusion of health promotion and prevention has continued their efforts into the current decade for *Healthy People 2020.*

Although the guide is intended to assist faculty in designing coursework directly linked to the Healthy People objectives, it can also be useful to faculty in other curriculum reform efforts and community activities; provide leaders in the community–campus partnership movement with the tools to build and sustain their partnership efforts; provide direction to students and residents on strategies for improving community service activities; equip community leaders and students with insight into the curriculum planning process and emphasize the important roles leaders and students play in student education and improving community health; equip faculty with new directions for evaluation and assessment of community-based courses and activities; and foster possible collaboration and sharing of resources with other leaders in the field around health, health disparities, and the Healthy People objectives.[53] Linking community-based education and service-learning activities with initiatives that address the healthcare needs of communities can successfully convey fundamentals of population health while improving health outcomes.

CHALLENGES AND BARRIERS TO HEALTH PROFESSIONS EDUCATION REFORM AND IMPLEMENTING CURRICULA IN POPULATION HEALTH

COMPOSITION OF THE POPULATION OF LEARNERS

Increasing Diversity

Attention to the composition of the future healthcare workforce, as well as to the geographic and specialty distribution of future healthcare professionals, is essential to efforts to eliminate health disparities, improve access and quality of care, adapt to changing demographics, and address recognized professional shortages. Making changes in education without substantially altering the composition and distribution of learners will most likely perpetuate current problems and fail to meet future demands.

Diversity in the healthcare workforce is associated with better access and quality of care for disadvantaged populations, greater patient choice and satisfaction, and better education experiences for students.[69] Of note, minority physicians are more likely to provide care for poor and underserved communities.[69-71]

During 2010–2011, the percentage of White matriculants exceeded all other racial and ethnic groups by a substantial amount (57.1% in 2010 and 57.5% in 2011), whereas Black or African American and Hispanic or Latino matriculants combined were just 15% of all matriculants. For both years, certain groups comprised less than 1% of the student body: American Indian or Alaska Native (0.3% and 0.2%), Native Hawaiian or Other Pacific Islander (0.1%), and Other Non-Hispanic or Latino Race (0.02%).[72] Steps to ensure a more diverse pool of physicians and other health professionals are pivotal for reducing health disparities and building a workforce that is attuned to the increasingly diverse population being served.[73]

In addition to the lack of diversity in regard to race and ethnicity, medical students have limited diversity with respect to economic and geographic backgrounds. In 2005, 55% of students came from families in the top quintile of family income, whereas about 5% came from families in the lowest quintile.[74] Nevertheless, at least 85% of medical students report substantial debt at graduation. The median total debt of medical school graduates in 2013 was reported at $176,348.[74] And, although geographic diversity is considered important for maintaining access to care across the United States, medical students tend to come disproportionately from urban areas.[72] Innovative methods to attract students from more diverse economic, ethnic, and geographic backgrounds, such as developing loan forgiveness policies, will be required to create a more diverse health professions workforce.

Increasing the Supply of Primary Care Providers

Countries in which primary care is the foundation of the healthcare system achieve better health outcomes at lower cost. Projections anticipate a growing shortage of primary care providers in the United States, where the supply may already be insufficient.[74] Recent results from the National Resident Matching Program (NRMP) document a disturbing decline in the number of medical students choosing primary care specialties (e.g., family medicine) since 2004 and an overall preference for subspecialties.[73] Student perceptions of the demands, rewards, and prestige of primary care specialties, as well as the influence of medical school faculty and curriculum, continue to affect career choice.[74] In the face of heavy debt upon exiting medical school, graduates are hard pressed to choose the less lucrative primary care specialties. Loan forgiveness to those who elect primary care careers may reverse the trend and entice a greater number of medical school graduates to enter primary care specialties. Clearly, educational institutions must play a vital role in increasing the number of health professionals choosing a career in primary care.

CHARACTERISTICS OF THE LEARNING ENVIRONMENT

Education in Transformed Models of Care

The MedPAC report on medical education in the United States aptly recognized that "residents and other health care professionals will best learn the skills needed to provide high-quality, efficient care when medical education occurs in settings where such care is actually performed."[3] Essentially, health professions education must occur in settings implementing innovative approaches to health care to equip students with the necessary knowledge and skills to effectively function in transformed systems. Investments in health professions education must reward healthcare institutions and practices that apply systems improvement and population health approaches to enhance learning opportunities.

The IOM Committee on Health Professions Education emphasized the need to support existing exemplary practice organizations, including academic health centers that are already delivering care utilizing innovative, population-based approaches. Such leading organizations should be provided with the resources necessary to serve as training models for other organizations and to test different methods for improving outcomes in clinical education. Some promising examples are described in the following sections.

Patient-Centered Medical Home The Patient-Centered Medical Home (PCMH) has been endorsed by several major medical professional societies and holds great promise for improving the health of populations. The National Committee for Quality Assurance (NCQA) has partnered with leading organizations and other stakeholders to support the Physician Practice Connections program, which recognizes practices as PCMHs if they meet specified criteria.[75,76] The PCMH concept is based on the provision of care that is accessible, continuous, comprehensive, coordinated, and culturally sensitive. Education and training of health professionals in such models of care may effectively impart desired knowledge, skills, and values.

Academic Chronic Care Collaborative An initiative of the Association of American Medical Colleges Institute for Improving Clinical Care and the Robert Wood Johnson Foundation national program Improving Chronic Illness Care, the Academic Chronic Care Collaborative (ACCC) initiative combines healthcare delivery reform with educational programs to improve the care of patients with chronic illness and to educate healthcare teams that provide care by facilitating the implementation of the Chronic Care Model.[77] The Chronic Care Model facilitates the creation of well prepared, proactive clinical teams by using clinical information systems, decision support, delivery system design, and self-management support, all of which are integrated into the community and healthcare system.[78]

Academic Health Department Another new system of care that combines population health education and healthcare delivery reform is the Academic Health Department (AHD) model, which is based on an affiliation between an academic institution and a public health practice organization and is designed to strengthen linkages between these entities with the goal of enhancing public health education, training, research, and service. Using an AHD model can expand training sites for students and professionals in clinical health sciences and help address the level of preparedness of undergraduate and graduate health professionals to meet local population health needs. The AHD model has been described as the "public health equivalent of the teaching hospital found between medical schools and hospitals."[79] In January 2011, the Council on Linkages Between Academia and Public Health Practice, with the support of the HRSA and the CDC, launched the Academic Health Learning Community to engage health professionals in a community of shared knowledge and experience in developing AHD relationships.[79]

FUTURE OPPORTUNITIES AND CHALLENGES

Education Utilizing Informatics

Although utilizing advanced information systems has been identified as a core competency for medical professionals and for the delivery of population health services, many healthcare organizations are not equipped with such systems. Even institutions that have invested in these systems and that provide related education and training often fail to integrate the technology into the delivery of care. Additional support will be required to widely implement information technology in healthcare organizations, universities, and delivery systems, and to retool current practices to improve clinical care and provide opportunities for students to develop related knowledge and skills.

Education in Community-Based Settings and Practices

Although the vast majority of health care in the United States occurs in community-based outpatient practices, graduate medical programs are largely based in inpatient, acute care teaching hospitals and offer very limited experiences in community-based medicine.[36] In addition, medical school curricula often place major emphasis on the delivery of tertiary services in the inpatient setting to individual patients.[80] Efforts to reform health professions education must consider "how the clinical setting of education prepares graduates to practice in modern health care settings."[80] Enhancing training and skills in nonhospital settings, including skilled nursing, rehabilitation, assisted living, and other outpatient and community-based practices, is crucial for understanding population health and affecting important health outcomes, as well as in reducing healthcare spending.

Family medicine residency training is the only postgraduate medical training to require community medicine as part of its core clinical curriculum content. All family medicine physician trainees receive curriculum in community medicine that includes experiential learning in community health assessment, program development to address community health priorities, community-based education, and structured interaction with the public health system. However, financing mechanisms for clinical education are largely based on hospital inpatient care and significantly limit incentives to provide education in outpatient settings.[3] In addition, students generally rate the quality of instruction in ambulatory settings lower than that in inpatient settings. Providing clinical education in outpatient, community-based settings will entail addressing graduate medical education funding policies that may be "out of synchrony with the public good"and developing high-quality training experiences in outpatient settings.[80]

Education and Interdisciplinary Teams

The division of health professions into silos poses an obstacle to achieving the higher levels of cooperation and coordination required to improve the quality, safety, effectiveness, and efficiency of healthcare delivery to populations. In practice, there is a general lack of understanding among health professions about what each profession does, the level of training and education required in each profession, and the existing or potential competencies of each profession.[1] The silo culture of health professionals is both created and reinforced by education settings that train health professionals in isolation. The ability to work in interdisciplinary teams has been identified as a core competency for all health professionals, but they are generally not educated together nor trained in team-based skills that would enhance their ability to work as part of interdisciplinary teams. Changes in education must contain specific aims and strategies to break down the silos of individual disciplines, as well as to develop and reward collaborative efforts in interdisciplinary education.

Interdisciplinary health professions education has yet to become the norm, despite the many examples of successful efforts to provide education about working in teams and in developing team-related skills.[81] Obstacles to implementing interdisciplinary education usually involve lack of funding and competition for scarce resources among disciplines, which inhibit collaboration. Accrediting bodies, which drive the educational agenda, often fail to set standards on core competencies and measurable outcomes pertaining to interdisciplinary education or collaborative performance. To stimulate population health curricular innovation, the HRSA instituted rounds of funding in 2009 to support the Interdisciplinary and Interprofessional Joint Graduate Degree program.[82] Funds may be used to plan, develop, and operate joint degree programs that provide interdisciplinary and interprofessional graduate training in public health and other health professions to provide training in environmental health, infectious disease control, disease prevention and health promotion, epidemiologic studies, and injury control. Currently, 16 national programs are implementing and evaluating these programs.

POPULATION HEALTH AND MEDICAL EDUCATION IN ACTION: TWO CASE STUDIES FROM ONE ACADEMIC MEDICAL CENTER

CASE 1: PATIENT-CENTERED MEDICAL HOME FOR REFUGEES

As of 2013, there were 10.4 million refugees worldwide, 58,000 of whom were resettled in the United States in 2012.[83] These refugee populations have resettled and become part of the population of roughly 40 million foreign-born immigrants living in the United States. As migrating populations are displaced from their countries of origin, they experience specific physical, psychological, and social challenges that have a profound effect on their health. Effectively training health professionals to care for immigrant and refugee populations, which in 2010 represented 13% of the U.S. population, presents unique challenges and opportunities for the integration of public health education and clinical training, specifically in several of the vital areas in the framework outlined by the IOM report titled *Who Will Keep the Public Healthy?: Educating Public Health Professionals for the 21st Century.*[46] Focusing educational efforts on the vital areas of communication, cultural competency, community-based participatory research, policy and law, and global health is imperative to providing safe, quality health care to these populations.

The Immigration and Nationality Act (INA) requires that medical screening examinations be performed overseas for all U.S.-bound immigrants and refugees that are valid for 1 year. Although there is state-by-state variability in postmigration screening, all refugees arriving in the United States must receive a screening health exam within 30 days of arrival. This screening exam is based on the 1995 medical screening protocol issued by the Office of Refugee Resettlement and includes a complete history and physical with a focus on geographic origin and path to host country, infectious disease, and trauma as well as screening labs, tuberculosis testing, immunizations, dental health, and mental health screening. All refugees are eligible for some form of financial support and medical insurance packages, most of which provide medical insurance coverage and benefits for 8 months. Public health systems in resettlement communities address these screening requirements through different care sites, including government-funded health centers, community health centers, and academic centers.

Refugee health clinics in primary care departments of academic health centers provide both the opportunity for the integration of population health education and clinical care across the continuum of medical training and a framework that directly links public health agencies, community-based social service organizations, and clinical care sites. One example of this integrated model of care and population health education is the Center for Refugee Health, which is housed within the Department of Family and Community Medicine (DFCM) at Thomas Jefferson University in Philadelphia. Established in 2007 as a partnership between the largest resettlement agency in Philadelphia and the DFCM, the Center for Refugee Health provides biweekly academic practice clinical sessions, a robust home visit program, and monthly community-based student-run clinics, during which health profession students and medical residents work directly with resettlement agency staff, social workers, and faculty to provide ongoing chronic disease management and preventive healthcare screenings in addition to required public health exams. Through these initiatives, the Center for Refugee Health at Thomas Jefferson University has developed a population-specific framework for clinical care and health professions education that employs several models of care, including the PCMH model and the Chronic Care Model, and provides essential training in communication, cultural competency, systems-based practice, health disparities, and global health.

As a case example that employs the principles outlined in the 2012 report of the IOM's Committee on Integrating Primary Care and Population Health[84] for successful integration of primary care and public health, this model provides the crucial link between primary care, public health practice, and population health education that results in higher quality health care and health professionals who are better prepared to meet the increasingly complex health needs of diverse populations.

CASE 2: POPULATION HEALTH MEDICAL SCHOOL CURRICULUM

The development of programmatic tracks that provide students with academic opportunities outside of the traditional medical curriculum represents a national trend in medical education. Enhancing medical student education with public health knowledge, skills, and attitudes has been recommended by many organizations. With the HRSA's Interdisciplinary and Interprofessional Joint Graduate Degree program's 5-year funding, the Department of Family and Community Medicine at Thomas Jefferson University created an Interprofessional Primary Care Dual Degree Program (IPCDDP), which builds on Jefferson Medical College's College within a College (CwiC) Scholarly Concentrations Program in Population Health. The mission of the IPCDDP is to provide training in primary care and population health to prepare primary care leaders to improve the health of vulnerable and underserved populations.

The CwiC program is an excellent example of increasing exposure to and knowledge of population health in medical education. Medical students have the option to choose a programmatic track that provides further training in population health outside of the traditional medical curriculum. Through a variety of methods (e.g., workshops, seminars, longitudinal research projects, mentorship from faculty advisers), students gain knowledge and skills. Students receive in-depth training and experience regarding community-based participatory research and the social determinants of health. In addition, students have the option to complete a master's in public health degree by transferring credits from medical school and completing the remaining coursework over the course of 1 year. Key CwiC components include the following:

- Year 1: Enhanced population health components of Introduction to Clinical Medicine, community immersions, twice-monthly seminars, and population health–related programs locally and globally during the summer
- Year 2: Case studies in Fundamentals of Clinical Medicine, twice-monthly seminars applying social and behavioral foundations of public health
- Year 3: Enhanced clerkship experiences with student presentations adding population health components to clinical cases (e.g., relevant Healthy People goals, Community Preventive Service Guidelines, utilization of community resources, quality improvement methods that may have prevented a hospital admission or more timely clinic visit)
- Year 4: Community-based electives and completion of a capstone project based on RMPHEC competencies

---

ORGANIZATION STRUCTURES AND SOURCE OF SUPPORT

OVERSIGHT OF HEALTH PROFESSIONS EDUCATION

Although the need for education reform is clear, several barriers have prevented the education system from changing. In particular, the IOM identified the lack of coordinated oversight across the continuum of education and between oversight processes, including accreditation, licensing, and certification within and among the various health professions.[1] Oversight systems hold one key to bringing about real change.

A concerted effort to enhance communication and collaboration between disciplines can provide a critical lever in competency development and education reform, yielding improvements in population health delivery. To address oversight challenges in health professions education, the IOM recommended that leading organizations develop an interdisciplinary effort focused on developing a common language to achieve consensus across the health professions on a core set of competencies that impact the delivery of population health programming (i.e., patient-centered care, interdisciplinary teams, evidence-based practice, quality improvement, and informatics). A shared set of competencies should be integrated into the health professions' oversight processes to align incentives and provide a catalyst for change. Further, those responsible for developing high-stakes tests and evaluations (i.e., admission, licensure, and certification) should make certain that their assessments support these shared competencies.

FINANCING SYSTEM OF HEALTH PROFESSIONS EDUCATION

The financing of health professions education has been identified as a key impediment to education reform, which is integrally linked to the overall healthcare financing system (see Box 4-1). The IOM committee strongly encourages Medicare and other payers to support changes and innovations in practice that will enhance patient care outcomes and provide productive training experiences for health professionals in population health.

Others have called on public and private entities to provide the funding necessary to support the evaluation and research to address education strategies and outcomes, as well as to disseminate successful innovations and approaches to population health.[16]

CHANGING THE CULTURE OF ORGANIZATIONS

The key goals of professional education are to transmit knowledge, impart skills, and inculcate the values of the profession.[69] Most students acquire their professional identities and norms of behavior by observing how respected role models interact with

BOX 4-1 CHALLENGES TO HEALTH PROFESSIONS EDUCATION REFORM

- Lack of funding to review curriculum and teaching methods and to acquire the resources required to make needed changes
- Too much emphasis on research and patient care in many academic settings, with little reward for teaching
- Lack of faculty and faculty development to ensure that faculty will be available at training sites and able to effectively teach students new competencies
- Fragmented responsibilities for undergraduate and graduate education and no coordinated oversight across the continuum of education
- No integration across oversight processes, including accreditation, licensing, and certification
- Lack of an evidence base assessing the effect of changes in teaching methods or curriculum
- A shortage of visionary leaders
- Silo structures and long-standing disciplinary boundaries among and across the professions
- Unsupportive culture and norms in health professions education
- Overly crowded curricula and competing demands
- Insufficient channels for sharing information and best practices[1]

Data from Institute of Medicine. *Health Professions Education: A Bridge to Quality.* Washington, DC: National Academies Press; 2003.

patients, staff, and others in the healthcare environment rather than in the classroom.[16] A variety of factors and historical trends, however, shape the attitudes and behaviors of faculty, which are ultimately passed on to students. The current culture of medicine has been characterized by the subordination of teaching to research, the intensifying pressure to increase clinical productivity, and the narrowing focus of medical education on biologic matters.[69] As Inui writes:

> And how are we faring as medical educators in preparing future physicians for professional roles in our complicated world? I would conclude that the "formative arc" of education today is strong on the acquisition of technical knowledge and weak-to-negative on the acquisition of values and moral formation. While preparing successfully to pass tests of knowledge, our students measurably move from being open-minded and curious to test-driven and minimalistic, from open-hearted and idealistic to self-centered and well-defended, and from altruistic to cynical. In the

course of their educational experience with us, they also move from taking notes and focusing on the explicit curriculum (what we say) to learning most from what we do. Here, then, is the greatest challenge of educating for professionalism. If we wish to change our students' preparation for their careers, we ourselves will need to change.[85]

In a complicated healthcare system, the values of health professionals and educators are becoming increasingly difficult for learners to discern. The call to reform healthcare delivery and health professions education is an opportunity to imbue professional values and the virtues of population health into our healthcare and education systems. Reframing education through the lens of population health to emphasize the social, economic, and political aspects of healthcare delivery is an essential step in transforming professional values. Support for the development of professionalism requires that institutions support appropriate "role model" faculty by giving them the time, opportunity, and professional development to learn, embrace, and impart intended virtues.

RECOMMENDATIONS

Despite existing innovative models, numerous updates to curricula, and proposals for reform, much work remains before we achieve the goal of a health professions workforce that can effectively deliver health care in the 21st century and implement the tenets of population health. Recommendations to facilitate this process for all schools teaching health professionals must include the following elements:

- Introduce education experiences that involve learners from more than one discipline. These experiences must be led or taught by teams of interprofessional faculty. Rigorous evaluation of interdisciplinary education efforts must be supported and should include qualitative and quantitative elements.
- Introduce curricula explicitly examining the roles, contributions, and skills of different health professionals. As an essential competency, effective participation in interdisciplinary teams should be rigorously assessed. Knowledge and skills pertaining to interdisciplinary teamwork should be included in formative examinations.
- Students must participate in a community experience that addresses the needs of a traditionally underserved population. These experiences must be designed and conducted in partnership with people who live in the community and work or live in the location that is the focus of the education experience.
- Integrate the knowledge and skills of public health into the fabric of health professions education.

- Integrate material relating the importance of social determinants of health in care delivery and outcomes.
- Integrate principles of quality improvement and patient safety into health professions education.
- Develop a population health steering group to formulate population health objectives and ensure that those objectives are routinely monitored and achieved.
- Support education research focusing on outcomes of population health curricula.

The product of these updates will be a healthcare workforce adequately prepared with the knowledge and skills to provide population-based care.

CONCLUSION

Flaws in health professions education both reflect and contribute to the failures in our current healthcare delivery system. Education for clinicians traditionally focuses on the medical conditions that acutely affect individuals and fails to incorporate principles of population health and prevention that are necessary to achieve a larger impact on our nation's health. Similar to healthcare reform, health professions education reform requires fundamental redesign. Multiple challenges and barriers to education reform exist, but the imperative to improve our healthcare delivery system and adequately prepare the healthcare workforce to successfully participate in the provision of care creates an unprecedented opportunity to overcome these obstacles.

SUGGESTED READINGS AND WEBSITES

READINGS

Association of American Medical Colleges. *Report II—Contemporary Issues in Medicine: Medical Informatics and Population Health*. Washington, DC: Association of American Medical Colleges; 1998.

Cohen JJ. Chairman's summary of the conference. In: Hager M, ed., *Revisiting the Medical School Educational Mission at a Time of Expansion*. Charleston, SC: Josiah Macy, Jr. Foundation; 2008.

Institute of Medicine. *Health Professions Education: A Bridge to Quality*. Washington, DC: National Academies Press; 2003.

Maeshiro R. Responding to the challenge: population health education for physicians. *Acad Med.* 2008;83(4):319-20.

Royeen CB, Jensen GM, Harvan RA. *Leadership in Interprofessional Health Education and Practice*. Sudbury, MA: Jones and Bartlett Publishers; 2009.

WEBSITES

Association for Prevention Teaching and Research: http://www.atpm.org
Community-Campus Partnerships for Health: https://ccph.memberclicks.net/
Institute for Healthcare Improvement, The Triple Aim: https://www.ihi.org/Topics/
    Triple Aim/Pages/default.aspx
Medicare Payment Advisory Commission: http://www.medpac.gov
National League for Nursing: http://www.nln.org

REFERENCES

1. Institute of Medicine. *Health Professions Education: A Bridge to Quality.* Washington, DC: National Academies Press; 2003.
2. Allan J, Barwick TA, Cashman S, et al. Clinical prevention and population health: curriculum framework for health professions. *Am J Prev Med.* 2004;27(5):471-6.
3. Medicare Payment Advisory Commission (MedPAC). *Report to the Congress: Improving Incentives in the Medicare Program.* Washington, DC: Medicare Payment Advisory Commission; 2009. http://www.ehidc.org/policy/fact-sheets/doc_download/158-reports-report-to-congress-improving-incentives-in-the-medicare-program-accountable-care. Accessed December 16, 2014.
4. Institute of Medicine. *Population Health Implications of the Affordable Care Act: Workshop Summary.* Washington, DC: The National Academies Press; 2013.
5. The Triple Aim. Institute for Healthcare Improvement. https://www.ihi.org/offerings/initiatives/tripleaim. Accessed October 1, 2014.
6. World Health Organization. *World Health Statistics 2009.* Geneva, Switzerland: WHO Press; 2009. http://www.who.int/whosis/whostat/2009/en/index.html. Accessed October 1, 2014.
7. Satcher D, Fryer GE Jr, Mccann J, et al. What if we were equal?: A comparison of the black–white mortality gap in 1960 and 2000. *Health Aff.* 2005;24(2): 459-64.
8. Institute of Medicine. *Coverage Matters: Insurance and Health Care.* Washington, DC: National Academies Press; 2001.
9. Institute of Medicine. *Crossing the Quality Chasm: A New Health System for the 21st Century.* Washington, DC: National Academies Press; 2001.
10. Association of American Medical Colleges. *Report I—Learning Objectives for Medical Student Education: Guidelines for Medical Schools.* Washington, DC: Association of American Medical Colleges; 1998.
11. Association of American Medical Colleges. *Report II—Contemporary Issues in Medicine: Medical Informatics and Population Health.* Washington, DC: Association of American Medical Colleges; 1998.
12. Association of American Medical Colleges. *Report V—Contemporary Issues in Medicine: Quality of Care.* Washington, DC: Association of American Medical Colleges; 2001.
13. Association of American Medical Colleges. *The Medical Home: Position Statement.* Washington, DC: Association of American Medical Colleges; 2008.
14. Association of American Medical Colleges. *Principles for U.S. Health Care Reform: A Guide for Policy Makers.* Washington, DC: Association of American Medical Colleges; 2008.
15. Swing S. R. (2007). The ACGME outcome project: retrospective and prospective. *Medical teacher, 29*(7), 648-54. https://www.paeaonline.org/index.php?ht=a/GetDocumentAction/id/110022
16. Institute of Medicine. *Who Will Keep the Public Healthy? Educating Public Health Professionals for*

the 21st Century. Washington, DC: National Academies Press; 2003.

17. Cohen JJ. Chairman's summary of the conference. In: Hager M, ed., *Revisiting the Medical School Educational Mission at a Time of Expansion*. Charleston, SC: Josiah Macy, Jr. Foundation; 2008.

18. Mead N, Bower P. Patient-centeredness: a conceptual framework and review of the empirical literature. *Soc Sci Med*. 2000;51(7):1087-110.

19. Beisecker AE, Murden RA, Moore WP, et al. Attitudes of medical students and primary care physicians regarding input of older and younger patients in medical decisions. *Med Care*. 1996; 34(2):126-37.

20. Beardsley RS. Communication skills development in colleges of pharmacy. *Am J Pharm Educ*. 2001;65(4):307-14.

21. Institute of Medicine. *Improving Palliative Care for Cancer*. Washington, DC: National Academies Press; 2001.

22. Peaceful death: recommended competencies and curricular guidelines for end-of-life nursing care. American Association of Colleges of Nursing. https://www.aacn.nche.edu/elnec/publications/peaceful-death. Accessed October 1, 2014.

23. Smedley BD, Stith AY, Nelson AR, eds. *Unequal Treatment: Confronting Racial and Ethnic Disparities in Health Care*. Washington, DC: National Academies Press; 2003.

24. Hall P, Weaver L. Interdisciplinary education and teamwork: a long and winding road. *Med Educ*. 2001;35(9):867-75.

25. Holmes DE, Osterweis M, eds. *Catalysts in Interdisciplinary Education: Innovation by Academic Health Centers*. Washington, DC: Association of Academic Health Centers; 1999.

26. Larson EL. New rules for the game: interdisciplinary education for health professionals. *Nurs Outlook*. 1995;43(4):180-5.

27. French P. The development of evidence-based nursing. *J Adv Med*. 1999;29(1):72-8.

28. Headrick LA, Knapp M, Neuhauser D, et al. Working from upstream to improve health care: the IHI interdisciplinary professional education collaborative. *Jt Comm J Qual Improv*. 1996; 22(3):149-64.

29. Henley E. A quality improvement curriculum for medical students. *Jt Comm J Qual Improv*. 2002; 28(1):42-8.

30. Mosher SA, Colton D. Quality improvement in the curriculum: a survey of AUPHA programs. *J Health Adm Educ*. 2001;19(2):203-20.

31. Buerhaus PI, Norman L. It's time to require theory and methods of quality improvement in basic and graduate nursing education. *Nurs Outlook*. 2001;49(2):67-9.

32. Carty B, Rosenfeld P. From computer technology to information technology: findings from a national study of nursing education. *Comput Nurs*. 1998;16(5):259-65.

33. Position statement: transforming nursing education. National League for Nursing. https://www.nln.org/aboutnln/positionstatements/transforming052005.pdf. Published May 9, 2005. Accessed October 1, 2014.

34. Nasca TJ, Philibert I, Brigham T, et al. The Next GME Accreditation System—Rationale and Benefits. *N Engl J Med*. 2012;36(6): 1051-56.

35. Cordasco KM, Horta M, Lurie N, et al. *How Are Residency Programs Preparing Our 21st Century Internists? A Review of Internal Medicine Residency Programs' Teaching on Selected Topics*. Santa Monica, CA: RAND Corporation; 2009. Doc. No. WR-686-MEDPAC. https://www.rand.org/pubs/working_papers/WR686. Accessed October 1, 2014.

36. Statement on health professions education in health reform. Federation of Associations of Schools of the Health Professions. https://www.asph.org/UserFiles/FASHPStatementOnHealthReform.pdf. Accessed November 19, 2013.

37. Kingdig DA, Asada Y, Booske B. A population health framework for setting national and state health goals. *JAMA*. 2008;299(17):2081-3.

38. Fielding JE, Teutsch SM. Integrating clinical care and community health: delivering health. *JAMA*. 2009;302(3):317-9.

39. Young TK. *Population Health: Concepts and Methods*. 2nd ed. New York, NY: Oxford University Press; 2005.

40. Kingdig D, Stoddart G. What is population health? *Am J Public Health*. 2003;93(3):380-3.

41. Lurie N, Fremont A. Building bridges between medical care and public health. *JAMA*. 2009; 302(1):84-6.

42. The New York Academy of Medicine. *Making an impact: annual report 2003*. http://www.nyam.org/news/docs/ar03.pdf. Accessed January 28, 2015.

43. Shortell SM, Swartzberg J. The physician as public health professional in the 21st century. *JAMA*. 2008;300(24):2916-8.

44. Institute of Medicine. *Training Physicians for Public Health Careers*. Washington, DC: National Academies Press; 2007.

45. Federman DD. *Healing and Heeling* [presentation]. Jordan J. Cohen Lecture at the AAMC annual meeting November 5, 2007. https://www.aamc.org/meetings/annual/2007/highlights/cohen_federman.pdf. Accessed December 10, 2013.

46. Institute of Medicine report. Who will keep the public healthy: educating public health professionals for the 21st century. https://www.iom.edu/Reports/2002/Who-Will-Keep-the-Public-Healthy-Educating-Public-Health-Professionals-for-the-21st-Century.aspx. Accessed October 20, 2014.

47. Association of American Colleges LEAP Initiative. http://www.aacu.org/leap/. Accessed October 1, 2014.

48. Riegelman, Richard. Undergraduate public health education: past, present, and future. *Am J Prev Med*. 2008;35(3):258-63.

49. Recommendations for public health curriculum—Consensus Conference on Undergraduate Public Health Education, November 2006. *MMWR*. 2007;56(1085-6). http://www.cdc.gov/mmwr/preview/mmwrhtml/mm5641a5.htm. Accessed October 1, 2014.

50. Maeshiro R. Responding to the challenge: population health education for physicians. *Acad Med*. 2008;83(4):319-20.

51. Finkelstein JA, McMahon GT, Peters A, et al. Teaching population health as a basic science at Harvard Medical School. *Acad Med*. 2008;83(4): 332-7.

52. Chamberlain LJ, Wang NE, Ho ET, et al. Integrating collaborative population health projects into a medical student curriculum at Stanford. *Acad Med*. 2008;83(4):338-44.

53. Kerkering KW, Novick LF. An enhancement strategy for integration of population health into medical school education: employing the framework developed by the Healthy People Curriculum Task Force. *Acad Med*. 2008;83(4):345-51.

54. Koo D, Thacker SB. The education of physicians: a CDC perspective. *Acad Med*. 2008;83(4): 399-407.

55. Johnson I, Donovan D, Parboosingh J. Steps to improve the teaching of public health to undergraduate medical students in Canada. *Acad Med*. 2008;83(4):414-8.

56. Michener JL, Yaggy S, Lyn M, et al. Improving the health of the community: Duke's experience with community engagement. *Acad Med*. 2008; 83(4):408-13.

57. Ornt DB, Aron DC, King NB, et al. Population medicine in a curricular revision at Case Western Reserve. *Acad Med*. 2008;83(4):327-31.

58. Riegelman RK, Garr DR. Evidence-based public health education as preparation for medical school. *Acad Med*. 2008;83(4):321-6.

59. Association for Prevention Teaching and Research. *Clinical Prevention and Population Health Curriculum Framework*. Washington, DC: Association for Prevention Teaching and Research; 2009.

60. American Association of Medical Colleges. Teaching for Quality: Integrating Quality Improvement and Patient Safety Across the Continuum of Medical Education, Report of Expert Panel. http://members.aamc.org/eweb/upload/Teaching%20for%20Quality%20Report.pdf. Accessed October 1, 2014.

61. Interprofessional Education Collaborative Expert Panel. *Core Competencies for Interprofessional Collaborative Practice: Report of an Expert Panel*. Washington, DC: Interprofessional Education Collaborative; 2011.

62. Institute of Medicine. *Population Health Implications of the Affordable Care Act: Workshop Summary*. Washington, DC: The National Academies Press; 2013.

63. Goodwin K, Tobler L. Community Health Workers: Expanding the Scope of the Healthcare Delivery System. National Conference of State Legislators. April 2008. https://www.ncsl.org/print/health/chwbrief.pdf. Accessed October 1, 2014.

64. The University of Arizona. National Community Health Worker Education Collaborative. http://www.chw-nec.org/. Accessed October 1, 2014.

65. Centers for Disease Control and Prevention.Promoting Policy and Systems Change to Expand Employment of Community Health Workers (CHWs) E-Learning Training Series. https://www.cdc.gov/dhdsp/pubs/chw_elearning.ht. Accessed October 1, 2014.

66. The University of Arizona. National Community Health Worker Education Collaborative. http://www.chw-nec.org. Accessed June 20, 2014.

67. Dumbald J, Kalichman M, Bell Y, et al. Case study in designing a research fundamentals curriculum for community health workers: a university-community clinic collaboration. *Health Promot Pract*. 2014;15:79-85.

68. Community-Campus Partnerships for Health. Advancing the Healthy People 2010 Objectives through Community-Based Education: A Curriculum Planning Guide. https://depts.washington.edu/ccph/guide-healthypeople.html. Accessed October 1, 2014.

69. Institute of Medicine. *In the Nation's Compelling Interest: Ensuring Diversity in the Health-Care Workforce*. Washington, DC: National Academies Press; 2004.

70. Cohen JJ, Gabriel BA, Terrell C. The case for diversity in the health care workforce. *Health Aff*. 2002;21(5):90-102.

71. Dill MJ, Salsberg ES. *The Complexities of Physician Supply and Demand: Projections Through 2025*. Washington, DC: Association of American Medical Colleges; 2008.

72. Castillo-Paige L. Diversity in Medical Education: Facts and Figures 2012. American Association of Medical Colleges. https://members.aamc.org/eweb/upload/Diversity%20in%20Medical%20Education_Facts%20and%20Figures%202012.pdf. Accessed October 1, 2014.

73. Diversity and Inclusion. American Association of Medical Colleges. https://www.aamc.org/initiatives/diversity/. Accessed October 1, 2014.

74. Association of American Medical Colleges. Medical Student Education: Debt, Cost, and Loan Repayment Fact Card. https://www.aamc.org/download/152968/data/debtfactcard.pdf. Accessed October 1, 2014.

75. Rabinowitz HK, Diamond JJ, Markham FW, et al. A program to increase the number of family physicians in rural and underserved areas: impact after 22 years. *JAMA*. 1999;281(3):255-60.

76. National Committee for Quality Assurance. Physician Practice Connections Programs. https://www.ncqa.org/portals/0/programs/recognition/PPC_web.pdf. Accessed October 1, 2014.

77. Improving Chronic Illness Care. Practice Change. http://www.improvingchroniccare.org/index.php?p=Practice_Change&s=3. Accessed October 1, 2014.

78. Improving Chronic Illness Care. The Chronic Care Model. http://www.improvingchroniccare.org/index.php?p=The_Chronic_Care_Model&s=2. Accessed October 1, 2014.

79. Public Health Foundation. Academic Health Department Learning Community. http://www.phf.org/programs/AHDLC/Pages/Academic_Health_Department_Learning_Community.aspx. Accessed October 1, 2014.

80. Newton WP, Du Bard CA. Shaping the future of academic health centers: the potential contributions of departments of family medicine. *Ann Fam Med*. 2006;4(Suppl 1):S2-11.

81. Cooke M, Irby DM, Sullivan W, et al. American medical education 100 years after the Flexner report. *N Engl J Med*. 2006;355(13):1339-44.

82. Interdisciplinary and Interprofessional Joint Graduate Degree. Health Resources and Services Administration. http://bhpr.hrsa.gov/grants/medicine/iijgd.html. Accessed October 1, 2014.

83. Utah State Legislature. 2014 General Session. Refugee assistance. Issue brief. http://le.utah.gov/interim/2013/pdf/00003191.pdf. Accessed January 30, 2015.

84. Institute of Medicine. Report brief: Primary care and public health: exploring integration to improve population health. March 2012. http://www.iom.edu/~/media/Files/Report%20Files/2012/Primary-Care-and-Public-Health/Primary%20Care%20and%20Public%20Health_Revised%20RB_FINAL.pdf. Accessed January 30, 2015.

85. Viewpoint: Educating for Professionalism in Medicine. http://professionalism.jefferson.edu/video8/2.cfm. Accessed January 28, 2015.

Chapter 5

THE POLITICAL LANDSCAPE IN RELATION TO THE HEALTH AND WEALTH OF NATIONS

C. ALAN LYLES

Executive Summary

The nation's wealth—a predictor of the population's health.

The health of a population is not an immutable fact, but rather is the result of inherent susceptibilities and multiple economic, political, and cultural influences. Political processes and the structures of government form the model under which policies to promote population health must be achieved. The health of a population has a strong but imperfect relationship to national wealth and to the proportion of the resources devoted directly to health services. The reciprocal is also true. The wealth of a nation is a by-product of its citizens' health status.

Even with metrics to measure and compare the health of the same population at different times or of different populations at the same time, the observed differences may be a consequence of multiple life experiences. Even the policies that affect health differ by domain (e.g., agricultural, educational, tax, immigration, and economic policies). The international economic crises that began in 2008 raise questions about the utility of narrowly focused measures of growth, particularly the measure of the gross domestic product (GDP) or even gross national income (GNI) and have prompted proposals for broader measures that would also assess well-being, social costs, and, particularly, sustainability.

The U.S. Constitution creates dual sovereignty between states and the federal government. Interest group politics influence the legislative agenda, substance, and outcomes for population health policies. Although there has been an expansion in federal powers related to the health of the population through preemption and legislation, many authorities remain at the state level. It may be efficient to have a central authority to oversee the health of the population, but the existing diversity of state and local entities that have responsibilities provides a natural laboratory for experimentation and innovation.

Learning Objectives

1. Describe the relationship between national wealth and population health and how it has evolved.
2. Illuminate the constitutional structures that influence population health policy.
3. Discuss the public and private sectors' interests in population health.
4. Explain the Preston curve and its implications.
5. Describe the public choice model as it applies to individual and special interest group political activity and voter behavior.

Key Terms

demographic transition
disability-adjusted life years
expected years of life
gross domestic product
gross national income
lobbying
Millennium Development Goals
per capita

preemption
Preston curve
prevention paradox
public choice model
purchasing power parity
quality-adjusted life years
years lived with disability

INTRODUCTION

The health of a population is not an immutable fact, but the result of multiple economic, historical and cultural influences. Political processes and the structures of government also influence a nation's health. In 1978, the International Conference on Primary Health Care called for all nations to protect and promote the health of their citizens. Named for the conference's location, the Alma-Ata Declaration proclaimed that "health is a fundamental human right . . . whose realization requires the action of many other social and economic sectors in addition to the health sector . . . [but] Governments have a responsibility for the health of their people which can be fulfilled only by the provision of adequate health and social measures."[1] In addition to the roles that governments may have, the health of a population has a strong but imperfect relationship to national wealth and to the proportion of the society's resources devoted directly to health services.[2]

In the years since the Alma-Ata Declaration, national variations in the distribution of health resources and the relative prominence of government in population health have persisted. These differences reflect values as well as differences in resources and technical capabilities. For example, consider how different national governments might respond to this question: Is access to health care a right of citizenship, a privilege of economic circumstances, or a negotiation among the public and private sectors and individuals? For the United States, a nation founded on individual liberties and strong protections for private property, what is the government's responsibility—and what are the limits on its authority—for the health of the population? For policies developed in the private sector, are resources used for healthcare costs or investments? The answers to these questions, in combination with differences in national resources, influence and reflect the political landscape of population health policies and innovations.

In the 20th century, the United States became concerned with population health when its experiences with conscription (a crude but useful proxy for assessing the health of a population) revealed alarming health deficiencies among men of age for military service. In World War I, roughly 15% of the approximately 3.8 million men who underwent a military draft physical were deemed unfit for military service, and almost half of the 2.7 million who did serve had physical impairments.[3] A quarter of a century later, a January 1944 draft proposal to President Roosevelt to improve access to medical care noted that "we are reaping today in wartime the consequences of our past neglect. Between 40 and 50 percent of those called in the military draft have been rejected on grounds of health."[4]

One way to view the political landscape is in terms of narrow self-interest and favoritism, with decisions determined by power rather than on their merit. However, while politics does concern authority relationships between individuals and governments and within levels of governments, it is more productive to understand politics as the legitimate processes and structures to manage and resolve competing interests where private interests, public life, and government intersect. Political outcomes reflect composite decisions about the appropriate roles of the individual, the private sector, and government. They are determined by national values, accidents of history, and legal and constitutional structures. Different nations approach the same issues with quite different expectations from, or constraints on, the actions of their central and subnational governments. Consequently, the political landscape sets the context for decisions about the generation and retention of wealth, direct and indirect public services that influence health and the rights and responsibilities of individuals, and the private sector and levels of government. These policy and political elements interact with differences in the inherent relative susceptibility of populations to disease, and the level and distribution of wealth and access to health services, which result in widely divergent comparative health levels and viable policies to improve them.

Constitutional provisions, legislation, case law, and in the private sector negotiations determine who receives which health services and who pays for them and how. Internationally, approaches to the organization, financing, and delivery of health services vary from those that are mainly market based to substantial central government roles. Because no nation has perfected a sustainable, comprehensive solution, comparative studies provide an opportunity to explore results from alternative approaches to identify potential best practices.

Even with metrics to measure and compare the health of the same population at different times or of different populations at the same time, wealth alone does not explain the variations that may be a consequence of multiple life experiences. Empiric research has established links between experiences across the life span: some protective and some that increase later health risks. Annual cross-sectional survey data can easily miss these associations. The life course health development model emphasizes these temporal connections between policies, access, and longer-term health status.[5] In other words, the health of an individual and of a population are the result of more than the consequences of health policies. Averages are convenient for quick, one-dimensional contrasts between populations, but they can obscure subgroup distinctions such as disparities in access; utilization; and outcomes by gender, age, race, or ethnicity.

Policies with consequences for human health seldom, if ever, have unanimous support. The direction and specifics of these policies are shaped through the political process and its leverage points for representing specific stakeholders. For example, Leonhardt explained stakeholder reactions to a proposed tax on more complete (and more costly) health insurance plans, even though the tax might lower overall healthcare costs for society: "By opposing the tax, the A.F.L.-C.I.O. [American Federation of Labor–Congress of Industrial Organizations, a leading federation of labor unions] is simply doing its job. It is defending the interests of its members who have such plans—just as business groups are defending the interests of their members. That is what special interests do: look out for their own constituents, even at the expense of the national interest."[6] Although it might seem that special interests are a relic of the past or represent the seedy underside of politics, they are one of the most visible expressions of pluralism in political life. The pursuit of a future population health system that considers everyone's interests equally would itself require organized interest groups. Effective advocacy of community-wide rather than narrow interests can influence policies and budgetary priorities only through the political process. Quixotic alternatives exist, but they are unlikely to achieve intended population health results.

Economics matter. Financial crises and business cycles also influence aggregate population health. M. Harvey Brenner received the American Public Health Association's Award for Excellence in 1996 for his lifetime of applied research into the lagged relationships between economic downturns, unemployment, and adverse consequences for health, including increased rates of suicide and mental disorders.[7]

MEASURING AND COMPARING POPULATION HEALTH AND WEALTH

As nations undergo economic development, there are identifiable patterns to their **demographic transitions**.[8] According to this process, high birth and high death rates are more commonly seen in agrarian societies, which have lower economic development. As industrialization and national development progress, death rates decline, as do birth rates. Although the net for each end of this process is a stable population, birth rates remain high and death rates decline during the transition period, producing population growth.[8]

HEALTH

Assessing a population's health requires sound metrics to determine its level and trends, and a process for evaluating the results of those measures against policy aims. Different metrics seek to measure specific aspects of the health of populations. Natural units, such as years of life, are often used for summary health statistics. However, unadjusted expected values, such as life expectancy at birth, represent the net result on health of numerous and often dissimilar factors (e.g., diet, sanitation, environment, access to primary health care, age pyramid, and the distribution of the population into socioeconomic strata). This issue is multifactorial (i.e., the same outcome can result from changes in different combinations of these factors). Consequently, multiple measures are required to understand the factors contributing to a population's health.

An encyclopedia of health measures exists, but one of the more commonly used indicators is the expectation for additional years of life beginning at a specific age. Each measure provides insight into the experience prior to the age referenced in the measure. In this way, the expectation of life at birth and the expectation of life at 1 year concern related but different contributing factors. Similarly, the infant mortality rate (IMR) is a summary indicator of prenatal care, nutrition, and environmental and related factors, and the maternal mortality rate is a crude comparator of the health system and of the general economic well-being among women.

Average life expectancy at birth in the United States has increased 18.4 years from 1930 to 2008 (Table 5-1). However, at every period for which data are reported, females had greater expected longevity than males, as did Caucasians over other ethnic groups. Disparities also exist among other races and ethnicities, age groups, and locations.[9]

Measurement of **expected years of life**, however, does not capture the variability within subgroups of the population. Additional measures that go beyond absolute years of life lived are useful in policy planning and evaluation, particularly in evaluating the health effect of technologies and policies. **Quality-adjusted life years** (QALYs), a measure commonly used in cost-utility or cost-effectiveness analyses, discount the years of life lived at less than full health. **Disability-adjusted life years** (DALYs), or **years lived with disability** (YLDs), quantify the gap between potential years of healthy life compared to years lived with less than full health and years of life lost to premature mortality. These measures provide objectivity and precision for contrasting the magnitude of disease and disability within and between populations. As a nation's income increases, it generally undergoes an epidemiologic transition. Acute infectious disease is more typical of the leading illnesses in low-income nations, whereas chronic illness and the consequences of lifestyle contribute more substantially to the burden of illness in high- and medium-income nations.[10]

Table 5-1 **Life Expectancy at Birth in the United States, Overall and by Gender and Race: 1930–2008**

	2008*	2006**	1996***	1986***	1976***	1966***	1935***	1930***
All races								
Both genders:	78.1	77.7	76.1	74.7	72.9		61.7	59.7
Female	80.6	80.2	79.1	78.2	76.8	73.9	63.9	61.6
Male	75.6	75.1	73.1	71.2	69.1	66.7	59.9	58.1
White								
Both genders:	78.5	78.2	76.8	75.4	73.6	71.1	62.9	61.4
Female	80.9	80.6	79.7	78.8	77.5	74.8	65.0	63.5
Male	76.1	75.7	73.9	71.9	69.9	67.5	61.0	59.7
Black								
Both genders:	74.0	73.2	70.2	69.1	67.2	64.2	53.1	48.1
Female	77.2	76.5	74.2	73.4	71.6	67.6	55.2	49.2
Male	70.6	69.7	66.1	64.8	62.9	60.9	51.1	47.3

Data from *Arias E. United States Life Tables, 2008. National Vital Statistics Reports. 2013;61(3):4. http://www.cdc.gov/nchs/data/nvsr/nvsr61/nvsr61_03.pdf; **Xu J, Kochanek KD, Tejada-Vera B. Deaths: Preliminary Data for 2007. *National Vital Statistics Reports.* 2009;58(1):27-8. Table 6 Expectation of life, by age, race, and sex: United States, final 2006 and preliminary 2007. http://www.cdc.gov/nchs/data/nvsr/nvsr58/nvsr58_01.pdf; ***Arias, E. United States Life Tables, 2001. *National Vital Statistics Reports.* 2004; 52(14):33-4. Table 12. Estimated life expectancy at birth in years, by race and sex: Death-registration States, 1900–28, and United States, 1929–2001. http://www.cdc.gov/nchs/data/nvsr/nvsr52/nvsr52_14.pdf.

A. R. Omran postulated three "Ages" to the epidemiologic profile of a population undergoing these changes: the Age of Pestilence and Famine, in which infectious disease and nutrition are more prominent sources of poor health; the Age of Receding Pandemics, in which increased life expectancy results in population growth and is associated with more chronic (noncommunicable) disease; and the Age of Degenerative and Man-Made Diseases, in which the chronic disease burden increases, yet infectious disease continues to be a population health concern.[11] Consequently, burden of illness determinations for populations are more useful if the epidemiologic profile includes details beyond the aggregate measures discussed so far (e.g., the leading specific conditions and their incidence and prevalence by the appropriate demographic categories).

Nations, nongovernmental organizations, and faith-based organizations each perform important roles in the politically charged environment of international development. As one measure of progress toward health goals, DALYs can be used as a planning and evaluation metric to align the activities of those who participate in international development and humanitarian assistance. In 2000, The United Nations Millennium Declaration set **Millenium Development Goals** (MDGs), including health, that would "free our fellow men, women and children from the abject and dehumanizing conditions of extreme poverty."[9] MDGs and relevant health targets include those described in Table 5-2.

The International Federation of Red Cross and Red Crescent Societies (IFRC) defines a noncommunicable disease (NCD) as one that "may result from genetic or lifestyle factors" but is not contagious, and it lists four principal NCD categories: cardiovascular, neoplastic, diabetic, and respiratory.[12] Not explicitly identified in the MDGs, NCDs have only recently become international priorities; therefore, NCD target identification, monitoring, and evaluation are being assessed in terms of a health systems approach.[13]

WEALTH

Health insurance is a critical factor in the effective demand for health services. Recent research indicates that lack of health insurance among people ages 17 to 64 may be responsible for as many as 45,000 excess deaths per year in the United States.[14] Just three of the 30 nation members of the Organisation for Economic Co-operation and Development (OECD) lack universal or near-universal health insurance: the United States, Turkey, and Mexico.[15] In reviewing these three countries, it is clear that the general economic level of a nation is not the determining factor for providing its citizens with health insurance. Instead, the proportion of a nation's population with health insurance coverage reflects cumulative societal decisions regarding the relative authorities and responsibilities between the public and private sectors, and with the individual members of a society.

Wealth disparities exist within as well as across nations. The GINI index can be used to compare nations over time and at a single point in time for different nations. The "GINI index measures the extent to which the distribution of income or consumption expenditure among individuals or households within an economy deviates from a perfectly equal distribution."[16] Its values range from zero (equality) to 100 (inequality), with gradations in the role that personal financial resources have in translating need and demand for healthcare services into effective demand.[17]

Table 5-2   Selected Population Health–Relevant Millennium Development Goals (MDGs)

MDG	Descriptor
MDG 4, Target 5	Reduce child mortality by two-thirds, between 1990 and 2015, the under-5 mortality rate
MDG 5, Target 6	Reduce by three-quarters, between 1990 and 2015, the maternal mortality ratio
MDG 6	Combat HIV/AIDS, malaria, and other diseases
MDG 6, Target 7	Have halted by 2015 and begun to reverse the spread of HIV/AIDS
MDG 6, Target 8	Have halted by 2015 and begun to reverse the incidence of malaria and other major diseases

Data from World Health Organization. Health and the Millennium Development Goals. Geneva. 2005. ISBN 92 4 156298 6 http://whqlibdoc.who.int/publications/2005/9241562986.pdf.

International comparisons reveal similarities and differences in economic and health status between countries. Unlike measures for health, there have been relatively few alternatives for quantifying the wealth of a nation until recently. Two conventional measures are used to compare wealth across nations:

- **Gross domestic product** (GDP) **per capita**, a measure of productivity that can be influenced by the relative value of different currencies, and one that is generally available for all nations
- GDP adjusted for **purchasing power parity** (PPP), which establishes a comparable monetary scale across currencies

The World Bank's lending policies reference **gross national income** (GNI). The income divisions that comprise GNI also prove useful in grouping nations for population health and health system performance comparisons. In 2012, the GNI for low-income countries was less than or equal to $1,035 per capita; for lower middle–income countries, $1,036–$4,085; for upper middle–income countries, $4,086–$12,615; and for high-income countries, greater than or equal to $12,616.[18,19]

The international economic crisis that began in 2008 raised questions about the utility of narrowly focused measures of growth, particularly GDP or even GNI, because tracking such measures failed to predict the economic failures. At the September 2009 conference of the G20 (the group of finance ministers and central bank governors from eight prominent industrialized nations, 11 emerging markets, and the European Union), President Nicolas Sarkozy presented the Report by the Commission on the Measurement of Economic Performance and Social Progress, which was authored by Nobel prize–winning economists Joseph Stiglitz and Amartya Sen and the commission's coordinator, Jean-Paul Fitoussi.[14] The report concluded that productivity alone is insufficient to assess the wealth of a nation and that GDP ignores too much of the collateral effects of economic development on individuals and nations. It proposed broader measures to assess well-being, social costs, and, particularly, sustainability.

Although not a tangible resource, social capital contributes to the health and vitality of a nation. It represents the informal networks that influence how and whether institutions flourish and whether the quality of life in a society is positive. Consider, for example, the roles of volunteers in terms of donated time to healthcare facilities, literacy tutoring programs, recreational councils, church activities, and 12-step programs.[20] Such voluntary activities vary considerably across and within communities.[21]

HEALTH AND DISPARITIES

A comparison of the relative, absolute, and mix of individual and public and private sector expenditures on health demonstrates stark contrasts between the United States and selected other nations with developed economies (Table 5-3). Although the United States ranks fifth in life expectancy at birth, it devotes a substantially greater percentage

Table 5-3 National Health Accounts: Life Expectancy at Birth (2011) and Health Expenditure Shares (2010)

	Canada	China	Ethiopia	France	Finland	Philippines	Russian Federation	United Kingdom	United States
Life expectancy at birth, years (2006)	82	76	60	82	81	69	69	80	79
Per capita total expenditures on health (US$ average exchange rate)	5,257	219	15	4,618	3,955	89	670	3,495	8,233
Health expenditures as % of GDP	11.4	5	4.8	11.7	9.0	4.1	6.5	9.6	17.6
Government expenditures as % of health expenditures	71.1	54.3	52.9	76.9	74.5	36.1	58.7	83.2	48.2
Private expenditures as % of health expenditures	28.9	45.7	47.1	23.1	25.5	63.9	41.3	16.8	51.8
Government health expenditures as % of all government expenditures	18.3	12.1	13.7	15.9	12.0	8.8	9.7	15.9	19.9

Data from World Health Organization. World Health Statistics 2013. http://www.who.int/gho/publications/world_health_statistics/2013/en/. Table I. Life expectancy and mortality; Table 7. Health Expenditures.

of its GDP to health expenditures. Most industrialized nations provide some level of government-funded health coverage for their entire population. This explains, in part, why U.S. government expenditures as a percentage of *all health expenditures* are the lowest among industrialized nations. However, health expenditures as a percentage of *total government expenditures* are highest for the United States (19.9%). That is, for comparable yet lower life expectancy at birth, the United States expends the highest percentage of its productivity on health-related costs. As a percentage of total health spending, private expenditures in the United States (i.e., employer-based coverage and consumer payments for individual coverage) are 83% higher than those of Canada and 308% more than those of the United Kingdom.

Since the mid-1960s, health expenditures under state and federal programs have been increasing while total national health expenditures from private sources have been decreasing (Table 5-4). When Medicare and Medicaid programs (enacted in 1965) became operational in 1966, 70% of national health expenditures were paid from private sources. In 1990, private sources of payment for national health expenditures had declined to 67.4%, and by 2011 they had decreased even further, to 55%. The change in composition is mainly attributable to increases in the share covered by the federal government.

National health expenditures alone do not produce health. A comparison of the United States and the United Kingdom (1970–2001) revealed that U.S. health expenditures consumed 9.5% of the U.S. GDP in 1970, compared to 5.6% in the United Kingdom. By 2001, health expenditures had grown to 13.9% of U.S. GDP, 6.3 percentage points higher than those of the United Kingdom. Despite spending a smaller share of its GDP on health, all-cause mortality (1974–2000) was lower in England and Wales than it was in the United States.[22]

Table 5-4   U. S. National Health Expenditures and Sources of Funds, 1990–2011

	2011	2007	2003	2000	1990
Total ($USD in billions)	2,701	2,298	1,775	1,377	724
Per capita ($USD)	8,680	7,536	6,121	4,878	2,854
Private (%)	55.0	59.4	61.3	64.5	67.4
Public (%)	45.0	40.6	38.7	35.5	34.1
Federal (%)	27.6	23.1	21.9	19.0	18.5
State and local (%)	17.4	17.5	16.8	16.5	15.6

Data from Centers for Medicare and Medicaid Services. Table 1. National Health Expenditures; Aggregate and Per Capita Amounts, Annual Percent Change and Percent Distribution: Selected Calendar Years 1960–2011. http://www.cms.gov/Research-Statistics-Data-and-Systems/Statistics-Trends-and-Reports/NationalHealthExpendData/downloads/tables.pdf. Accessed October 2, 2014.

The relationship between national wealth and life expectancy showed a similar but improved nonlinear pattern in the 1960s compared with that in the 1930s. Because only 16% of the estimated 12.2 years of improvement in life expectancy at birth during that period could be explained by changes in average national income, multiple factors are clearly at work.[23] The curvilinear relationship (**Preston curve**) still held when data from 196 countries were compared for 1975 and 2005[24] (Figure 5-1). Although increasing average wealth does not explain much of the increase in average life expectancy, it has a stronger association at the lowest income levels with decreasing marginal returns at higher income levels.

The aggregate mean life expectancy at birth (Table 5-1) in the United States has been increasing over the period displayed (1930–2008), yet differences persist by gender and by race. Caucasian women consistently had the greatest mean life expectancy at birth, and African American males had the lowest.

It is possible that differences by levels of national wealth might be attenuated by the diffusion of medical advances from the more affluent to the less wealthy countries. Conversely, increases in health may come first, resulting in healthier students and more productive workers, who also live longer, which in turn raises the average wealth of a nation.[25] An area of active interest is determining whether the unequal distribution, and not just the average income, within a nation is associated with differential life expectancy. The instruments to assess this are blunt, and the findings to date are either inconsistent or inconclusive.

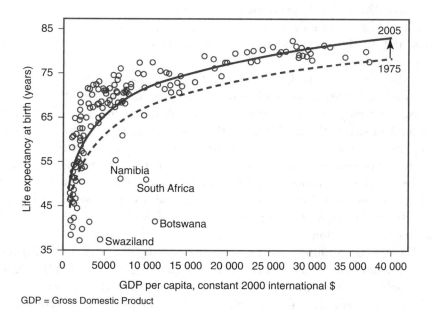

GDP = Gross Domestic Product

Figure 5-1   GDP per capita and life expectancy at birth in 169 countries,[a] 1975 and 2005.
Reproduced from World Health Organization. The World Health Report 2008. Primary Health Care, Now More Than Ever. WHO Press, Geneva, Switzerland. 2008. ISBN 978 92 4 156373 4. http://www.who.int/whr/2008/whr08_en.pdf.

FEDERALISM, POLITICS, AND POPULATION HEALTH

Understanding how federal and state health policies function in the United States requires a short review of constitutional history. The U.S. Constitution created a republic: "a government which derives all of its powers directly or indirectly from the great body of the people; and is administered by persons holding their office during pleasure, for a limited period, or during good behavior."[26] The delegates wrote the Constitution to ensure that it protects individual liberties and balances federal authority with necessity, while retaining state powers as much as feasible. The Constitution also implements a coherent set of political values: representative democracy; individual liberty in which the rights of minorities are respected by the majority; rule of law; separation of powers among the legislative, executive, and judicial branches; federalism; judicial independence; and civilian control of the military. Collectively, these values represented the national identity of that time. The authorities and limitations on governmental powers they created stretch across the centuries to influence current health policy initiatives.

A brief historical review is required to place the U.S. model for federalism in context, specifically the division of authorities between states and the national government. It begins with the independent former colonies, which operated as a confederation during and immediately following the American Revolution. As such, each state ceded only the most modest authorities to the central government, which prevented its functioning effectively. The national government lacked a common currency, trade was impeded by taxes levied on commerce between states, and treaties were signed between individual states and foreign powers—to the disadvantage of those relatively less powerful individual states.

It did not work. The Constitutional Congress that met in the summer of 1787 to draft a written constitution had to overcome these deficiencies, but it was not able to impose a central government upon the states. Authority began with and resided in the independent states. The final form of the new government and the specific partitioning of authorities between the states and the central government relied on each state's voluntarily relinquishing some authorities to the federal government. It was uncertain whether a balance acceptable to all could be achieved and whether such efforts could lead to a constitution that would be ratified and accepted by the newly independent states. It may be helpful to consider the analogy of the European Union's challenges with ratifying a constitution.

Through compromise and an elaborate system of checks and balances on power within the new federal government and between that government and each of the states, a workable though fragile constitution was created. Since the Constitution replaced the Articles of Confederation in 1789, the size and scope of the federal government's role in health care has grown through legislation and case law—slowly at first but more rapidly in the 20th and 21st centuries.

In response to concerns that the powerful British government that had been defeated in the revolution should not be replaced with a powerful domestic central government, a set of 10 amendments was offered and ratified 2 years after the Constitution itself. Within the Constitution and its amendments, there are enumerated powers for the federal government, and denied[27] and implied powers for the state governments. The enumerated powers of the federal government mainly remedy the shortcomings of the Articles of Confederation. Because state constitutions at that time predated the U.S. Constitution, the primacy clause in the U.S. Constitution asserted the limited form of federalism that was being created: "This Constitution, and the Laws of the United States which shall be made in Pursuance thereof; and all Treaties made, or which shall be made, under the Authority of the United States, shall be the supreme Law of the Land; and the Judges in every State shall be bound thereby, any Thing in the Constitution or Laws of any State to the Contrary notwithstanding."[28]

However, according to the Tenth Amendment, "The powers not delegated to the United States by the Constitution, nor prohibited by it to the States, are reserved to the States respectively, or to the people."[29] Police powers, as the term was understood in the 18th century, were retained by the state: notably, *health*, education, law enforcement, and welfare. Writing to encourage states to ratify the constitution, Alexander Hamilton specifically noted that "the proposed constitution . . . leaves in their [state government's] possession certain exclusive, and very important, portions of the sovereign power."[30] There are, however, circumstances for which federal law preempts state law:

- Under *express **preemption***, federal law restricts specific state regulatory actions, though a "savings clause" may remove some state actions from the prohibition.[31]
- *Field preemption* applies when federal law regulates a matter to such an extent that there is no opportunity for state law to be introduced without conflicting with it (e.g., employee benefit plans).
- *Conflict preemption* occurs when state and federal laws actually conflict or when the state law impedes achieving the intent of the federal law. Where the state law concerns the health or safety of the public, the U.S. Supreme Court has a strong presumption against preemption unless achieving the explicit intent of Congress requires that preemption.[31]

Interpretations of two other provisions in the Constitution have, over time, supported expanded federal authorities:

- The Commerce Clause,[32] which provides the federal government with the authority to regulate interstate commerce
- The Necessary and Proper Clause,[33] which is quite elastic, giving the federal government the power to make laws that may be required to implement or achieve the other powers that it has been given

The expansion is not a full transfer of authority from states to the federal government regarding population health law. Consequently, the United States does not have a national health policy, nor can it. Indirect means are used to influence healthcare quality, safety, and access where direct federal authority is lacking.

INTEREST GROUPS: THE FIRST AMENDMENT, PLURALISM, AND POLITICAL CAMPAIGN FINANCING

James Madison, an influential delegate to the Constitutional Convention of 1787 and a key contributing author to the Constitution, warned against "the mischiefs of factions"[34] (as political parties were then called). He cautioned that conflicts between rival parties lead to the neglect of the public good. Nonetheless, Madison also asserted that "among the numerous advantages promised by a well constructed Union, none deserves to be more accurately developed, than its tendency to break and control the violence of faction." Despite this optimism, political parties developed in the early years of the nation and have continued to evolve. People with similar interests also form associations that directly and indirectly seek to advance their interests through government actions. Between the associations and the elected members of political parties, there is a third group of people who work to influence government's decisions: lobbyists. The flow of money was deemed to be sufficiently large and regular that Congress passed the Federal Regulation of Lobbying Act (FRLA) in 1946,[35] which required registration and financial disclosure. The FRLA was amended and subsequently repealed by the Lobbying Disclosure Act of 1995,[36] though regulation of **lobbying** activities, particularly financial activities, continues to trail the evolution of these activities and to be less than effective in achieving their intended outcomes.

The political values of pluralism, respect for the rights of minorities within the majority rule, and effective checks on power require certain freedoms. The First Amendment to the Constitution declares these rights: "Congress shall make no law . . . abridging the freedom of speech, or of the press; or the right of the people peaceably to assemble, and to petition the Government for a redress of grievances."[37] Organizing into political parties to develop policies that express the political philosophy and interests of its members is a natural consequence of this.

The organization, financing, and delivery of health services partially represent a response to incentives, but interest groups influence these incentives through the political process. As explained by the **public choice model**,[38] the costs and gains from political activity to influence legislation and regulation do not fall equally on everyone. The costs of political activity tend to be high for individuals because of the relatively low frequency of events of potential interest or relevance to them and the low probability of an individual's position prevailing when such issues arise. Additionally, the time and opportunity cost of staying informed is relatively high for individuals versus an interest group or other organized stakeholders as a result of the many issues that arise versus the few issues that would be relevant for them.

According to the public choice model, general voters are rationally uninformed and politically inactive based on their expected individual gains versus the costs of their potential political activity. By contrast, other stakeholders have more enduring interests and are more likely to be affected by government policies and regulations in their focused area of interest. Interest groups organize to influence the distributional effects of governmental policies that would influence these stakeholders. For them, it is rational to commit the resources necessary to remain engaged in attempting to influence the probability of a preferred outcome. The result can be to the advantage of the interest group even at the expense of the greater good. As Watkins and Bazerman observed, "Through a combination of focused contributions to reelection campaigns, well-connected lobbyists, nurtured relationships with committee chairpersons and selected staff members, and intimate knowledge of leverage points in key processes, special interest groups routinely stall or torpedo policy changes, even when there is broad consensus that action is needed."[39]

The **prevention paradox** is a population health corollary to the public choice model. Changes in population health measures are influenced less by intervening with high-risk individuals than by even modestly changing exposure to risk factors by the population as a whole. This prevention paradox, that "a preventive measure that brings much benefit to the population offers little to each participating individual,"[40] suggests that effective long-term preventive changes for population health will require some public role. Fluoridation clearly illustrates the application of an insight into controlling the incidence of dental caries in populations; however, it was the focus of intense political opposition.[41]

Major interest groups in health care include the American Medical Association, America's Health Insurance Plans, the National Alliance on Mental Illness, and the National Business Group on Health, to name a few. These groups represent the interests of healthcare providers, insurers, employers, patient advocacy groups, and consumers. The amounts and methods of payment for lobbying and donations for political campaigns have the potential to exert substantial influence on legislation.[42] During the period from 1998 to 2013, five of the top-spending lobbying clients were from the health sector, and they spent a combined $1,241,765,824 to influence legislation (Table 5-5). To counter the risks that such sums may pose, the Bipartisan Campaign Reform Act of 2002 (the McCain-Feingold Act)[43] established categories and limits for monies that could be raised beyond those amounts specified under campaign finance law.

PUBLIC AND PRIVATE SECTOR ARRANGEMENTS IN HEALTH CARE

The development of the means to detect disease at an earlier stage stimulated screening of healthy individuals, transforming the traditional reliance on more urgent medical services once a person became ill. As the number of tests grew, U.S. health departments began offering screenings. Then, in an efficiency reorganization, "multiphasic" screenings were introduced, which enabled multiple screenings to be completed at one encounter. As these services were implemented, there was resistance from physicians who argued that

Table 5-5 Lobbying Payments, 1998–2013

Rank	Lobbying client	Amount ($)	Totals ($)
1	U.S. Chamber of Commerce		1,018,910,680
3	American Medical Association	295,057,500	
4	American Hospital Association	249,433,008	
5	Pharmaceutical Research & Manufacturers of America	246,386,420	
7	AARP	229,932,064	
8	Blue Cross/Blue Shield	220,956,832	
Subtotal Health Sector			1,241,765,824
Total			2,260,676,504

Data from Center for Responsive Politics, as of November 14, 2013. Washington, DC. http://www.opensecrets.org/lobby/top.php.

the "multiphasic screening concept placed a government agency between them and their patients . . . that primary responsibility for disease prevention rested with them and not the health department. They insisted that the individual not go first to the health center for tests and then to the doctor: the order must be reversed."[44] In its strong opposition to government initiatives such as public health clinics' performance of multiphasic screenings,[3] inclusion of national health insurance in the Social Security Act of 1935,[45] and subsequent versions of healthcare reform, the American Medical Association has consistently promoted its interest in maintaining strict physician autonomy in the practice of medicine.

The division of healthcare authorities between state and federal government and the vibrant role that voluntary associations play in American life have resulted in a variety of mechanisms to influence healthcare delivery, insurance, medical quality, and health practitioners' credentialing.

The Joint Commission is a private, not-for-profit organization that reviews and accredits healthcare entities. The Medicare and Medicaid programs require participating entities to continually meet eligibility requirements, though they do not directly assess or certify such standards. Instead, the entities can meet deemed status either by a state agency survey or through accreditation by The Joint Commission.

Accreditation of schools of medicine, a requirement for participation in Department of Education programs and funding, is performed by the Liaison Committee for Medical Education (LCME), a joint private entity comprising the American Medical Association and the Association of American Medical Colleges.

The National Association of Insurance Commissioners (NAIC) offers a similar model. Each state has authority over regulation of insurance within the state; however, national or multistate employers have a strong interest in consistent laws and regulations in each of the states in which they have employees. State insurance commissioners meet through the NAIC and draft model acts, which then are acted upon within each state. In this way state authority is maintained, but coherence is improved.

Establishing national goals for the health of the nation is not an authority of the federal government. However, in 1979 the U.S. Surgeon General issued the first of the decennial Healthy People reports. The reports provide a snapshot of the health of Americans, both baseline and quantitative goals for improvement over the following decade; the intent is to align autonomous entities toward jointly developed goals and to track achievements. *Healthy People 2020*[46] consists of 42 topic areas and 1,200 measures. These focus areas and objectives were collaboratively developed by hundreds of private organizations, state and federal agencies, and individuals—not dictated by the federal government. To sharpen the focus, 12 topics carrying the highest priority for improvement were identified as leading health indicators (Box 5-1).

BOX 5-1: *HEALTHY PEOPLE 2020* LEADING HEALTH INDICATORS: 12 TOPICS

- Access to health services
- Clinical preventive services
- Environmental quality
- Injury and violence
- Maternal, infant, and child health
- Mental health
- Nutrition, physical activity, and obesity
- Oral health
- Reproductive and sexual health
- Social determinants
- Substance abuse
- Tobacco

Data from *Healthy People 2020* Leading Health Indicators: Twelve Topics, Retrieved from http://healthypeople .gov/2020/LHI/2020indicators.aspx.

Similarly, the National Strategy for Suicide Prevention (NSSP) provides a framework of goals and objectives to improve efforts at suicide prevention, but it is the responsibility and decision of each state as to whether and how it will modify, adopt, and implement its own plan based on the NSSP.

These public and private sector arrangements in health care strive to set standards for health (Healthy People), reduction of harm (NSSP), quality in facilities (The Joint Commission), and medical education (LCME), and consistency in health insurance regulation (NAIC). These particular structures are necessary as a consequence of the form of federalism in the United States, evolving policies, legislation, and case law. Consequently, they are not all working to achieve population health goals (NAIC), but their work does influence population health goals.

CONCLUSION

The health of a population is not an immutable fact but rather a consequence of multiple economic, political, and cultural influences. The curvilinear relationship between wealth and expected length of life at birth holds true today as it did for data from the 1930s. The Preston curve implies that the largest gains can be achieved at the low end of GDP per capita, with decreasing marginal results at higher income levels. Over time, however, the Preston curve has shifted upward. Modeling the relationship for observed versus expected changes in life expectancy at birth for different nations yields the surprising result that most of the observed increase in life expectancy is due to factors other than income per se.

Policies to influence the organization, financing, and delivery of healthcare are strongly influenced by each nation's history, culture, political values, structures, and processes. The political process and structures of government in the United States are inefficient. This inefficiency is by design and continues in order to protect core values such as checks and balances on governmental authorities, pluralism, individual freedom, and the rights of states. The organization of stakeholders into special interest groups gives voice to these values, yet it can result in perverse results or inaction when change or innovations are introduced. Over time, the political landscape is an evolving rather than a fixed map. Opportunities and constraints and interests and capacities change, but the path for public expression provides enduring boundaries and processes for resolving the competing and conflicting interests of the nation's population.

STUDY AND DISCUSSION QUESTIONS

1. What are the relative merits of alternative measures for measuring the health of a population?
2. What is the relationship between the health and wealth of a population? Is increased wealth always associated with increased health? Explain why or why not.
3. When might measures other than economic productivity be appropriate?
4. What is the relationship between the political process and access to health services in the United States? How might policies other than those directly concerning health care influence the health of a population?
5. There are differences between countries in population health, but why are there differences in the health of subgroups within countries?

SUGGESTED READINGS AND WEBSITES

READINGS

Acs ZJ, Lyles A (eds). *Obesity, Business and Public Policy*. Cheltenham, UK: Edward Elgar Publishing; 2007.

Blumenthal D, Morone J. *The Heart of Power: Health and Politics in the Oval Office.* Berkeley and Los Angeles: University of California Press; 2009.

Field RI. *Mother of Invention: How the Government Created "Free Market" Health Care.* New York: Oxford University Press; 2013.

Fisher ES, Bynum JP, Skinner JS. Slowing the growth of health care costs—lessons from regional variation. *N Engl J Med.* 2009;360(9):849-52.

Patel K, Rushefsky ME. *Health Care in America: Separate and Unequal.* New York: M. E. Sharpe; 2008.

Redman E. *The Dance of Legislation.* Seattle: University of Washington Press; 2001.

Starr P. *The Social Transformation of American Medicine.* New York: Basic Books; 1982.

WEBSITES

Centers for Disease Control and Prevention, Health, United States (updated annually): http://www.cdc.gov/nchs/hus.htm

Healthy Communities Program: http://www.cdc.gov/healthycommunitiesprogram/

Morbidity and Mortality Weekly Report: http://www.cdc.gov/mmwr/

Center for Global Health and Economic Development: http://cghed.ei.columbia.edu/

Center for Responsive Politics: http://www.opensecrets.org/index.php

The Commonwealth Fund: http://www.commonwealthfund.org/

Healthy People: http://www.healthypeople.gov/

The Joint Commission: http://www.jointcommission.org/

Kaiser Family Foundation (not associated with Kaiser Permanente or Kaiser Industries): http://www.kff.org

Patient-Centered Outcomes Research Institute: http://www.pcori.org/

Preventing Chronic Disease: Public Health Research, Practice and Policy http://www.cdc.gov/pcd/

The World Bank, World Development Indicators: http://data.worldbank.org/products/wdi

World Health Organization: http://www.who.int/en/

World Health Organization, World Health Statistics: http://www.who.int/gho/publications/world_health_statistics/en/

REFERENCES

1. Declaration of Alma-Ata: International Conference on Primary Health Care, Alma-Ata, USSR, 6–12 September 1978. http://www.who.int/publications/almaata_declaration_en.pdf. Accessed October 2, 2014.

2. World Health Organization. *World Health Statistics 2009.* Geneva, Switzerland: World Health Organization; 2009. http://www.who.int/gho/publications/world_health_statistics/EN_WHS09_Full.pdf?ua=1. Accessed October 2, 2014.

3. Reiser SJ. The emergence of the concept of screening for disease. *Milbank Mem Fund QHealth Soc.* 1978;56(4):403-25.

4. Milton Handler, memo to Judge Rosenman, January 28, 1944, Papers of Samuel I. Rosenman, Subject File: Health, Legislative Proposal, Box 1, Truman Library. *Cited in* Blumenthal D and Morone JA. *The Heart of Power: Health and Politics in the Oval Office.* Berkeley and Los Angeles: University of California Press; 2009.

5. Halfon N, Hochstein M. Life course health development: an integrated framework for developing health, policy, and research. *Milbank Q.* 2002; 80(3):433-79.

6. Leonhardt D. 'Cadillac tax' offers opportunities. *New York Times.* September 30, 2009: B1.7.

7. Brenner MH. *Society and Health.* New York: Oxford University Press; 1995.

8. Bongaarts J. Human population growth and the demographic transition. *Philos Tran R Soc Lond B Biol Sci*, 2009; 364(1532):2985-90.

9. Patel K, Rushefsky ME. *Health Care in America: Separate and Unequal.* New York: M. E. Sharpe; 2008.

10. McKeown RE. The epidemiologic transition: changing patterns of mortality and population dynamics. *Am J Lifestyle Med.* 2009;3(1 Suppl):19S-26S. http://www.ncbi.nlm.nih.gov/pmc/articles/PMC2805833/pdf/nihms134943.pdf. Accessed October 2, 2014.

11. Omran AR. The epidemiologic transition: a theory of the epidemiology of population change. *Milbank Q.* 2005;83(4):731-57.

12. The International Federation of Red Cross and Red Crescent Societies. Noncommunicable disease. http://www.ifrc.org/what-we-do/health/diseases/noncommunicable-diseases/. Accessed October 2, 2014.

13. World Health Organization. Global Health Observatory. Health system response and capacity to address and respond to NCDs. http://www.who.int/gho/ncd/health_system_response/en/. Accessed October 2, 2014.

14. Stiglitz JE, Sen A, Fitoussi J-P. Report by the Commission on the Measurement of Economic Performance and Social Progress. Paris, France. http://www.stiglitz-sen-fitoussi.fr/en/index.htm. Accessed October 31, 2014.

15. Organisation for Economic Co-operation and Development. Health at a glance 2007: OECD indicators; page 96. http://vorige.nrc.nl/redactie/binnenland/oecd.pdf. Accessed October 2, 2014.

16. The World Bank. GINI index. http://data.worldbank.org/indicator/SI.POV.GINI. Accessed October 2, 2014.

17. Berndt DJ, Fisher JW, Rajendrababu RV, et al. Measuring healthcare inequities using the Gini index. Proceedings of the 36th Hawaii International Conference on System Science; 2003. http://www.hicss.hawaii.edu/HICSS36/HICSSpapers/HCDMG03.pdf. Accessed October 2, 2014.

18. The World Bank. Country and lending groups. http://data.worldbank.org/about/country-and-lending-groups. Accessed October 2, 2014.

19. The World Bank. A short history. http://go.worldbank.org/U9BK7IA1J0. Accessed October 2, 2014.

20. Lyles A. Improving long-term weight management: social capital and missed opportunities [commentary]. *Popul Health Manag.* 2009; 12(6):293-5.

21. Putnam RD. *Bowling Alone: The Collapse and Revival of American Community.* New York: Simon & Schuster; 2000.

22. Pritchard C, Galvin K. A comparison of British and US mortality outcomes. *Nurs Times.* 2006;102(48):33-4.

23. Preston SH. The changing relation between mortality and level of economic development. *Popul Stud.* 1975;29(2):231-48. Reprinted in *Int. J Epidemiol.* 2007;36:484-90.

24. World Health Organization. *The World Health Report 2008. Primary Health Care, Now More Than Ever.* Geneva, Switzerland: WHO Press; 2008.

25. Bloom DE, Canning D. Commentary: The Preston curve 30 years on: still sparking fires. *Int J Epidemiol.* 2007;36:498-9.

26. James Madison, "Federalist #39," in The Federalist Papers. Bantam Books.

27. U.S. Constitution, art. 1, sec. 10.

28. U.S. Constitution, art. 6, cl. 2.

29. U.S. Constitution, amend. 10.

30. Alexander Hamilton, "Federalist #9," in The Federalist Papers. Bantam Books.

31. Mermin SE, Graff SK. A legal primer for the obesity prevention movement. *Am J Public Health* 2009;99:1799-805.

32. U.S. Constitution, art. 1, sec. 8, cl. 3: "To regulate Commerce with foreign Nations, and among the several States, and with the Indian Tribes."

33. U.S. Constitution, art. 1, sec. 8, cl. 18: "To make all Laws which shall be necessary and proper for carrying into Execution the foregoing Powers, and all other Powers vested by this Constitution in the Government of the United States, or in any Department or Officer thereof."

34. James Madison, "Federalist #10," in The Federalist Papers. Bantam Books.

35. Federal Regulation of Lobbying Act 2 U.S.C. 261 et seq.

36. Lobbying Disclosure Act of 1995, Pub. L. No. 104-65, 109 Stat. 691 (1995).

37. U.S. Constitution, amend. 1: "Congress shall make no law respecting an establishment of religion, or prohibiting the free exercise thereof; or abridging the freedom of speech, or of the press; or the right of the people peaceably to assemble, and to petition the Government for a redress of grievances."

38. Jensen GA, Morrisey MA. Employer-sponsored health insurance and mandated benefit laws. *Milbank Q.* 1999;77(4):425-59.

39. Watkins MD, Bazerman MH. Predictable surprises: the disasters you should have seen coming. *Harv Bus Rev.* March 2003:72-80.

40. Rose G. Strategy of prevention: lessons from cardiovascular disease. *Br Med J.* 1981;282:1847-51.

41. Gamson WA. The fluoridation dialogue: is it an ideological conflict? *Public Opin Q.* 1961;251:526-37.

42. Lyles A. Chapter 24: Politics, public policy, and national healthcare reform: Medicare and the Medicare Modernization Act of 2003. In: Navarro RP. *Managed Care Pharmacy Practice*, 2nd ed. Sudbury, MA: Jones and Bartlett Publishers; 2009.

43. Bipartisan Campaign Reform Act of 2002. Pub. L. No. 107-155.

44. Smillie WG. "Multiphasic" screening tests. *JAMA* 1951;145(16):1254-6.

45. Starr P. *The Social Transformation of American Medicine.* New York: Basic Books; 1982.

46. *Healthy People 2020.* http://www.healthypeople.gov/2020/default.aspx. Accessed October 2, 2014.

BEHAVIOR CHANGE

JAMES O. PROCHASKA AND
JANICE M. PROCHASKA

Executive Summary

Behavior change—an essential component of a well-being system.

Health risk behaviors, such as smoking, inactivity, unhealthy diets, nonadherence to prescribed therapies, and ineffectively managed stress, significantly contribute to a population's morbidity, disability, mortality, reduced productivity, and escalating health-care costs. To have a significant and sustainable effect on these behaviors, a model of behavior change is needed to address the needs of entire populations, not just the minority who are motivated to take immediate action. The Transtheoretical Model of Behavior Change (TTM) is founded on stages of change, which categorize segments of populations based on where they are in the process of change. Principles and processes are applied to initiate movement through the stages of change. Interventions tailored to specific needs allow programs to be interactive and broadly applicable for treatment of entire populations. Computer-tailored interventions (CTIs) delivered through various modalities, such as clinical guidance, telephonic counseling, and the Internet, greatly affect both single and multiple behaviors for disease prevention and management. These interventions involve new paradigms that complement existing ones, such as proactive stage-matched interventions for multiple behaviors delivered to homes via computers, with evidence based on population trials that use impact metrics. These integrated paradigms have the potential to provide the foundation for a well-being system, which will complement the existing sick-care system.

Learning Objectives

1. Identify the major constructs of the transtheoretical model of behavior change (TTM).
2. Select and apply TTM principles at each stage of change when working with patients and populations.
3. Understand the critical assumptions of the TTM.
4. Realize the importance of multiple behavior changes.
5. Describe the provider's role in understanding and managing the behaviors of patient populations.

Key Terms

multiple behavior changes   stages of change
processes of change   transtheoretical model of behavior change

INTRODUCTION

Healthcare providers and patients have a shared responsibility for population health. As the ultimate authority on their personal health, patients have responsibility for sharing health-related information with their providers. Healthcare providers are responsible for listening to patients' concerns and providing advice accordingly. This shared responsibility is essential for all patient populations and is especially important for those dealing with chronic conditions. Behaviors affect morbidity, and unhealthy behaviors may lead to mortality. Understanding what causes patients to exhibit certain behaviors and what motivates them to change provides information that can be broadly applied to populations with similar characteristics.

In this chapter, we focus on the provider's role in understanding and managing the behaviors of patient populations. Behavior change is important in several domains of chronic care management: (1) in personal health care, when providers work with a patient to change the behaviors that are contributing to or exacerbating the patient's disease; (2) in quality and safety, as they relate to advising patients on the risks of smoking, including fires, for example; and (3) in public health activities, in advising older populations to receive pneumonia vaccinations for protection. Behavior affects three of the four pillars of population health, demonstrating that it is a key driver in population health management (Box 6-1). It is the healthcare provider's role to advise patients on the risks of their behaviors and the benefits of changing unhealthy ones. Providers can follow the **transtheoretical model of behavior change** in advising patients, guiding them, and working with them wherever they are at in their readiness to change. While this model has traditionally been applied to individuals, it can also be used with populations.

BOX 6-1 FOUR PILLARS OF POPULATION HEALTH

Chronic care management   Health policy

Quality and safety   Public health

THE TRANSTHEORETICAL MODEL OF BEHAVIOR CHANGE

The TTM uses stages to integrate principles and **processes of change** derived from major theories of intervention—hence, the name "transtheoretical." This model emerged from a comparative analysis of leading theories that are grounded in psychotherapy and behavior change. Because more than 300 psychotherapy theories were found, the TTM developers determined that there was a need for systematic integration.[1] Ten processes of change emerged, including consciousness raising from the Freudian tradition, reinforcement management from the Skinnerian tradition, and helping relationships from the Rogerian tradition.

In an empirical analysis of self-changers compared to smokers in professional treatments, researchers assessed how frequently each group used each of the 10 processes.[2] Research participants indicated that they used different processes at different times in their struggles with smoking. These naive subjects revealed a phenomenon that was overlooked in the multitude of therapy theories, specifically that behavior change unfolds through a series of stages.[3] From these initial studies of smoking, the stage model rapidly expanded in scope to include investigations and applications to a broad range of physical health and mental health behaviors. Examples include alcohol and substance abuse, stress, bullying, delinquency, depression, eating disorders and obesity, high-fat diets, HIV/AIDS prevention, mammography screening, medication compliance, family planning, smoking during pregnancy, radon testing, sedentary lifestyles, and sun exposure. Over time, behavior studies have expanded, validated, applied, and challenged the core constructs of the TTM.

CORE CONSTRUCTS

Stages of change lie at the heart of the TTM. Studies of change have found that people move through a series of stages when modifying behavior. While the time a person stays in each stage is variable, the tasks required to move to the next stage are not. Certain principles and processes of change work best at each stage to reduce resistance, facilitate progress, and prevent relapse. These include decisional balance, self-efficacy, and processes of change. Only a minority (usually less than 20%) of a population at risk is prepared to take action at any given time. Thus, action-oriented advice misserves individuals in the early stages. Guidance based on the TTM results in increased participation in the change process, because it appeals to the whole population rather than the minority ready to take action.

STAGES OF CHANGE

The stage construct represents a temporal dimension. Although change implies phenomena occurring over time, none of the leading theories of therapy contained a core construct representing time. Traditionally, behavior change was construed as an event (e.g., quitting smoking, drinking, or overeating.) In contrast, TTM recognizes change as a process that unfolds over time, involving progress through a series of stages.

Precontemplation
People in the precontemplation stage do not intend to take action in the foreseeable future, usually defined as the next 6 months. Being uninformed or underinformed about the consequences of one's behavior may cause a person to be in the precontemplation stage. Multiple unsuccessful attempts at change can lead to demoralization about the ability to change. Both the uninformed and underinformed tend to avoid reading, talking, or thinking about their high-risk behaviors. They are often characterized in other theories as resistant, unmotivated, or unready for health promotion programs. The fact is that traditional population health promotion programs were not prepared for such individuals and were not designed to meet their needs.

Contemplation
Contemplation is the stage in which people intend to change in the next 6 months. They are more aware of the pros of changing but are also acutely aware of the cons. In a meta-analysis across 48 health risk behaviors, the pros and cons of changing were equal. This weighting between the costs and benefits of changing can produce profound ambivalence, causing some people to remain in this stage for long periods of time. This phenomenon is often characterized as chronic contemplation or behavioral procrastination. Individuals in the contemplation stage are not ready for traditional action-oriented programs that expect participants to act immediately.

Preparation
Preparation is the stage in which people intend to take action in the immediate future, usually measured as the next month. Typically, they have already taken some significant action in the past year. These individuals have a plan of action, such as joining a health education class, consulting a counselor, talking to their physician, buying a self-help book, or relying on a self-change approach. These are the people who should be recruited for action-oriented programs.

Action
Action is the stage in which people have made specific overt modifications in their lifestyles within the past 6 months. Because action is observable, the overall process of behavior change often has been equated with action. But in the TTM, action is only

one of six stages. Typically, not all behavior modifications count as action in this model. In most applications, people have to attain a criterion that scientists and professionals agree is sufficient to reduce risk of disease. For example, reduction in the number of cigarettes or switching to low-tar and low-nicotine cigarettes were formerly considered acceptable actions toward smoking cessation. Now the consensus is clear—only total abstinence counts.

Maintenance

Maintenance is the stage in which people have made specific overt modifications in their lifestyles and are working to prevent relapse; however, they do not apply change processes as frequently as do people in the action stage. While in the maintenance stage, people are less tempted to relapse and grow increasingly more confident in their ability to continue their behavior changes. Based on temptation and self-efficacy data, researchers have estimated that maintenance lasts from 6 months to about 5 years. While this estimate may seem somewhat pessimistic, longitudinal data in the 1990 Surgeon General's report support this temporal estimate.[4] After 12 months of continuous abstinence, 43% of individuals returned to regular smoking. It was not until 5 years of continuous abstinence that the risk for relapse dropped to 7%.[4]

Termination

Termination is the stage in which individuals are not tempted; they have 100% self-efficacy. Whether depressed, anxious, bored, lonely, angry, or stressed, individuals in this stage are sure they will not return to unhealthy habits as a way of coping. It is as if their new behavior has become an automatic habit. Examples include adults who have developed automatic seat belt use or who automatically take their antihypertensive medication at the same time and place each day. In a study of former smokers and alcoholics, researchers found that less than 20% of each group had reached the criteria of zero temptation and total self-efficacy.[5] The criterion of 100% self-efficacy may be too strict, or it may be that this stage is an ideal goal for population health efforts. In other areas (e.g., exercise, consistent condom use, weight control), the realistic goal may be a lifetime of maintenance. Termination has not been given as much emphasis in TTM research because it may not be a practical reality for populations and it occurs long after interventions have ended.

PROCESSES OF CHANGE

Because processes of change are the experiential and behavioral activities that people use to progress through the stages, it is important for practitioners of population health to understand these progressions. By providing important guides for intervention programs, they serve as independent variables that are applied to move from stage to stage. The following 10 processes have received the most empirical support in our research to date.

Consciousness Raising

Consciousness raising involves increased awareness about the causes, consequences, and cures for a particular problem behavior. Healthcare provider interventions that can increase awareness include feedback, interpretations, and reading materials. Sedentary patients, for example, may not be aware that their inactivity can have the same risk as smoking a pack of cigarettes a day.

Dramatic Relief

Dramatic relief initially produces increased emotional experiences followed by reduced affect or anticipated relief if appropriate action is taken. Healthcare providers can provide health risk feedback and success stories to move people to be inspired by how others have changed.

Environmental Reevaluation

Environmental reevaluation combines both affective and cognitive assessments of how the presence or absence of a personal habit affects one's social environment (e.g., the effect of smoking on others). It can also include the awareness that one can serve as a positive or negative role model for others. Providers can help by suggesting that patients ask others about their behavior or by offering family interventions that lead to such reassessments.

Self-Reevaluation

Self-reevaluation combines both cognitive and affective assessments of one's self-image with and without a particular unhealthy habit, such as one's image as a couch potato versus an active person. Values clarification, identifying healthy role models, and imagery are techniques that healthcare providers can use to move patients toward self-reevaluation. During an interaction with a patient, the provider might ask, "Imagine you were free from smoking. How would you feel about yourself?"

Self-Liberation

Self-liberation is both the belief that one can change and the commitment, or recommitment, to act on that belief. Encouraging patients to make New Year's resolutions, public testimonies, or contracts are ways of enhancing resolve. The provider might say, "Telling others about your commitment to take action can strengthen your willpower. Who are you going to tell?"

Social Liberation

Social liberation requires an increase in social opportunities or alternatives, especially for patients who are relatively deprived or oppressed. For example, advocacy, empowerment procedures, and appropriate policies can produce increased opportunities for health promotion, particularly for minority (social, racial, ethnic), underserved, and/or impoverished segments of the population. The same procedures can be used to help populations change (e.g., smoke-free zones, salad bars in school cafeterias, easy access to condoms and other contraceptives). Healthcare providers can promote changes in society by encouraging healthy lifestyles and making them easier to achieve.

Counterconditioning

Counterconditioning requires learning and adopting healthy behaviors as substitutes for problem behaviors. Examples of counterconditioning include healthcare provider recommendations for use of nicotine replacement as a safe substitute for smoking and walking as a healthy alternative to comfort foods for coping with stress.

Helping Relationships

Helping relationships combine caring, trust, openness, and acceptance, as well as support, for healthy behavior change. Rapport building, a therapeutic alliance, supportive calls, and buddy systems are sources of social support that may be offered by healthcare providers. SilverSneakers, an exercise program often covered by Medicare, is an example of a program that providers might suggest to their patients.

Reinforcement Management

Reinforcement management provides supportive consequences for taking steps in a positive direction. We have found that self-changers rely on reward much more than on punishment. We recommend that healthcare providers emphasize reinforcement to work in harmony with how people change naturally. Because patients expect to be reinforced by others more frequently than this generally occurs, they should be encouraged to reinforce themselves through self-statements like "Nice going—you handled that temptation." Patients also need to treat themselves at milestones as a way to provide reinforcement and to increase the probability that healthy responses will be repeated.

Stimulus Control

Stimulus control removes cues for unhealthy habits and adds prompts for healthier alternatives. Healthcare providers can help by recommending removing of all the ashtrays from the house and car or removing high-fat foods that are tempting cues for unhealthy eating.

DECISIONAL BALANCE

The process of reflecting and weighing the pros and cons of changing is termed *decisional balance*. According to Janis and Mann, sound decision making requires the consideration of the potential gains (pros) and losses (cons) associated with a behavior's consequences.[6] For example, after telling patients that there are more than 65 scientific benefits of regular physical activity, providers can encourage patients to make a list of all the pros they can identify. They can also list the cons. The more the list of pros outweighs the cons, the better prepared patients will be to take effective action.

SELF-EFFICACY

Self-efficacy is the situation-specific confidence that people have while coping with high-risk situations without relapsing to their unhealthy habit. This construct was integrated from Bandura's self-efficacy theory.[7]

TEMPTATION

Temptation reflects the intensity of urges to engage in a specific risky habit while in the midst of difficult situations. Typically, three factors reflect the most common types of tempting situations: negative affect or emotional distress, social situations, and craving. Asking patients how they will cope with emotional distress without relying on a cigarette or comfort foods can help them cope more effectively and thereby build their confidence or self-esteem.

CRITICAL ASSUMPTIONS

The TTM is also based on critical assumptions about the nature of behavior change and population health interventions that can best facilitate such change. The following set of assumptions drives TTM theory, research, and practice:

- Behavior change is a process that unfolds over time through a sequence of stages, and providers and health population programs should be designed to assist patients as they progress over time.
- Stages are both stable and open to change, just as chronic behavioral risk factors are both stable and open to change.
- Population health initiatives can motivate change by enhancing the understanding of the pros and diminishing the value of the cons.
- The majority of at-risk populations are not prepared for action and will not be well served by traditional action-oriented prevention programs. Helping patients set realistic goals, like progressing to the next stage, will facilitate the change process.
- Specific principles and processes of change need to be emphasized at specific stages for progress through the stages to occur. Table 6-1 outlines which principles and processes to apply at each stage.

These critical assumptions must be taken into consideration when developing an effective population-based approach to behavior change and facilitating progress through the stages.

EMPIRICAL SUPPORT AND CHALLENGES

Each of the core constructs has been the subject of a number of studies across a broad range of behaviors and populations.

Table 6-1 Principles and Processes of Change That Facilitate Progression Between the Stages of Change

Precontemplation	Contemplation	Preparation	Action	Maintenance
	Consciousness raising			
	Dramatic relief			
	Environmental reevaluation			
		Self-reevaluation		
		Social liberation		
			Self-liberation	
				Counterconditioning
				Helping relationships
Increase pros				Reinforcement
	Reduce cons			Management
				Stimulus control
		Increase self-efficacy		

STAGE DISTRIBUTION

If interventions are to match the needs of entire populations, it is important to know the stage distributions of specific high-risk behaviors. A series of studies on smoking in the United States clearly demonstrated that less than 20% of smokers are in the preparation stage in most populations.[8,9] Approximately 40% of smokers are in the precontemplation stage, and another 40% are in the contemplation stage. In countries without a long history of tobacco control campaigns, the stage distributions are even more challenging. In Germany, about 70% of smokers are in precontemplation, and about 10% of smokers are in preparation,[10] while in China, more than 70% are in precontemplation, and about 5% are in preparation.[11] With a sample of 20,000 members of a health maintenance organization (HMO) across 15 health risk behaviors, only a small portion were ready for action.[12]

INTEGRATION OF PROS AND CONS AND STAGES OF CHANGE ACROSS 12 HEALTH BEHAVIORS

Stage is not a theory; it is a construct. TTM is a theory and thus requires systematic relationships between a set of constructs, ideally culminating in mathematical relationships. Systematic relationships were found between stages and the pros and cons of changing in studies of 12 health behaviors.

In all 12 studies, the pros of changing were higher than the cons for people in precontemplation,[13] and the pros increased between precontemplation and contemplation. From contemplation to action for all 12 behaviors, the cons of changing were lower in action than in contemplation. In 11 of the 12 studies, the pros of changing were higher than the cons for people in action. These relationships suggest that to progress from precontemplation, the pros of changing must increase; to progress from contemplation, the cons must decrease; and to progress to action, the pros must exceed the cons.

PRINCIPLES OF PROGRESS

Practical implications of these principles for population health programs are that for change to occur, the pros of changing must increase about twice as much as the cons must decrease.[14,15] Twice as much emphasis should be placed on raising the benefits as on reducing the costs or barriers. For example, if a couch potato in precontemplation can list only five pros of exercise, then being too busy will be a big barrier to change, whereas if a patient learns to appreciate the 65+ benefits for 150 minutes of exercise a week, being too busy becomes a relatively smaller barrier.[16]

RELATIONSHIPS BETWEEN STAGES AND PROCESSES OF CHANGE

One of the earliest empirical integrations was the discovery of systematic relationships between the stage of change and the processes that applied, a discovery that allowed integration of processes from theories that were typically seen as incompatible and in conflict. For example, the Freudian theory relied almost entirely on consciousness raising for producing change. This theory was viewed as incompatible with Skinnerian theory, which relied on reinforcement management for modifying behavior. But self-changers were unaware of this theoretical incompatibility; their behavior revealed that processes from different theories needed to be emphasized at different stages of change. This new understanding suggests that in early stages of population health management, efforts should support the application of cognitive, affective, and evaluative processes to progress through the stages. In later stages, programs should focus more on commitments, conditioning, rewards, environmental controls, and support to progress toward maintenance or termination.

Table 6-1 has important practical implications for population health projects. To help people progress from precontemplation to contemplation, processes such as consciousness raising and dramatic relief must be applied. Applying reinforcement management, counterconditioning, and stimulus control processes in precontemplation would constitute a theoretical, empirical, and practical mistake. Conversely, such strategies would be optimally matched for people in the action stage.

APPLIED STUDIES

A large, diverse body of evidence on the application of TTM has revealed several trends. The most common application involves TTM tailored interventions (CTIs), which match guidance to an individual's particular needs[17,18] across all TTM constructs. Tailored interventions that combine the best of population health with clinical best practice can be individualized and prescribed by providers to their patients. For example, individuals in precontemplation would receive feedback designed to increase their pros of changing to help them progress to contemplation. Applications have been developed for delivery in clinic settings; at work sites; in schools; or at home via computers, tablets, and smartphones. To see a demo, go to http://www.prochange.com/stressdemo.

TTM is being applied in patient-centered medical homes, hospitals, accountable care organizations,[19,20,21] churches,[22] campuses,[23] and communities.[24] Increasingly, employers and health plans are making such TTM-tailored programs available to entire employee or subscriber populations. As part of the change process initiated through the clinical relationship, providers can recommend that eligible patients access such programs.

A recent meta-analysis of tailored print communications found that TTM and the stages of change model were the most commonly used theory across a broad range of behaviors[25] (i.e., 35 of the 53 studies). In terms of effectiveness, significantly greater effect sizes were produced when tailored communications included each of the following TTM constructs: stages of change, pros and cons of changing, self-efficacy, and processes of change.[25] In contrast, interventions that included the non-TTM construct of perceived susceptibility had significantly worse outcomes. Tailoring on non-TTM constructs (e.g., social norms, behavioral intentions) did not produce significant differences.[25]

These unprecedented effects push for scientific and professional shifts in our approach to population health:

- From an action paradigm to a stage paradigm
- From reactive to proactive recruitment of participants
- From expecting patients to match the needs of our programs to having our programs match their needs
- From clinic-based to community-based behavioral health programs that apply the field's most powerful individualized and interactive intervention strategies
- From assuming some groups do not have the ability to change to making sure that all groups have accessibility to evidence-based programs that provide stage-matched tailored interventions. Without such access, behavior change programs may not serve entire populations.

MULTIPLE BEHAVIOR CHANGE PROGRAMS: INCREASING IMPACTS

One of the greatest challenges for the application of any theory is to continually raise the bar, thereby increasing the theory's effect on enhancing health. Our original impact equation was Impact = (Reach × Efficacy). Then we raised the bar to Impact = (Reach × # of behaviors changed).

One way to increase the effect of TTM is by using it to treat multiple behaviors. Populations with multiple behavior risks are also at greatest risk for both chronic disease and premature death, and account for a disproportionate percentage of healthcare costs.

The best estimates are that about 60% of healthcare costs are generated by about 15% of populations with multiple behavior risks and medical conditions.[26] Until recently, the research literature indicated that attempting to change multiple behaviors on a population basis would be a particularly risky test. This was, in part, because studies conducted on **multiple behavior changes** were limited by reliance on the action paradigm and lacked application of the most promising interventions (e.g., interactive and individualized TTM-tailored communications).[27] From a TTM perspective, action is the most demanding stage, and applying an action paradigm to two or more behaviors simultaneously would indeed risk overwhelming a population. Among individuals with four health behavior risks (e.g., smoking, diet, sun exposure, and sedentary lifestyles), less than 10% of the population was ready to take action on two or more behaviors.[28] The same was true for populations with diabetes who needed to change four behaviors.[29]

IMPACT OF TTM RECENT STUDIES

Johnson and colleagues applied the first strategy for multiple behavior change with a population of 1,277 overweight and obese patients proactively recruited in the United States. In this modular approach, participants received a separate TTM CTI module for each of their risk behaviors related to healthy weight management. The treatment groups reported significant positive changes at 24 months with respect to low-fat eating, exercise, and emotional eating. This study was the first to report results showing significant changes in fruit and vegetable intake even though the treatment did not focus on this behavior. Also, this study reported a mean of 0.8 behaviors changed per participant in the TTM group, 60% greater than the 0.5 behaviors changed in the control group.[30]

An exciting development in our knowledge of simultaneously changing multiple behaviors is the phenomena of coaction. Coaction is the increased probability that if individuals take effective action on one behavior (e.g., exercise), they are more likely to take action on a secondary behavior (e.g., diet). The weight management study was one of the first to show that significant coaction typically occurs only in TTM treatment groups and not in control groups, a strong indication that it is treatment induced.[30-32]

Prochaska and colleagues' study made available online modular TTM CTIs for each of four behaviors (smoking, inactivity, body mass index [BMI] > 25, and stress) and three motivational interviewing telephonic or in-person sessions.[33] Participants (1,400 employees in a major medical setting) chose which behaviors to target and how much time and effort to spend on any behavior. At 6 months, both interventions outperformed the health risk intervention, which included feedback on the person's stage for each risk and guidance on how he or she could progress to the next stage.

In another study with a population of 1,800 students recruited from eight high schools in four states, Mauriello and colleagues applied a second-generation strategy, with exercise as the primary behavior with three online sessions of fully tailored CTIs.[31] The secondary behaviors of fruit and vegetable intake and limited TV watching alternated between moderate and minimal (stage only) tailoring. Over the course of the 6-month treatment, there were significant treatment effects in each of the three behaviors, but only changes in fruit and vegetable intake were sustained at 12 months. Significant coaction was found for each pair of behaviors in the treatment group but none in the control group.

Prochaska and colleagues recruited 3,391 at-risk adults from 39 states for an exercise and stress management program.[32] This study applied a third-generation strategy for multiple tailored behavior change. Two treatment groups were formed:

- Group 1 received a fully tailored TTM CTI online for the primary behavior of stress management and was stage matched for exercise.
- Group 2 received three sessions of optimally tailored telephonic coaching for exercise and was stage matched for stress. This group also received SMART (specific, measurable, attainable, realistic, and time bound) goals for exercise based on four effects that predict long-term success across very different types of behaviors (i.e., treatment, stage, severity, and effort).[34]

The four effects mentioned in group 2 are (1) those in treatment are significantly more successful than controls, (2) those in preparation are more successful than those in contemplation who are more successful than those in precontemplation, (3) those with less severe problems are more likely to progress to action or maintenance for their problems, and (4) those making better efforts (e.g., on the pros and cons of changing) at baseline are more likely to change. These four effects can produce smarter goals early on to help patients complete the intervention, progress from precontemplation to contemplation to preparation, reduce severity, make better efforts on using the TTM change variables, and make more progress across multiple behaviors.

In another Prochaska et al. study, the TTM exercise coaching outperformed the TTM online stress management, which outperformed the controls.[33] Also, the exercise coaching produced significant effects on healthy eating and depression management, which were not part of the treatment intervention. The mean number of behaviors changed per participant was 1.18 for exercise coaching, 0.8 for online stress management, and 0.5 for controls. The last two results were remarkably similar to the findings in the Velicer et al. study.[8] Finally, the same order of effective treatment was found for enhancing five domains of well-being (i.e., emotional health, physical health, life evaluation, thriving, and overall well-being). This study demonstrates the greatest effect to date on decreasing multiple health risk behaviors and increasing multiple domains of well-being.

FUTURE RESEARCH

Although research results are encouraging, much remains to be done to advance practical behavior change through evidence-based efforts such as the TTM. Basic research must incorporate other theoretical variables (e.g., processes of resistance, problem severity) to determine whether such variables relate systematically to the stages and whether they predict progress across particular stages. More research is needed on the structure or integration of the processes and stages of change across a broad range of behaviors (e.g., acquisition behaviors, such as exercise, and extinction behaviors, such as smoking cessation).[35] Modifications are needed for specific types of behaviors (e.g., fewer processes for infrequent behaviors such as mammography screening).

Because tailored communications represent the most promising interventions for applying TTM to entire populations, more research is needed to compare the effectiveness, efficiency, and impacts of alternative technologies. The Internet is excellent for individualized interactions at low cost, but it has not produced the high participation rates generated by person-to-person outreach via telephone or visits to primary care practitioners. Increasingly, employers are incentivizing employee populations to participate in more integrated Internet, telephone, and provider programs. Interventions that were once seen as applicable only on an individual basis are being applied as high-impact programs for population health.

How do diverse populations respond to stage-matched interventions and to high-tech systems? How could programs best be tailored to meet the needs of diverse populations? Could menus of alternative intervention modalities (e.g., telephone, Internet, neighborhood or church leaders, person to person, or community programs) empower diverse populations to best match health-enhancing programs to their particular needs?

Changing multiple behaviors represents special challenges, in particular, the large number of demands placed on participants and providers. Alternative strategies that go beyond the sequential (one at a time) and simultaneous (all treated intensely at the same time) must be tried.

Integrative approaches are promising. For example, with bullying prevention, there are multiple behaviors (e.g., hitting, stealing, ostracizing, mean gossiping, labeling, damaging personal belongings) and multiple roles (bully, victim, and passive bystander) that are best addressed by an integrated approach within the given time constraints.

If behavior change is construct driven (e.g., by stage or self-efficacy), what is a higher-order construct that could integrate all of these more concrete behaviors and roles? A study wherein relating with mutual respect was used as a higher-order construct yielded significant and important improvements across roles and behaviors for elementary, middle, and high school students.[36] As with any theory, effective applications may be limited more by our creativity than by the ability of the theory to drive significant research and effective interventions.

FUTURE PRACTICE

Applying TTM on a population basis to change multiple health risks has required the use of innovative paradigms that complement established paradigms. Table 6-2 illustrates how a population paradigm that uses proactive outreach to homes complements the

Table 6-2   Inclusive Care from Two Clusters of Paradigms for Individual Patients and Entire Populations

Patient health	Complemented by	Population health
1. Individual patients		Entire populations
2. Passive reactance		Proactive
3. Acute conditions		Chronic conditions
4. Efficacy trials		Effectiveness trials
5. Action oriented		Stage based
6. Clinic based		Home based
7. Clinician delivered		Technology delivered
8. Standardized		Tailored
9. Single-target behavior		Multiple-target behaviors
10. Fragmented		Integrated

individual patient paradigm, which passively reacts when patients seek clinical services. The use of the stage paradigm complements the action paradigm, which assumes that because patients are seeking services, they are prepared to take action. The use of CTIs complements the traditional reliance on clinicians, and the treatment of multiple behaviors complements the established clinical wisdom of treating one behavior at a time. The population-theme paradigm based on impacts (reach × efficacy × # of behaviors changed) complements individualized clinical trials with select samples that rely on efficacy. Integrating these new paradigms can produce the foundation for a well-being system that complements the established sick-care system. Combining the two systems would enhance the health and well-being of many more people than are currently being helped, by healing the sick while maximizing wellness for all.

CONCLUSION

The TTM is a dynamic theory of change, and it must remain open to modifications and enhancements as more students, scientists, and practitioners apply the stage paradigm to a growing number of diverse theoretical issues, public health problems, and at-risk populations.

STUDY AND DISCUSSION QUESTIONS

1. What is the transtheoretical model of behavior change (TTM)?
2. What are the stages of change included in the TTM?

3. What is your role, as a healthcare provider, in helping a patient who is in precontemplation realize the benefits of changing?

4. If you are encountered by a smoker with multiple health behavior risks, how would you help manage this patient's need for multiple behavior changes?

SUGGESTED READINGS AND WEBSITES

READINGS

Hall KL, Rossi JS. Meta-analytic examination of the strong and weak principles across 48 health behaviors. *Prev Med.* 2008;46(3):266–74.

Prochaska JO, DiClemente CC, Norcross JC. In search of how people change: applications to addictive behaviors. *Am Psychol.* 1992;47(9):1102–14.

Prochaska JO, Norcross JC, DiClemente CC. *Changing for Good.* New York: Morrow; 1994.

Prochaska JO, Velicer WF, Redding C, et al. Stage-based expert systems to guide a population of primary care patients to quit smoking, eat healthier, prevent skin cancer, and receive regular mammograms. *Prev Med.* 2005;41(2):406–16.

WEBSITES

Basic Transtheoretical Model Training: contact elearning@prochange.com

Cancer Prevention Research Center: http://www.uri.edu/research/cprc

Coaches' Guide for Using the TTM with Clients: contact info@prochange.com

Pro-Change Behavior Systems, Inc.: http://www.prochange.com

REFERENCES

1. Prochaska JO, Norcross JC. *Systems of Psychotherapy: A Transtheoretical Analysis.* 8th ed. Belmont, CA: Brooks/Cole, Cengage Learning; 2013.

2. DiClemente CC, Prochaska JO. Self-change and therapy change of smoking behavior: a comparison of processes of change in cessation and maintenance. *Addict Behav.* 1982;7(2):133-42.

3. Prochaska JO, DiClemente CC. Stages and processes of self-change of smoking: toward an integrative model of change. *J Consult Clin Psychol.* 1983;51(3):390-5.

4. U.S. Department of Health and Human Services. *The Health Benefits of Smoking Cessation: A Report of the Surgeon General.* Washington, DC: U.S. Department of Health and Human Services; 1990. DHHS Publication No. (CDC) 90-8416.

5. Snow MG, Prochaska JO, Rossi JS. Stages of change for smoking cessation among former problem drinkers: a cross-sectional analysis. *J Subst Abuse.* 1992;4(2):107-16.

6. Janis IL, Mann L. *Decision Making: A Psychological Analysis of Conflict, Choice, and Commitment.* London: Cassel & Collier Macmillan; 1977.

7. Bandura A. Selfefficacy mechanism in human agency. *Am Psychol.* 1982;37(2):122-47.

8. Velicer WF, Fava JL, Prochaska JO, et al. Distribution of smokers by stage in three representative samples. *Prev Med.* 1995;24(4):401-11.

9. Wewers ME, Stillman FA, Hartman AM, et al. Distribution of daily smokers by stage of change: Current Population Survey results. *Prev Med.* 2003;36(6):710-20.

10. Etter JF, Perneger TV, Ronchi A. Distributions of smokers by stage: international comparison and association with smoking prevalence. *Prev Med.* 1997;26(4):580-5.

11. Yang G, Ma J, Chen A, et al. Smoking cessation in China: findings from the 1996 National Prevalence Survey. *Tob Control.* 2001;10(2):170-4.

12. Rossi JS. Stages of change for 15 health risk behaviors in an HMO population. Paper presented at the 13th meeting of the Society for Behavioral Medicine; 1992; New York, NY.

13. Prochaska JO, Velicer WF, Rossi JS, et al. Stages of change and decisional balance for 12 problem behaviors. *Health Psychol.* 1994; 13(1):39-46.

14. Prochaska JO. Strong and weak principles for progressing from precontemplation to action on the basis of twelve problem behaviors. *Health Psychol.* 1994;13(1):47-51.

15. Hall KL, Rossi JS. Meta-analytic examination of the strong and weak principles across 48 health behaviors. *Prev Med.* 2008;46(3):266-74.

16. Johnson SS, Paiva AL, Cummins CO, et al. Transtheoretical model-based multiple behavior intervention for weight management: effectiveness on a population basis. *Prev Med.* 2008;46(3): 238-46.

17. Kreuter MW, Strecher VJ, Glassman B. One size does not fit all: the case for tailoring print materials. *Ann Behav Med.* 1999;21(4):276-83.

18. Skinner CS, Campbell MD, Rimer BK, et al. How effective is tailored print communication? *Ann Behav Med.* 1999;21(4):290-8.

19. Goldstein MG, Pinto BM, Marcus BH, et al. Physician-based physical activity counseling for middle-aged and older adults: a randomized trial. *Ann Behav Med.* 1999;21(1):40-7.

20. Hoffman A, Redding CA, Goldberg DN, et al. Computer expert systems for African-American smokers in physicians' offices: a feasibility study. *Prev Med.* 2006;43(3):204-11.

21. Hollis JF, Polen MR, Whitlock EP, et al. Teen REACH: outcomes from a randomized, controlled trial of a tobacco reduction program for teens seen in primary medical care. *Pediatr.* 2005;115(4): 981-9.

22. Voorhees CC, Stillman FA, Swank RT, et al. Heart, body, and soul: impact of church-based smoking cessation interventions on readiness to quit. *Prev Med.* 1996;25(3):277-85.

23. Prochaska JM, Prochaska JO, Cohen FC, et al. The transtheoretical model of change for multilevel interventions for alcohol abuse on campus. *J Alcohol Drug Educ.* 2004;47(3):34-50.

24. The CDC AIDS Community Demonstration Projects Research Group. Community-level HIV intervention in 5 cities: final outcome data from the CDC AIDS Community Demonstration Projects. *Am J Public Health.* 1999;89(3):336-45.

25. Noar SM, Benac CN, Harris MS. Does tailoring matter? Meta-analytic review of tailored print health behavior change interventions. *Psychol Bull.* 2007;133(4):673-93.

26. Edington DW. Emerging research: a view from one research center. *Am J Health Promot.* 2001;15(5):341-9.

27. Prochaska JO, Velicer WF, Fava JL, et al. Counselor and stimulus control enhancements of a stage-matched expert system for smokers in a managed care setting. *Prev Med.* 2000;32:39-46.

28. Prochaska JO, Velicer WF. The transtheoretical model of health behavior change. *Am J Health Promot.* 1997;12(1):38-48. doi:10.4278/0890-1171-12.1.38.

29. Ruggiero L, Glasgow R, Dryfoos JM, et al. Diabetes self-management: Self-reported recommendations and patterns in a large population. *Diabetes Care.* 1997;20(4):x568-76. doi:10.2337/diacare.20.4.568.

30. Johnson SS, Paiva AL, Cummins CO, et al. Transtheoretical model-based multiple behavior intervention for weight management: effectiveness on a population basis. *Prev Med.* 2008;46:238-46. doi:10.1016/y.ypmed.2007.09.010.

31. Mauriello LM, Ciavatta MMH, Paiva AL, et al. Results of a multi-media multiple behavior obesity prevention program for adolescents. *Prev Med.* 2010;51:451-6. doi:10.1016/j.ypmed.2010.08.004.

32. Prochaska JO, Ever KE, Castle PH, et al. Enhancing multiple domains of well-being by decreasing

multiple health risk behaviors. *Popul Health Manag.* 2012;15:276-86.

33. Prochaska JO, Butterworth S, Redding CA, et al. Initial efficacy of MI, TTM tailoring and HRIs with multiple behaviors for employee health promotion. *Prev Med.* 2008;45:226-31. doi:10.1016/j. ypmed.2007.11.007.

34. Blissmer B, Prochaska JO, Velicer WF, et al. Common factors predicting long-term changes in multiple health behaviors. *J Health Psychol.* 2010;15:201-14. doi:10.1177/1359105309345555.

35. Rosen CS. Is the sequencing of change processes by stage consistent across health problems? A meta-analysis. *Health Psychol.* 2000;19(6):593-604.

36. Evers KE, Prochaska JO, Van Marter DF, et al. Transtheoretical-based bullying prevention effectiveness trials in middle schools and high schools. *Educational Research.* 2007;49:397-414.

PATIENT ENGAGEMENT: ENGAGING PATIENTS IN THE CARE PROCESS BY LEVERAGING MEANINGFUL USE GOALS

CHRISTY CALHOUN, LESLIE KELLY HALL, AND DON KEMPER

Executive Summary

Patient engagement is becoming a dominant theme in health care today. Many now see the patient as the greatest, and most valuable, untapped resource in health care—and patient engagement is the focal point. This chapter explores patient engagement and its evolution across philosophies, information technologies, government policies, and health-care economics.

Given that patient engagement crosses all aspects of the care continuum, we will use a collaboratively developed patient engagement framework to provide context for our study of patient engagement. The framework was first created to inform policy and industry leaders on patient engagement within the meaningful use (MU) rules for certified electronic health record (EHR) technology in the United States.

The five stages of the framework provide a pathway for strengthening the provider–patient relationship through the lens of health information technology. Each of the following stages builds upon previous stages:

- Inform Me: This stage makes it easier for providers to help patients find and understand care information.
- Engage Me: This stage supports provider interaction with patients to improve care.
- Empower Me: This stage enables patients to become an integral part of the care team.
- Partner with Me: This stage facilitates the provider–patient partnership through shared care planning.
- Support My e-Community: This stage expands the network of patient support to include the community.

This chapter describes how a patient engagement road map can add value for hospitals, clinicians, and patients. It explores the use and application of various tools and methodologies that support engagement as a part of policy efforts, including MU. **Meaningful use** is defined as the provision of financial incentives for providers who "meaningfully use" certified EHR technology to improve results over time. Grounding patient engagement in such important policy initiatives will help guide the development of future population health and patient engagement strategies, and strengthen the provider–patient relationship across the continuum of care.

Learning Objectives

1. Understand how a patient engagement road map can add value for hospitals, clinicians, and patients.
2. Explore the use and application of various tools and methodologies that support patient engagement as part of meaningful use and health reform.
3. Identify opportunities to leverage the patient engagement framework to support population health and health information technology.

Key Terms

health information technology	patient engagement
meaningful use	patient engagement framework
online tools	population health

INTRODUCTION

When Asclepius and the other Greek gods of medicine inspired Hippocrates and his physician followers to establish the science of Western medicine, there was no mention of patient engagement. Some even interpret the original text of the Hippocratic Oath as directing physicians to "keep secret and never reveal" their medical knowledge to their patients or anyone else. Nonetheless, patient engagement is not a new idea. Even the term "doctor" comes from the Latin word *docere*, meaning "to teach." Teaching and engaging patients to do more for themselves has been a key part of most physicians' daily duties ever since.

Today, patient engagement is spiraling up to a whole new level of importance. Almost simultaneously, hospitals, professionals, and health organizations have come to see the patient as the greatest untapped resource in health care—and patient engagement has become the focal point. This chapter explores the emergence of patient engagement—from its simplest definition to its evolution across philosophies, information technologies, government policies, and healthcare economics.

Over time we have seen a groundswell of interest in patient engagement. The call for patient-centered care in the Institute of Medicine's (IOM's) *Crossing the Quality Chasm* report made this apparent in 2001 by specifying 10 rules for redesigning health care. Many of these clearly reflect a movement toward putting the patient at the center of care:

- Care is based on continuous healing relationships.
- Care is customized according to patient needs and values.
- The patient is the source of control.
- Knowledge is shared and information flows freely.
- Decision making is evidence based.
- Safety is a system property.
- Transparency is necessary.
- Needs are anticipated.
- Waste is continuously decreased.
- Cooperation among clinicians is a priority.[1]

Other forces that have shaped patient engagement include the Patient Protection and Affordable Care Act (ACA). As part of the ACA, the Centers for Medicare and Medicaid Services (CMS) is fostering incentive-based pilot projects to encourage new forms of practice, which range from accountable care organizations (ACOs) to patient-centered medical homes (PCMHs). In this movement away from fee-for-service medicine to value-based care, the demand for an engaged patient has become vital. As healthcare costs rise and access to digital health innovations becomes increasingly common, we will continue to see patients demand the opportunity to have access to their health records and be active partners in their care, which ultimately changes the nature of the patient–provider relationship.

Although patient engagement encompasses all aspects of the patient–provider relationship and beyond, we will discuss it in the context of a framework first developed to inform patient engagement within the MU rules for certified EHR technology and other health reforms in the United States. The patient engagement framework reflects an expanding partnership between the patient and his or her care team. Progressively expanding patient engagement by leveraging **health information technology** (HIT) is critical both to meet MU requirements and to achieve the Institute for Healthcare Improvement's Triple Aim—better care, better health, and lower cost.

In a simple sense, **patient engagement** is any effort to involve a person in his or her own health or health care. Simple is good, a concept that may be helpful throughout the course of one's studies. Yet, to understand the depth, power, and promise of HIT-powered patient engagement and the ways in which innovative organizations are reinventing it, a good deal more is needed. For that we will rely on the patient engagement framework.[2]

THE PATIENT ENGAGEMENT FRAMEWORK

The **patient engagement framework** (Figure 7-1) is a five-phase continuum used by hospitals and other care providers to gradually expand the methods and tools for informing, engaging, empowering, and partnering with patients and their communities to improve both the quality of the care they receive and their overall quality of health. An early form of the framework was drafted by the authors in partnership with the National eHealth Collaborative (NeHC). By means of a collaborative process, the NeHC helped refine the framework and gained consensus around it through the NeHC Consumer Consortium. Since its first publication by NeHC in 2012, the framework has been downloaded over 20,000 times (according to Kate Barry, former CEO of NeHC, in communication sent February 3, 2014). (NeHC merged with the HIMSS Foundation on December 23, 2013.) It is increasingly considered the definitive structure for patient engagement—at least as it applies in the world of HIT.

The framework has special value to hospitals and clinicians for two primary reasons. First, the framework provides a pathway toward fully integrating the individual into his or her own health care. Beginning with small, easy steps that require little change to the clinical workflow, it progressively adds meaningful ways for the patient to become a full member of his or her own care team. The framework also aligns patient engagement to the patient-facing requirements of the MU rules that the U.S. federal government has set forth. These rules allow hospitals and clinicians to receive reimbursement for HIT investments initially and to avoid penalties in the future when that technology is used in ways that enhance the experience and quality of care. Achievement of all four main MU goals largely depends on successful patient engagement, and goal number two spells it out explicitly. The goals for MU include:

- Improve quality of care and safety.
- Engage patients and their families in care.
- Improve care coordination.
- Improve **population health**.

Each phase of MU emphasizes each of these areas.[3] MU presents new functionality first as an optional, or "menu," item. These menu items are not required, but they send important signals for future requirements. Starting in a modest way, both in the achievement of thresholds and in the complexity of use, the menu items gradually move into mandatory, or "core," requirements in future stages. MU stage 3 builds upon menu items from MU stages 1 and 2, to move into more robust requirements and thresholds for use, as reflected in Figure 7-2 on MU stage 3 priorities.[4]

If approved, the implementation of MU state 3 is estimated to occur in 2017. Several MU recommendations under consideration for stage 3 reflect a commitment to public and population health. Examples of such recommendations follow:

- Patient-generated health data
- Advance directives in the patient record

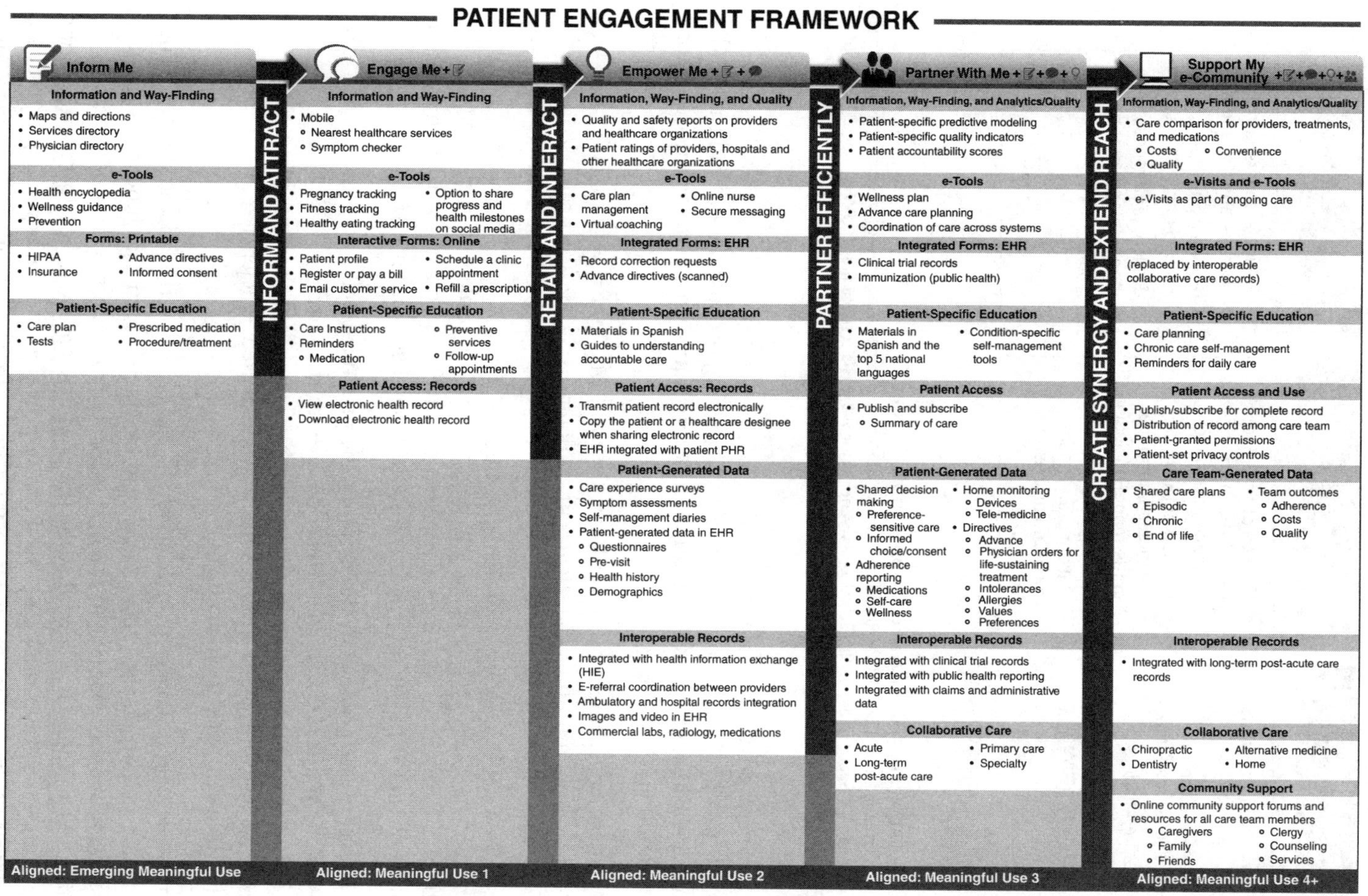

PATIENT ENGAGEMENT FRAMEWORK

Inform Me

Information and Way-Finding
- Maps and directions
- Services directory
- Physician directory

e-Tools
- Health encyclopedia
- Wellness guidance
- Prevention

Forms: Printable
- HIPAA
- Insurance
- Advance directives
- Informed consent

Patient-Specific Education
- Care plan
- Tests
- Prescribed medication
- Procedure/treatment

Aligned: Emerging Meaningful Use

Engage Me + ✓

Information and Way-Finding
Mobile
- Nearest healthcare services
- Symptom checker

e-Tools
- Pregnancy tracking
- Fitness tracking
- Healthy eating tracking
- Option to share progress and health milestones on social media

Interactive Forms: Online
- Patient profile
- Register or pay a bill
- Email customer service
- Schedule a clinic appointment
- Refill a prescription

Patient-Specific Education
- Care Instructions
- Reminders
- Medication
- Preventive services
- Follow-up appointments

Patient Access: Records
- View electronic health record
- Download electronic health record

Aligned: Meaningful Use 1

Empower Me + ✓ + ●

Information, Way-Finding, and Quality
- Quality and safety reports on providers and healthcare organizations
- Patient ratings of providers, hospitals and other healthcare organizations

e-Tools
- Care plan management
- Virtual coaching
- Online nurse
- Secure messaging

Integrated Forms: EHR
- Record correction requests
- Advance directives (scanned)

Patient-Specific Education
- Materials in Spanish
- Guides to understanding accountable care

Patient Access: Records
- Transmit patient record electronically
- Copy the patient or a healthcare designee when sharing electronic record
- EHR integrated with patient PHR

Patient-Generated Data
- Care experience surveys
- Symptom assessments
- Self-management diaries
- Patient-generated data in EHR
  - Questionnaires
  - Pre-visit
  - Health history
  - Demographics

Interoperable Records
- Integrated with health information exchange (HIE)
- E-referral coordination between providers
- Ambulatory and hospital records integration
- Images and video in EHR
- Commercial labs, radiology, medications

Aligned: Meaningful Use 2

Partner With Me + ✓ + ● + ◆

Information, Way-Finding, and Analytics/Quality
- Patient-specific predictive modeling
- Patient-specific quality indicators
- Patient accountability scores

e-Tools
- Wellness plan
- Advance care planning
- Coordination of care across systems

Integrated Forms: EHR
- Clinical trial records
- Immunization (public health)

Patient-Specific Education
- Materials in Spanish and the top 5 national languages
- Condition-specific self-management tools

Patient Access
- Publish and subscribe
  - Summary of care

Patient-Generated Data
- Shared decision making
- Preference-sensitive care
- Informed choice/consent
- Adherence reporting
  - Medications
  - Self-care
  - Wellness
- Home monitoring
  - Devices
- Tele-medicine
- Directives
  - Advance
  - Physician orders for life-sustaining treatment
  - Intolerances
  - Allergies
  - Values
  - Preferences

Interoperable Records
- Integrated with clinical trial records
- Integrated with public health reporting
- Integrated with claims and administrative data

Collaborative Care
- Acute
- Long-term post-acute care
- Primary care
- Specialty

Aligned: Meaningful Use 3

Support My e-Community + ✓ + ● + ◆ + ▦

Information, Way-Finding, and Analytics/Quality
- Care comparison for providers, treatments, and medications
  - Costs
  - Convenience
  - Quality

e-Visits and e-Tools
- e-Visits as part of ongoing care

Integrated Forms: EHR
(replaced by interoperable collaborative care records)

Patient-Specific Education
- Care planning
- Chronic care self-management
- Reminders for daily care

Patient Access and Use
- Publish/subscribe for complete record
- Distribution of record among care team
- Patient-granted permissions
- Patient-set privacy controls

Care Team-Generated Data
- Shared care plans
  - Episodic
  - Chronic
  - End of life
- Team outcomes
  - Adherence
  - Costs
  - Quality

Interoperable Records
- Integrated with long-term post-acute care records

Collaborative Care
- Chiropractic
- Dentistry
- Alternative medicine
- Home

Community Support
- Online community support forums and resources for all care team members
  - Caregivers
  - Family
  - Friends
  - Clergy
  - Counseling
  - Services

Aligned: Meaningful Use 4+

Row bands: **INFORM AND ATTRACT** · **RETAIN AND INTERACT** · **PARTNER EFFICIENTLY** · **CREATE SYNERGY AND EXTEND REACH**

Figure 7-1 The patient engagement framework.
Reproduced from National eHealth Collaborative. The patient engagement framework. http://www.nationalehealth.org/patient-engagement-framework. Accessed January 24, 2014.

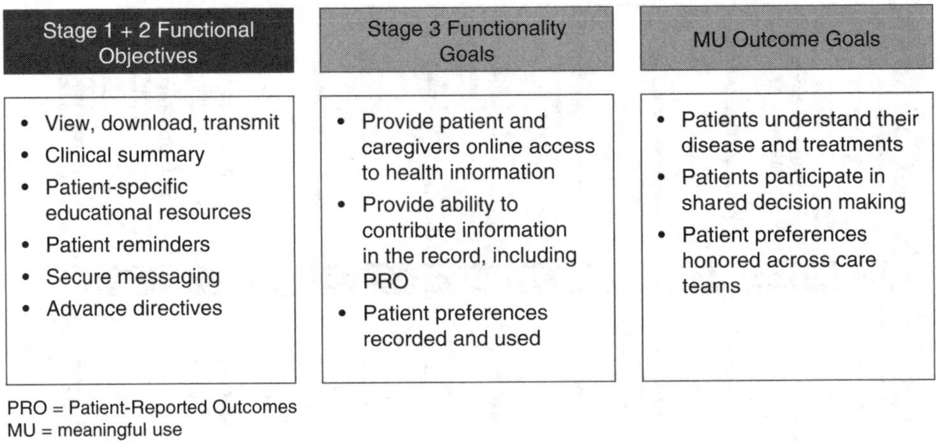

Stage 1 + 2 Functional Objectives	Stage 3 Functionality Goals	MU Outcome Goals
• View, download, transmit • Clinical summary • Patient-specific educational resources • Patient reminders • Secure messaging • Advance directives	• Provide patient and caregivers online access to health information • Provide ability to contribute information in the record, including PRO • Patient preferences recorded and used	• Patients understand their disease and treatments • Patients participate in shared decision making • Patient preferences honored across care teams

PRO = Patient-Reported Outcomes
MU = meaningful use

Figure 7-2 Engaging patients and families in their care.
Reproduced from Tang P, Hripcsak G. Meaningful use workgroup stage 3 update. Report presented at: Health IT Policy Committee meeting; September 4, 2013. http://www.healthit.gov/facas/sites/faca/files/MUWG_Stage3_13_Sep_4_FINAL_0.pdf. Accessed January 16, 2014.

- Family history available to patients
- Commitment to addressing disparities by capturing occupation and industry codes, gender identity and sexual orientation, disability status, and preferred mode of communication and language

The patient engagement framework goes beyond MU but is very much in line with industry discussions and direction. At recent conferences of the American Medical Informatics Association and Healthcare Unbound, speakers outlined their work, using the framework as a guidepost and road map.

The framework's five levels of patient engagement are explained in the sections that follow from the provider's and the patient's perspectives. As you study the framework in the context of the examples presented, there are a few key concepts to note:

- Each level of the framework builds upon the previous level.
- No functions are ever dropped from one level to the next.
- Each new level generally requires more sophisticated HIT infrastructure.
- Each new level provides opportunities for increased efficiencies, better care, and higher levels of patient engagement.

Notice that the patient engagement concepts in each level overlap. Because patient engagement is not a clearly defined science, the way in which a particular function is delivered can differ from one environment to the next, depending on the mix of people, technology, economics, and attitudes. It follows that the framework is a guide rather than a prescription.

The framework has a dual purpose. For the provider, the framework's purpose is to tap the power of the patient–provider relationship,[5,6] to better achieve the Triple Aim of better care, better health, and lower cost. For the patient, the framework's purpose is empowerment by better understanding how to achieve the health outcomes that matter most to him or her. Its implementation empowers people to do as much as they can to improve their health, to ask for the care they need, and to say no to care that is not right for them.

LEVEL 1: INFORM ME

The "Inform Me" level of patient engagement is about providing patient information (Box 7-1). It involves basics that most people would expect from any other sector of society. For the patient, the benefits can range from modest to life saving.

BOX 7-1

Level 1: Inform Me

Provider: Make it easy for me to point my patients to information I want them to access and understand.

Patient: Make it easy for me to find accurate, up-to-date information relevant to my health, my care, and my medical needs.

"Give me access to good information. Make it easy for me to find out about my care." Most healthcare systems address the "Inform Me" need through their patient and marketing portals. They can often license for their patients information similar to what the patient might find on WebMD or other health portals, but without the bias of pharmaceutical or medical device ads that contribute to the health portal business model. Providing health information through the hospital's website adds a degree of authenticity that leads patients to trust the information and feel more comfortable sharing what they've learned with their trusted clinicians. One example is PatientConnection, a secure website that gives patients access to health *information* from their electronic medical records through Peace Health Medical Group, a provider system serving populations in Oregon, Washington, and Alaska.[7]

"Give me clear directions on where to go, where to park, and what to wear." This sounds simple enough until you try to find your way around a busy hospital, even when you are feeling well—but especially when you are sick. Hospitals that respond with maps, way-finding tips, and explicit directions on how to prepare for procedures save the patient frustration, embarrassment, and exhaustion.

From the provider's perspective, the "Inform Me" level of the framework provides modest benefit without disrupting clinician workflow. Electronic offerings such as maps of the provider's location, a health encyclopedia, instructions, and information on providers and services assure consistency of information and can help patients be better prepared for their visits. Even though some patients may come in with more questions for the clinician, using **online tools** helps to ensure that patients are informed, an essential first step to developing engaged patients and building strong patient–provider relationships. In a fee-for-value model that focuses on better care, better health, and lower costs, engaged patients and trusted clinical relationships are critical.

Even before HIT, progress was made with respect to educating patients at the "Inform Me" level. For years, Kaiser Permanente encouraged patients to self-assess their symptoms and practice self-care using the Kaiser Permanente Healthwise Handbook.[8] The U.S. Department of Veterans Affairs continues a similar strategy across many of its regions. Such tools have been critical in helping patients to determine when and where they should seek care, if at all, and to decide whether home treatment and self-care are sufficient to manage symptoms. In some cases, a patient's use of clear, understandable health information has helped the patient seek life-saving treatments.[9] Printed health education materials, in addition to HIT-enabled tools, can contribute to greater patient engagement and loyalty.

LEVEL 2: ENGAGE ME

The "Engage Me" level takes the patient a step beyond information (Box 7-2). It requires some level of interaction and provides value to both patient and clinician. To do that, "Engage Me" brings a set of e-health tools, incentives, and health coaching into the patient engagement solution.

BOX 7-2

Level 2: Engage Me

Provider: Help me interact with my patients and recommend steps they can take to improve their health.

Patient: Make it easy for me to understand my provider's instructions so I can do self-care well.

"Honor my time as if it had value. Don't make me fill out the same form twice." One of the most irksome aspects of medical care is the clipboard experience. People don't mind filling out forms for the first time, but they dislike being asked to provide the same demographic and personal health information at every visit. It's becoming more common to standardize forms and prepopulate them with answers that are already known, as exemplified in a Multnomah County Health Department case study.[10] If Amazon doesn't make you retype your address for every order, why should your doctor or hospital? Leveraging HIT to make the patient workflow more efficient demonstrates that the patient's time is valued, which contributes to greater levels of patient satisfaction and engagement.

The symptom checker is a good example of "Engage Me." Symptom checkers are often linked to service locators that direct patients to the closest place for needed care and sometimes even report the current wait time at that location—as exemplified by the Group Health mobile app.[11] For the patient, there is real value in the help that a symptom checker provides:

- "Help me decide if my new pain or symptom is something that needs a doctor's care."
- "Help me make a good decision about whether self-care or watchful waiting might be enough."
- "Help me know if I need to go to the emergency department [ED] on Sunday night or if it is safe to wait for my doctor's office to open Monday morning."

For the provider, there is real value as well. When a patient uses a symptom checker and then calls a nurse coach, the call is more efficient and effective. A person who has gone through the symptom checker's set of questions can help the clinician get to the heart of the problem. Symptom checkers also save lives. Mobile symptom checker tools have helped patients recognize dangerous symptoms and seek care immediately.[12]

"Engage Me" also brings a set of e-tools to help patients do more for themselves:

- Fitness and healthy eating tracker tools help people set goals and track their progress.
- Stress tracking apps help people assess stress levels, evaluate trends, and learn what helps improve stress management.
- Pregnancy trackers provide a weekly guide through the common concerns of pregnancy, with educational tips for improving the chances of a healthy birth.

"Engage Me" almost always includes convenience features for the patient:

- "Help me refill my prescription online."
- "Let me e-mail questions regarding my appointment or my bill."
- "Help me match my schedule with my doctor's availability for my next appointment."

Of course, "Engage Me" need not be all Web-based or virtual. Healthcare navigators and care coaches are often used to reach out to people whose active engagement is needed to achieve improved outcomes.

At this level there is also an expectation that the patient will be proactively informed. "Information Therapy"[13] is the prescription of the right information to the right person at the right time to help the person make a better health decision or improve a health behavior. Within the MU rules, it is described as "patient-specific educational resources." Printed or e-delivered patient instructions should become a part of most, if not all, clinic visits. After-visit summaries help patients understand their diagnoses, their care plans, and their self-care instructions. As a consequence, this improves engagement and care treatment outcomes.

"Engage Me" includes many automated nudges and interactive tools to help patients remember what's next and why it is important. The effects on treatment adherence and satisfaction can be quite powerful. In one study, patients suffering from depression were given interactive engagement tools. These patients showed a 33% increase in antidepressant medication adherence and lower overall depression scores, resulting in a 61% increase in satisfaction with treatment.[14] In another study, patients with diabetes who used an online patient portal to refill medications increased their medication adherence and improved their cholesterol levels.[15] Patient reminders can help patients keep their upcoming appointments (reducing no-show rates for providers) and assist them in remembering preventive cancer screenings[16] or flu shots,[17] thus improving scores on quality measures for providers.

Patients at the "Engage Me" level can also view and download their electronic medical records. With access to their records, patients can step up to informed roles on their own healthcare teams, and they may be able to spot errors before they are consequential. The knowledge gained can also inspire them to do more for themselves in terms of medical self-care and adherence to their health and lifestyle goals.

LEVEL 3: EMPOWER ME

The "Empower Me" level of patient engagement offers the individual greater status and influence as a member of his or her own care team (Box 7-3). At the "Empower Me" level, the patient is considered a sufficient "source of truth," and patient-generated data can become an important part of the clinical record. The "Empower Me" level also enables patients to interact with the record digitally—either directly or through their own personal health record—which may ultimately be more comprehensive than the electronic medical record.

BOX 7-3

Level 3: Empower Me

Provider: The information I learn from my patients helps me provide better care.

Patient: Make it easy for me to be a part of my healthcare team.

In proposed MU stage 3 objectives, structured and semistructured questionnaires will be gathered in a systematic and highly interoperable method. This allows for information generated and entered by the patient to be included in the record. Previsit questionnaires, surveillance device data, and experience of care assessments are just a few of the anticipated uses.

The Previsit and Secure Messaging

"Empower Me" technology gives birth to the previsit, which can "flip the visit" in the same way that the Kahn Academy and other massive open online courses "flip the classroom" in education. In the flipped classroom, lectures and tests to evaluate comprehension and mastery happen online, while homework is done in class with help from the teacher or from other students who have already mastered the lesson.

In the medical previsit, the patient responds online to an interactive questionnaire developed by clinical experts to probe symptoms, concerns, and preferences around a specific health problem or condition. Responses to the questionnaire trigger patient education prescriptions for the person to review before visiting the clinician. When the patient arrives, the clinician quickly reviews a summary of the questionnaire responses, probes uncertainties, and then engages the patient in shared development of the treatment plan.

When the patient–provider relationship is strong, the previsit experience resolves the issue for the patient with a minimum of secure messaging exchange. As this new idea becomes easier and more efficient for all, the use of the previsit will likely become routine. Some organizations already recognize the previsit as an important part of a telemedicine strategy. For instance, Zoomcare, Inc.,[18] an Oregon-based primary and specialty care service, offers "take-out" functions that allow the patient to interact in secure messaging and Skype sessions. In this case, the previsit interaction may be the only "visit" needed.

Secure messaging is a primary work tool in the "Empower Me" level. This safe, two-way communication extends the patient–provider relationship in two important ways. First, it adds the time dimension to the relationship, allowing the patient to report on how a treatment is working or to ask questions about issues that were not evident during the visit. When symptoms worsen or improve, that two-way communication can be both life saving and cost saving by allowing quick adjustments to the treatment plan. At Geisinger Health System, patients involved in a study accessed their medication lists and provided feedback online to providers through the patient portal. As a result, providers reported that they were able to keep medication lists updated more efficiently. Patients were "eager to provide feedback on medication data and felt that it enabled them to track their medications in a more effective manner." Pharmacists made patient-suggested medication changes in 80% of the cases, and providers found that the online communication with patients resulted in time savings. Further, patients indicated that previsit online messaging improved the quality of communication with providers during office visits.[19]

The second way that secure messaging expands the relationship is in how it allows the full care team to become involved. Nurses, care coordinators, and others are often able to monitor the messages and respond to some without involving the primary clinician. This provides the advantage of a quick reply and gives the patient confidence that his or her response will be reviewed at a later point in the clinician's workflow. Both clinicians and patients have observed the benefits of secure messaging tools. As noted in an MU case study, "It actually cuts down on the phone calls and the back and forth" (Tracy Morris, Primary Health Medical Group).[20]

Campaigns

Perhaps even more important to the future of patient engagement is a tool sometimes called a campaign. A patient engagement campaign is a series of educational experiences presented to a select group of people who are facing a common health problem or moment in care. A campaign for a person recently diagnosed with diabetes could include all of the following, presented over a 6-week period (see Figure 7-3).

With patient empowerment comes a degree of patient accountability. The technology needed to deliver previsit questionnaires and condition-specific patient empowerment campaigns can also track the individual's responses to each opportunity for engagement. Calculating a patient engagement score is not difficult, and it can help the care team assess the effectiveness of the campaign in increasing levels of patient understanding and engagement.[21] As the patient's role on the care team expands, his or her engagement becomes more important and influential. Encouragement and rewards are often used to help support this increased role.

In selected areas, "Empower Me" promotes the use of patient decision aids to support shared decision making. Patient decision aids are tools that help people become involved in decision making by making explicit the decision that needs to be made, providing information about the options and outcomes, and clarifying personal values.[22] Most tools help guide people through a series of steps to help them get the facts, compare their options, share their feelings, and express their decision preference to their clinicians.

Including decision support and patient decision aids can be a natural part of a patient engagement campaign. For example, a patient engagement campaign for knee pain could begin with first-aid responses (e.g., ice, rest, elevation); include guidelines for over-the-counter medications; and introduce the patient to helpful programs in strengthening exercises, weight loss, and healthy eating. Later, if symptoms do not improve, the campaign would present a patient decision aid for the consideration of knee surgery. After comparing the benefits of surgery to the risks, the patient's preferences, concerns, and uncertainties would then be automatically sent to the care team to help in the shared decision making about surgery.

For the patient who chose surgery, the focus of the campaign would shift toward successfully preparing for and recovering from surgery and would include patient safety tips that benefit both the patient (e.g., exercise, healthy weight, and other advice aimed at keeping healthy) and the hospital (e.g., help meet critical quality measures). For the patient who decided to forgo surgery, the campaign would guide the person toward efforts that would help make the nonsurgical selection successful. In each case, the campaign would target the outcomes that matter most to the patient (e.g., pain-free mobility). Involving patients in shared decision making about treatment options is critical to patient engagement and satisfaction.[23]

"Empower Me" should also resolve the clipboard experience for the patient because online questionnaires allow things already known about the patient to be preloaded into every questionnaire and form. "Empower Me" technology also allows clinically valuable questionnaires (e.g., the Patient Health Questionnaires [PHQ-12 and PHQ-2] used by clinicians to monitor depression risks or assessments used to determine functional status)

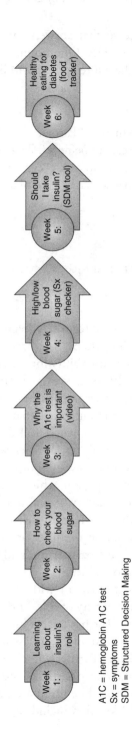

A1C = hemoglobin A1C test
Sx = symptoms
SDM = Structured Decision Making

Figure 7-3   Sample campaign for diabetes.

to be sent to the patient in advance so that answers can be scored and analyzed, and a summary automatically posted in the EHR. Questionnaire fatigue will be greatly reduced for both patient and provider, and their interactions will be much more meaningful.

LEVEL 4: PARTNER WITH ME

In the fourth level of patient engagement—"Partner with Me"—the role of the patient is elevated from being a recipient of the care to being a full partner with the provider (Box 7-4). As the "Partner with Me" concept is embraced, every clinical decision becomes a shared decision, and every care plan becomes a shared care plan.

> **BOX 7-4**
>
> **Level 4: Partner with Me**
> Provider and Patient: Help us clarify and record what we know and do together to manage my health.

At this level, the patient and the care team have shared accountability for achieving the outcomes that matter most to the patient. The patient engagement scores discussed in level 3 would be combined with accountability for setting and working toward chronic condition self-management and health-behavior goals. Increased accountability on the care team side would come from greater transparency into cost and quality measure scores—particularly as they relate to the outcomes that matter to the individual.

Just as secure messaging is the primary work tool for "Empower Me," the personal care plan becomes the primary work tool for "Partner with Me." A personal care plan brings together—with one voice and one view—all of the care plans, wellness goals, and supporting resources available to help a person achieve the outcomes that matter to him or her. Aided by the increasing interoperability of health information systems, the personal care plan enables each member of the care team to see the patient's progress toward outcome goals and to contribute information useful to achievement of the goal. As shown in Figure 7-4,[3] MU stage 3 supports this partnership and recognizes the pivotal role that care planning plays in the coordination of care.

A personal care plan integrates the patient with the care team members chosen by the patient. This team participates in a variety of roles and responsibilities, with the patient highly integrated at the center of care. The patient's values, goals, and health status inform the process and the participants in a fluid and seamless way.

Advance directives are essential for "Partner with Me" patient engagement. Personal preferences and values are needed to balance the risks and benefits of late-life treatments. Patients and their family caregivers should be given a clear view of the benefits and risks of each proposed treatment. Those risks often include an increased likelihood of dying in

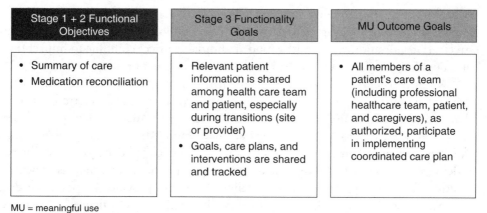

MU = meaningful use

Figure 7-4   Improving care coordination.
Reproduced from the Office of the National Coordinator for Health Information Technology. Meaningful use definition and objectives. HealthIT.gov website. http://www.healthit.gov/providers-professionals/meaningful-use-definition-objectives. Accessed January 24, 2014.

a hospital, connected to tubes and surrounded by machines and strangers, instead of in the familiarity and comfort of one's own home. Yet most people would prefer to avoid such treatment at the end of life. As noted by the Dartmouth Institute for Health Policy and Clinical Practice, "More than 80% of patients say that they wish to avoid hospitalization and intensive care during the terminal phase of illness."[24]

Health systems will need more sophisticated analytics to support the "Partner with Me" level of patient engagement, whereby each patient's most probable illness trajectories can be used to trigger patient engagement campaigns that provide both learning and action options for the individual. The descriptive analytics now used to select patients to participate in "Empower Me" campaigns will be replaced by predictive analytics that forecast each person's future health challenges and proactively prescribe approaches that have been shown to help in similar situations.

LEVEL 5: SUPPORT MY E-COMMUNITY

The fifth and final level of patient engagement is all about community (Box 7-5). Here, providers go outside of their walls and networks to incorporate the social determinants

BOX 7-5

Level 5: Support My e-Community

Provider/Patient: Expand and include the coproducers of health of the patient.

Community: Make it easy for me to support the patient.

of health for the populations they serve. There is no reason to wait for the completion of levels 1 to 4 before engaging the community. Employment, education, clean air, safe streets, transportation, and healthy food at affordable prices combine to impact the health of a population far more than the health care the population receives.

When providers and hospitals invest in social workers who team with patients to strengthen community-based systems and positively affect social determinants of health, they can reduce readmissions and unnecessary emergency department visits. Researchers at New York City's Mount Sinai Hospital[25] have found that "patients' relationships with care providers and their ratings of the quality of their care all depend . . . on the way care is delivered."[26] And care delivery encompasses an array of factors, such as patients' use of health information technology, the quality of patient–provider rapport, the degree of connectedness patients feel to their care facility, patients' confidence in their decision-making ability, and how informed patients feel about their health.

These predictors of quality of care are powerful factors influencing the overall health and well-being of patients within their communities. Use of HIT has been shown to reduce gaps in care that exist between higher- and lower-income populations. The use of e-communication between patient and provider—via text messages and e-mails—has increased patient satisfaction in care, despite disparities in income level and social determinants of health, thus leveling the playing field in the quality of care.[26]

Innovative health systems will help connect people to others who can support their goals through social networks or neighborhood actions. They will also find ways to partner with the safety net social agencies at work in every community. Geographic information systems placing each patient in a specific neighborhood will help to tailor patient engagement support to neighborhood characteristics. As provider systems learn more about a patient's social determinant data, e-communication and health information campaigns can be targeted to address those social determinants and can bring the care team and invited stakeholders (providers, family, and friends) into the e-health community. The Network of Care data provided by Trilogy Integrated Resources,[27] for example, allows hospitals or public health districts to understand trends by ZIP code and to target at-risk populations with tailored HIT-enabled health information (i.e., using data to tailor patient engagement support).

Population health improvement is a community effort. MU stage 3 highlights the need for integration of health records with the public service ecosystem to better improve the health of the population at large (Figure 7-5).[3]

Although the efforts supported by MU stage 3 emphasize the public service community, it is envisioned and recognized in the framework that "community" will be further defined by the patient. Family members, nontraditional caregivers, pharmacy, dentistry, and social media groups may all contribute to the well-being and health of any individual.

As emphasized in recommendations from the Robert Wood Johnson Foundation's "Health and Health Care in 2032," we have an obligation to "address social and economic barriers that prevent many Americans from realizing the 'pursuit of happiness' proclaimed

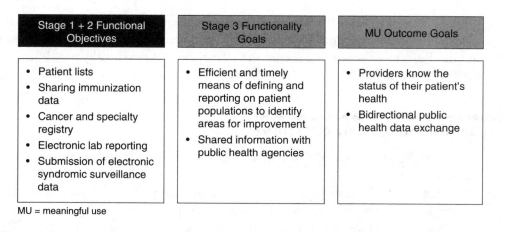

Stage 1 + 2 Functional Objectives	Stage 3 Functionality Goals	MU Outcome Goals
• Patient lists • Sharing immunization data • Cancer and specialty registry • Electronic lab reporting • Submission of electronic syndromic surveillance data	• Efficient and timely means of defining and reporting on patient populations to identify areas for improvement • Shared information with public health agencies	• Providers know the status of their patient's health • Bidirectional public health data exchange

MU = meaningful use

Figure 7-5   Improving care coordination.
Reproduced from the Office of the National Coordinator for Health Information Technology. Meaningful use definition and objectives. HealthIT.gov website. http://www.healthit.gov/providers-professionals/meaningful-use-definition-objectives. Accessed January 24, 2014.

in the nation's founding document."[28] Poor health is tied to disparities in housing, education, economic opportunity, race and ethnicity, public safety, and other socioeconomic factors. To improve population health, the social determinants of health must be addressed as a fundamental part of engaging the patient through his or her digital and physical community, thereby creating cultures of wellness.

CONCLUSION

It is imperative that efforts to improve population health and patient engagement operate through a coordinated framework supporting HIT and MU. As we become progressively more interconnected through e-tools in most other aspects of our lives, so must the healthcare system facilitate access to information electronically. The five stages of the patient engagement framework offer a collaboratively developed path for implementation that benefits providers, patients, and communities.

The tools discussed here that support each of the five stages can positively effect change and influence the achievement of better care, better health, and lower cost—tools like shared decision making and tailored patient education. Patients receiving care from providers with whom they shared in decision making showed a 12.5% reduction in hospital admissions, as well as lower costs.[29] And the delivery of clear, easy-to-understand patient education has been shown to reduce readmissions for heart failure.[30] Ultimately, more engaged patients incur lower costs, while less engaged patients can generate up to 21% more health costs.[31]

Greater public and provider education about the value of the patient engagement framework is necessary to help key players understand their changing roles within the system. Redefining roles with clear communication is fundamental so that key stakeholders—patients, providers, care teams, and loved ones—can contribute optimally in care. Readers are urged to consider the roles they might eventually play in enhancing patient engagement.

STUDY AND DISCUSSION QUESTIONS

1. How can innovative application of HIT tools impact and improve population health?
2. What are the benefits of aligning population health efforts with a framework that supports meaningful use, for both patients and providers?
3. How might future tools evolve to more fully support MU stage 3 and the "Partner with Me" and "Support My e-Community" stages?
4. Why is it important to engage the community in the pursuit of better health and the Triple Aim?

SUGGESTED READINGS AND WEBSITES

READINGS

Oldenberg J, Chase D, Christensen KT, et al., eds. *Engage! Transforming Healthcare Through Digital Patient Engagement*. Chicago, IL: HIMSS; 2013.

WEBSITES

Health information technology: http://www.healthit.gov/
National eHealth Collaborative: http://www.himss.org/ResourceLibrary/genResourceDetailPDF
.aspx?ItemNumber=28305

REFERENCES

1. Committee on Quality of Health Care in America, Institute of Medicine. *Crossing the Quality Chasm: A New Health System for the 21st Century*. Washington, DC: National Academies Press; 2001.
2. National eHealth Collaborative. The patient engagement framework. http://www.nationalehealth.org/patient-engagement-framework. Accessed January 24, 2014.
3. Office of the National Coordinator for Health Information Technology. Meaningful use definition and objectives. http://www.healthit.gov/providers-professionals/meaningful-use-definition-objectives. Accessed October 3, 2014.
4. Tang P, Hripcsak G. Meaningful use workgroup stage 3 update. Report presented at Health IT Policy Committee meeting; September 4, 2013.

http://www.healthit.gov/facas/sites/faca/files/ MUWG_Stage3_13_Sep_4_FINAL_0.pdf. Accessed October 3, 2014.

5. Frazee SG, Kirkpatrick P, Fabius R, et al. Leveraging the trusted clinician: documenting disease management program enrollment. *Dis Manage.* 2007; 10(1):16-29. doi:10.1089/dis.2006.629. Accessed May 7, 2014.

6. Frazee SG, Sherman B, Fabius R, et al. Leveraging the trusted clinician: increasing retention in disease management through integrated program delivery. *Popul Health Manage.* 2008;11(5):247-54. doi:10.1089/pop.2008.0010. Accessed May 7, 2014.

7. About PatientConnection. http://www.peacehealth .org/phmg/Pages/default.aspx. Accessed October 3, 2014.

8. Kemper DW. *Healthwise Handbook: Take Charge of Your Health.* Ellig E, ed. Husney A, Romito K, medical eds. 18th ed. Owensville, MO: Healthwise, Inc.; 2013.

9. Healthwise. Healthwise success story: Healthwise for Life helps people make better health decisions. http://www.healthwise.org/docs/document/2076 .pdf. Accessed October 3, 2014.

10. Office of the National Coordinator for Health Information Technology. Customizing EHR implementation to capture patient and clinical information for quality measurement and reporting. http:// www.healthit.gov/providers-professionals/ multnomah-county-health-department-case-study. Accessed October 3, 2014.

11. Group Health Cooperative. Group Health's mobile app. https://www1.ghc.org/html/public/ mobile/. Accessed October 3, 2014.

12. Runyon B. Personal testimonial on the value of mobile symptom triage tool to direct patients to the right level of care at the right time. Interviewed by Christy Calhoun, January 2014.

13. Kemper DW, Mettler M. *Information Therapy: Prescribed Information as a Reimbursable Medical Service.* Boise, ID: Healthwise; 2002.

14. Simon GE, Ralston JD, Savarino J, et al. Randomized trial of depression follow-up care by online messaging. *J Gen Intern Med.* 2011;26(7):698-704. doi:10.1007/s11606-011-1679-8.

15. Sarkar U, Lyles CR, Parker MM, et al. Use of the refill function through online patient portal is associated with improved adherence to statins in an integrated health system [published online ahead of print December 26, 2013]. *Med Care.* doi:10.1097/MLR.0000000000000069.

16. Wilkinson C, Champion JD, Sabharwal K. Promoting preventive health screening through the use of a clinical reminder tool: an accountable care organization quality improvement initiative. *J Healthc Qual.* 2013;35(5):7-19. doi:10.111/jhq .12024.

17. Stockwell MS, Westhoff C, Kharbanda EO, et al. Influenza vaccine text message reminders for urban, low-income pregnant women: a randomized controlled trial. *Am J Public Health.* 2014;104 (supp 1):e7-12. doi:10.2105/AJPH.2013.301620.

18. Barney L, Barney and Associates. ZoomCare—changing the model for delivering health care. Bio Quarterly. https://www.oregonbio.org/news/bio-quarterly/88-bio-quarterly/475-zoomcare. Accessed October 3, 2014.

19. Deering MJ. Issue brief: patient-generated health data and health IT. Report presented at The Office of the National Coordinator for Health Information Technology meeting; December 20, 2013. http://www.healthit.gov/sites/default/files/pghd_ brief_final122013.pdf. Accessed October 3, 2014.

20. Office of the National Coordinator for Health Information Technology. Patient portal benefits patient care and provider workflow. http://www .healthit.gov/providers-professionals/patient-portal-benefits-patient-care-and-provider-workflow. Accessed October 3, 2014.

21. Solomon M, Wagner SL, Goes J. Effects of a web-based intervention for adults with chronic conditions on patient activation: online randomized controlled trial. *J Med Internet Res.* 2012;14(1):e32. doi:10.2196/jimr.1924.

22. Patient decision aids. Ottawa Hospital Research Institute website. https://decisionaid.ohri.ca/. Updated May 7, 2013. Accessed October 3, 2014.

23. Barry MJ, Edgman-Levitan S. Shared decision making—pinnacle of patient-centered care. *N Engl J Med.* 2012;366(9):780-1. doi:10.1056/ NEJMp1109283.

24. Dartmouth Institute for Health Policy and Clinical Practice. Inpatient days per decedent during the last six months of life, by gender and level of care intensity. http://www.dartmouthatlas.org/data/topic/topic .aspx?cat=18. Accessed October 3, 2014.

25. Advisory Board Company. How a hospital used social workers to cut readmission. *Daily Briefing.* September 30, 2013. http://www.advisory.com/ daily-briefing/2013/09/30/how-a-hospital-used-social-workers-to-cut-readmissions. Accessed October 3, 2014.

26. Blue Shield of California Foundation. Health care in California: leveling the playing field. http:// www.blueshieldcafoundation.org/sites/default/ files/publications/downloadable/BCSF_leveling_ the_playing_field.pdf. Published November 2013. Accessed October 3, 2014.

27. Network of Care for public health assessment and wellness. Network of Care website. http://ph .networkofcare.org/. Accessed October 3, 2014.

28. Institute for Alternative Futures. *Health and Health Care in 2032: Report from the RWJF Futures Symposium, June 20-21, 2012.* Alexandria, VA: Institute for Alternative Futures; 2012.

29. Carman KL, Dardess P, Maurer M, et al. Patient and family engagement: a framework for understanding the elements and developing interventions and policies. *Health Aff.* 2013; 32(2):223–31. doi:10.1377/hlthaff.2012.1133.

30. Heart failure education reduces readmissions [news release]. Robert Wood Johnson Foundation Newsroom; February 26, 2013. http://www .rwjf.org/en/about-rwjf/newsroom/newsroom-content/2013/02/heart-failure-education-reduces-readmissions.html. Accessed October 3, 2014.

31. Hibbard JH, Green J, Overton V. Patients with lower activation associated with higher costs; delivery systems should know their patients' "scores." *Health Aff.* 2013;32(2):216-22. doi:10.1377/hlthaff.2012.1064.

Chapter 8

BEHAVIORAL ECONOMICS

JIN LEE

Executive Summary

Behavioral economics can influence population health by motivating and nudging people toward healthier decisions.

Behavioral economics is the study of the effects of social and cognitive factors on an individual's economic decision-making process. Rooted in psychology and economics, behavioral economics theories can be applied in population health to help influence and change health outcomes. Physicians, patients, and health insurance companies exhibit a set of common behavioral economic heuristics. Understanding these rule-of-thumb practices can help healthcare administrators make better choices regarding their employee wellness programs and support positive patient behaviors, such as medication adherence and substance avoidance. Reinforced by corresponding legislation, behavioral economics has the potential to move our society toward improved population health outcomes.

Learning Objectives

1. Understand the core elements of behavioral economics.
2. Describe some behavioral economics heuristics.
3. Apply heuristics to influence/change individual health decisions.
4. Understand the limitations of behavioral economics.

Key Terms

behavioral economics

behavioral intervention

heuristics

patient behavior

physician behavior

INTRODUCTION

Studies consistently reveal that a large percentage of the deaths in the United States could be avoided through behavioral modifications. Approximately half of the 2 million deaths in the United States in 1990 were attributable to or associated with external factors that could have been prevented.[1] In 2000, 36% of deaths were related to smoking, poor diet, physical inactivity, and alcohol consumption.[2] In 2009, the World Health Organization linked smoking, one of the most deadly behaviors, to 18% of deaths; excess body weight and physical inactivity were associated with 8% of deaths.

Unhealthy behavior is also highly correlated with morbidity; obesity is associated with high risk of arthritis and type 2 diabetes,[3] and smoking is linked to lung cancer, emphysema, and chronic obstructive pulmonary disease.[4]

Behavioral economics incorporates economic, cognitive, and social psychology disciplines to determine how individuals and institutions make economic decisions. Traditional economics assumes that humans are rational; behavioral economics recognizes that humans are innately impulsive and irrational, and exhibit inconsistent patterns in decision making based on emotions, social environment, and immediate circumstance.

Many scientists hypothesize that human decision making is governed by a two-tiered process in the brain. Although long-term planned behavior is directed by the prefrontal cortex, short-term impulsive behavior is controlled by the primitive and autonomic limbic system.[5] External stimuli often act upon the limbic system in the center of the brain before deliberate cognitive processing occurs. This partly explains why the careful planning of the prefrontal cortex is sometimes overwhelmed by the emotions generated in the limbic system.

The study of patients with structural brain damage has confirmed that these areas are critical to decision making. People with impaired limbic systems are less able to learn gradually or respond to conditioned emotions, and people with deficient prefrontal cortexes struggle with decision making, especially with respect to long-term goals.[6]

Prospect theory is one of the better known theories of behavioral economics. First formulated by Daniel Kahneman in 1979,[7] it was expanded in 1992.[8] Kahneman's work marked him as one of the founding fathers of behavioral economics and later won him the 2002 Nobel Prize in Economics. Prospect theory explains the human propensity to make economical, irrational decisions with respect to reward preferences. For example, because humans are averse to losses, they tend to overvalue low-probability options. Kahneman also hypothesized that our biological two-tiered decision-making process is clear evidence of humans' limited mental capacity.[9]

ROLE OF BEHAVIORAL ECONOMICS IN HEALTH CARE

Michael Grossman, an expert in health economics, suggests that an individual's health depends on his or her genetic makeup, unique environmental factors, and personal decisions regarding resource allocation.[10] Understanding this decision-making process and the human tendency to commit cognitive errors, behavioral economists can influence population health by motivating and nudging people toward healthier decisions and thus healthy behaviors.

In 2008, Peter Orszag, director of the U.S. Office of Management and Budget, called for an increased effort to incorporate behavioral economics into health care, in particular, by improving decision making by both doctors and patients.[11] Because applying behavioral economics requires only minimal change to existing programs and participants, its principles have great potential for making significant impacts on individual well-being and population health.

BEHAVIORAL ECONOMICS HEURISTICS

Behavioral economics recognizes that people make decisions based on certain **heuristics**, or rules of thumb, in particular situations. These heuristics include the following.

PHYSICIAN BEHAVIORS

Anchoring

Anchoring means to start from a reference point and make (usually inappropriate) adjustments[12] when making decisions and/or answering questions. Primary care physicians have an average of 7 to 15 minutes to evaluate a patient. Time constraints and decision fatigue often lead physicians to base treatment recommendations and prescriptions on their mental reference points (i.e., giving patients what they have habitually prescribed in like circumstances). Likewise, patients are anchored in past behaviors (e.g., individual exercise habits at specific times and places, with similar friends, and performing the same exercise routines).

Status Quo Bias

Status quo bias is the failure to proactively change a default stance. Physicians often prescribe the same medications to patients with similar symptoms. Research has shown that both physicians and patients are reluctant to change drugs, even when the new medication is comparably effective to an existing one and lower in cost,[13] such as generic alternatives to brand-name medicines.

Bandwagon Effect

The bandwagon effect refers to conforming to social norms and carrying out certain actions because others do.[14] In working with other medical professionals, physicians often comply with certain informal norms and rules of behavior. Doctors often make treatment choices based on the weighted average of prior actions in their social environments. Studies have shown that doctors overvalue information immediately available to them, while undervaluing available scientific data on a treatment's medical merit.[15] By unconsciously conforming to these local norms, an individual physician may decrease the chance of malpractice suits by doing "everything" as others have done.[16]

PATIENT BEHAVIORS

Hyperbolic Discounting

Hyperbolic discounting occurs when someone is presented with two comparable rewards, and he or she prefers the one that comes sooner to the one that comes later, thus "discounting" the value of the later reward.[17] Furthermore, the greater the uncertainty of the reward in the future, the greater the preference for the earlier reward.

Present Bias

Present bias occurs when someone pays greater attention to immediate costs and benefits than to those anticipated in the future.[18] When applying the notions of hyperbolic discounting and present bias, one begins to understand why it is difficult for drug addicts to quit. They are focused on immediate gratification rather than on the health consequences that likely will arise in the future. The inability to fully appreciate future outcomes also helps to explain why people procrastinate when it comes to establishing healthy behaviors. One way to combat present bias is to immediately and frequently reward the desired behavior, for example, giving a cash reward to a patient whenever she refills her medication on time,[19] quits smoking,[20] or loses weight.[21]

Law of Small Numbers

The law of small numbers refers to the overinterpretation of information that is based on an insufficiently small number of observable events.[22] This can cause a family member to avoid needed surgery because a loved one died on the operating table in the past.

Relativity and Choice

Relativity and choice pertain to making decisions based on what is currently present versus other available alternatives.[23] When choosing a healthcare provider, 70% of patients rely on family and friends rather than on national surveys and other published data. People tend to base judgments more heavily on easily accessible, "trusted," subjective evidence even when more objective sources of data are available.[24] Moreover, studies reveal that patient-reported quality of care ratings are not reliable because their opinions are highly skewed toward a physician's respectfulness, courtesy, and office cleanliness. One way to take advantage of this bias is to have a lottery system that encourages the continuity of the desired behavior (e.g., the widely televised lottery winner will create a positive impact encouraging all the participants to enter the lottery).

Message Framing

Message framing refers to the way information is communicated, for instance, the manner in which a doctor presents information frames the patient's decision regarding treatment options. In one study, patients were increasingly compliant when positive messages were displayed. For example, a doctor may tell a patient either "choosing radiation will result in a 95% increased chance of success" or "not choosing radiation will result in a 5% increased chance of failure." Although both statements describe the same outcome, more patients choose the radiation option when told in the first manner. Another study found that most people do not understand statistical references, especially when weighing different types of treatment options.[25] Hence, it is preferable for a physician to explain treatment plans in frequencies rather than in probabilities. Framing becomes especially important when discussing treatment options for a patient undergoing end-of-life care.

HEALTH INSURANCE COVERAGE AND OTHER HEALTH-RELATED DECISIONS

Mental Accounting

Mental accounting is when someone has difficulty with compartmentalizing complex decisions. Health insurance information is complex and often contains jargon that is unfamiliar to consumers. When choosing plans, a member weighs the trade-off between the cost of the insurance and the likelihood of future illness or trauma. Amos Tversky and Daniel Kahneman, two leaders in behavioral economics, have shown that probability-related decisions are especially difficult to make.[26] Furthermore, it has been demonstrated that an overabundance of available choice options decreases consumers' motivation and satisfaction when making a decision.[27]

Unnecessary complexity heightens the hurdle in the decision-making process and causes consumers to default to their status quo. To counter the bias, some companies provide their employees with limited health plan choices regarding quality, price, and covered services.[28] Compared with selecting an insurance plan on the open market, the limited-option approach places less of a cognitive burden on their employees or consumers.

More choices do not always lead to better decisions. The 2010 Patient Protection and Affordable Care Act mandates that all chain restaurants with 20 locations or more must list calories on their menus. Yet studies show that information alone does not change consumer dietary decisions,[29] especially when consumers lack appropriate knowledge regarding what is considered to be a healthy quantity of calories.[30] Similarly, studies suggest that providing more data on hospital quality and medical errors to consumers has led to few changes in their decisions to choose one over another.[31]

Choice Architecture

Choice architecture refers to the context in which a choice is presented. Humans have limited cognitive ability and limited attention when making individual choices. When choosing from many different options, we experience decision fatigue, lose a sense of priority among the choices, and sometimes avoid making a choice altogether.[32] This explains why patients often want their doctors to make key treatment decisions for them.[33]

Loss Aversion

Loss aversion occurs when someone prefers loss avoidance to acquiring gains. Humans detest losses at about twice the rate they like gains[34] (i.e., losses have twice the psychological power of gains). Further, elevated anxiety levels have been shown to affect one's desire for new information, tests, or treatments.[35] Therefore, it is more effective to penalize than reward when one is designing incentives.

A penalty can sometimes appear fairer than financial rewards. After financial rewards were shown to be effective in smoking cessation at a U.S. company, the company instituted a financial penalty on nonsmoking employees who begrudged smokers for receiving rewards.[36] Loss aversion can also be a powerful tool in employee wellness programs. After Blue Shield of California incorporated loss aversion to their Healthy Lifestyle Rewards, they increased the participation rate while decreasing program expenses.[37] Because of the perceived disadvantage of losing what we already have, people have a strong tendency to maintain their status quo.

BEHAVIORAL INTERVENTIONS USING BEHAVIORAL ECONOMICS PRINCIPLES

Understanding the behavior heuristics of patients, doctors, and health coverage can inform health services providers, professionals, and policy makers in creating more effective programs.

WORKPLACE/EMPLOYEE WELLNESS PROGRAMS

A 2007 study of 500 employers representing approximately 5 million workers found that about 73% of the companies offer workplace or employee wellness programs to incentivize engagement in healthy behavior.[38] It is estimated that companies can save $3 for every dollar invested in its employees.[39] Recognizing the reality of choice fatigue, companies often set the healthiest choice as their default option: In cafeterias, for example, water is offered rather than soda, or whole wheat instead of white bread. These organizations display the healthier food option early in the waiting queue at lunch and move energy-dense items to less-convenient areas.[40] Acting upon the herd behavior concept, insurance companies like Humana leverage peer pressure to launch step challenges, which encourage their employees to remain active.

Research regarding the effectiveness of financial incentives is mixed. For example, Microsoft rewarded each employee $50 for having an annual health checkup in 2013. Dr. David Anderson's group was able to show a direct correlation between the amount of monetary incentives used and the degree of participation in health risk appraisals.[41] On the other hand, a RAND study showed that financial incentives generate only modest behavioral change and therefore little cost savings.[42]

MEDICATION ADHERENCE

Medication nonadherence is estimated to incur an annual cost of $100 billion in the United States.[43] The mean adherence rate to appointments, screenings, and medication remained at a low 25% from 1948 to 1998,[44] and this low adherence rate has had a significant impact on clinical outcomes. The 63 studies on 19,000 patients (1968–1998) indicated that those who were adherent had a 26% greater improvement in their clinical outcomes than the nonadherent population. This difference is even more pronounced when chronic illnesses are compared with acute diseases.[45]

Barriers to adherence include patient, medical, and healthcare system challenges. A study of 1,433 patients taking statins found that past prescription-refill behavior is a better predictor of medication adherence than prospective health beliefs. The strongest indicator was the impact of the medication regimen on a patients' daily routine.[46]

Express Scripts, one of the largest pharmacy benefit management organizations, understands that most people resort to familiar, default options. The company provides an opt-in option for mail-order delivery to ensure that chronic medication arrives at the subscriber's door every 90 days. To foster healthy habits, many healthcare startups are leveraging behavioral economics principles, using "gamification" and refill reminders to encourage medication adherence among their subscribers. A review of 11 studies has shown that financial incentives improve adherence, especially for chronic diseases.[47] However, while copay reduction increased pharmacy costs, its overall savings (especially in emergency room usage) remains controversial.[48,49]

SUBSTANCE ABUSE AND OTHER FORMS OF IMPULSIVE BEHAVIOR

Developed countries are burdened with excess consumption of alcohol, tobacco, high-calorie fast food, and other addictive goods. Humans' strong preference toward immediate gratification, even at the expense of larger, delayed rewards such as better health, is an example of the aforesaid hyperbolic inconsistency.[50] Some people—gamblers, in particular—are insensitive to risky outcomes; others underestimate the harmful effects of risky behaviors like smoking[51] or binge drinking.[52]

Whether it be an addiction to drugs, fast food, or risky behavior, studies have shown that these activities trigger cues that act directly on the emotional limbic system rather than on the long-term decision-making prefrontal cortex.[53] To better understand the effect of circumstances and choice, a study on school nutrition found that decreasing portion size had a positive effect on lowering the obesity rate.[54] Another study suggested that school-based activities are the best format for changing risky behaviors in younger people, whereas mass media and legislative intervention have little to moderate effect,[55] perhaps because of the bandwagon effect.

One way to decrease substance abuse and other forms of impulsive behavior is to ask people to precommit to an action. For example, when a smoker announces that his New Year's resolution is to quit smoking, he is using social pressure to precommit and reinforce healthier behavior.[56] The same mechanism applies to a suffering alcoholic who joins Alcoholics Anonymous. More intrusive methods of a self-imposed, precommitment strategy include bariatric surgery (used to physically limit the amount of food intake) and the drug Antabuse (used by alcoholics to trigger a nauseating response to alcohol consumption).[57] The precommitment tactic becomes more effective when combined with financial incentives. Such programs are effective for drug abuse even with small financial rewards (e.g., $2.50 for a single negative test for cocaine).[58] However, these programs have been shown to be less effective for tobacco use[59] and weight loss,[60] which suggests that sustained behavior changes may require more time and intervention.

FUTURE CHALLENGES

PREDICTION

Because humans are inconsistent in their choices, decision prediction is incredibly difficult. As previously noted, our preconceived mental schemas alter our perceptions, our interpretations of our senses, and our decisions. However, humans appear to be predictably influenced by heuristic rules of thumb.

Physicians' attitudes toward their patients depend on the heuristics they use in the context of meeting with each patient.[61] For example, doctors may evaluate and prescribe different treatments on the basis of a patient's skin color.[62] Because an individual's choices change over time, any decision prediction must be performed constantly and in real time to be beneficial. Yet, influences on collective behavior on a population level may be easier to predict.

INCENTIVES

Different incentives can be used to influence others toward preferred behaviors. Dr. Maxine Stitzer, professor of psychiatry and behavioral science at Johns Hopkins University, suggests that social reinforcement provides a longer lasting effect than external, tangible incentives.[63] The success of an incentive depends on its size, frequency, trigger, duration, and execution. Evaluation of an incentive depends on the desired outcome, but it often includes participation or engagement rates, clinical effectiveness, cost savings, acceptability, sustainability, and change over time.

SCALABILITY

Understanding behavioral principles can help change people's decisions and guide them toward healthy behaviors. However, because the heuristics are person focused, scaling the effect of behavioral economics remains a challenge. Peoples' motivations to change vary depending on career progression, culture, finances, and many other factors. For behavioral economics–focused health programs to be successful, framing, timing, incentives, distribution, customization, and measurement will be key.

VARIABLES

To better leverage behavioral economics in population health, one clearly needs to understand the effect of unhealthy behavior on health outcomes and, conversely, the effect of poor outcomes on unhealthy behavior. One also needs to investigate confounding factors, such as low level of education and socioeconomic status, which affect both unhealthy behavior and poor outcomes.[64] Other variables to consider include social relationships, intrinsic motivation, individual behavior, and personal responsibility.

ETHICS

Behavioral economics is sometimes construed as a practice of new or libertarian paternalism.[65] In the popular nonfiction book *Nudge*, authors Richard Thaler and Cass Sunstein[66] explain that unlike libertarian paternalists, behavior experts and "nudgers" help people make better decisions without explicitly forcing them. The final decision is up to the individual to make and carry out.

Nevertheless, there are ethical issues in play when leveraging behavioral economics in health interventions. For example, what level of intervention would be considered too intrusive at the individual, family, or community level? What is the best approach to maximize program effectiveness while not seeming too paternalistic? What role should legislation play in health nudging? To what extent should employers influence the health decisions of their workforce?

CONCLUSION

Humans are myopic and impulsive. We make inconsistent decisions using certain rules of thumb in particular situations. Behavioral economics acknowledges that these natural tendencies underlay the ubiquity of our unhealthy behaviors. Rather than emphasizing how humans should behave, behavioral economics accepts that we make choices based on specific biological, cognitive, and social contexts at the moment of decision making.

A more effective way of promoting healthy behavior is to take into account the patient and his or her family, healthcare advocates, community, and state—the entire social ecosystem. Behavioral economics encourages only slight modifications to existing programs and mindsets and minimal change from its participants, yet it may have a substantial potential effect. With proper legislation and appropriate technology to empower individual responsibility and decision making, behavioral economics has the potential to help individuals and society as a whole to achieve improved health outcomes.

STUDY AND DISCUSSION QUESTIONS

1. What is behavioral economics?
2. List five heuristics.
3. How can behavioral economics principles be used to improve your health? The health of your family?
4. What are some of the limitations or challenges of behavioral economics?

SUGGESTED READINGS AND WEBSITES

READINGS

Ariely D. *Predictably Irrational: The Hidden Forces That Shape Our Decisions*. New York: HarperCollins; 2008.

DiClemente RJ, Salazar LF, Crosby RA. *Health behavior theory for public health*. Burlington, MA: Jones & Bartlett Learning; 2013.

Frank RG. Behavioral economics and health economics. Working Paper 10881, National Bureau of Economic Research; 2004.

Kahneman D. Maps of bounded rationality: psychology for behavioral economics. *Am Econ Rev.* 2003;1449-62.

Thaler RH, Sunstein C. *Nudge: improving decisions about health, wealth, and happiness*. New Haven, CT: Yale University Press; 2008.

WEBSITES

Center for Behavioral Economics in Child Nutrition Programs, Cornell University: http://ben.cornell.edu/

Center for Health Incentives and Behavioral Economics at the Leonard David Institute, University of Pennsylvania: http://chibe.upenn.edu/

Dan Ariely: http://danariely.com

Vermont Center on Behavior and Health, University of Vermont: http://www.uvm.edu/medicine/behaviorandhealth/

REFERENCES

1. McGinnis JM, Foege, WH. Actual causes of death in the United States. *JAMA.* 1993;270(18): 2207-12.

2. Mokdad AH, Marks JS, Stroup DF, et al. Actual causes of death in the United States, 2000. *JAMA.* 2004;291(10):1238-45.

3. Dixon JB. The effect of obesity on health outcomes. *Mol Cell Endocrinol.* 2010;316:104-8.

4. U.S. Department of Health and Human Services. The health benefits of smoking cessation: A report of the Surgeon General. Atlanta: U.S. Dept. of Health and Human Services, Public Health Service, Centers for Disease Control, Center for Chronic Disease Prevention and Health Promotion, Office on Smoking and Health; 1990.

5. Thaler RH, Shefrin HM. An economic theory of self-control. *J Polit Econ.* 1981;89(2):392-406.

6. Loewenstein GF, O'Donoghue T. Animal Spirits: Affective and Deliberative Processes in Economic Behavior. 2004; Working Paper 04-14, Center for Analytic Economics, Cornell University.

7. Kahneman D, Tversky A. Prospect theory: An analysis of decision under risk. *Econometrica.* 1979;47(2):263-92.

8. Tversky A, Kaheman D. Advances in prospect theory: cumulative representation of uncertainty. *J Risk Uncertain.* 1992;5(4):297-323.

9. Kahneman D. Maps of bounded rationality: psychology for behavioral economics. *Am Econ Rev.* 2003;93(5):1449-62.

10. Grossman M. On the concept of health capital and the demand for health. *J Pol Econ.* 1972; 80(2):223-4.

11. Hansen F, Anell A, Gerdtham U, et al. The future of health economics: the potential of behavioral and experimental economics. Working Paper 20, Department of Economics, Lund University; 2013.

12. Kahneman D. Reference points, anchors, norms, and mixed feelings. *Organ Behav Hum Dec.* 1992;51(2):296-312.

13. Wolfe MW. Overview and comparison of the proton pump inhibitors for the treatment of acid-related disorders. UpToDate. 2013. http://www.uptodate.com/contents/overview-and-comparison-of-the-proton-pump-inhibitors-for-the-treatment-of-acid-related-disorders. Accessed October 4, 2014.

14. Leibenstein H. Bandwagon, snob, and veblen effects in the theory of consumers' demand. *Q J Econ.* 1950;64(2):183-207.

15. Frank RG. Behavioral economics and health economics. 2004; Working Paper 10881, National Bureau of Economic Research.

16. Thaler R. Toward a positive theory of consumer choice. *J Econ Behav Organ.* 1980;1(1):39-60.

17. Ainslie G. Derivation of 'rational' economic behavior from hyperbolic discount curves. *Am Econ Rev.* 1991;81(2):334-40.

18. O'Donoghue T, Rabin M. The economics of immediate gratification. *J Behav Dec Making.* 2000;13:233-50.

19. Volpp KG, Loewenstein G, Troxel AB, et al. A test of financial incentives to improve warfarin adherence. *BMC Health Serv Res.* 2008;8:272.

20. Volpp KG, Troxel AB, Pauly MV, et al. A randomized, controlled trial of financial incentives for smoking cessation. *N Engl J Med.* 2009;360: 699-709.

21. Volpp KG, John LK, Troxel AB, et al. Financial incentive-based approaches for weight loss: a randomized trial. *JAMA.* 2008;300:2631-7.

22. Rabin M. Inference by believers in the law of small numbers. *Q J Econ.* 2002;117(3):775-816.

23. Ariely D. *Predictably Irrational: The Hidden Forces That Shape Our Decisions.* New York: HarperCollins; 2008.

24. Tversky A, Kahneman D. Judgment under uncertainty: heuristics and biases. *Science.* 1974;185(4157): 1124-31.

25. Gigerenzer G, Gaissmaier W, Kurz-Milcke E, et al. Helping doctors and patients make sense of health statistics. *Psychol Sci Public Interest.* 2007;8(2):53-96.

26. Tversky A, Kahneman D. Judgment under uncertainty: heuristics and biases. *Science.* 1974; 185(4157):1124-31.

27. Iyengar SS, Lepper MR. When choice is demotivating: can one desire too much of a good thing? *J Pers Soc Psychol.* 2000;79:995-6.

28. Liebman J, Zeckhauser R. Simple humans, complex insurance, subtle subsidies. In: Aaron HJ, Burman LE, eds. *Using Taxes to Reform Health Insurance, Pitfalls and Promises.* Washington DC: Brookings Institution Press; 2008:230-62.

29. Loewenstein G. Confronting reality: pitfalls of calorie posting. *Am J Clin Nutr.* 2011;93:679-80.

30. Chernev A. The dieter's paradox. *J Consumer Psychology.* 2011;21(2):178-83.

31. Schneider EC, Epstein AM. Use of public performance reports: a survey of patients undergoing cardiac surgery. *JAMA.* 1998;279:1638-40.

32. Johnson EJ, Hershey J, Meszaros J, et al. Framing probability distortions, and insurance decisions. *J Risk Uncertain.* 1993;7:35-51.

33. Beaver K, Bogg JB, Luker KA. Decision-making role preferences and information needs: a comparison of colorectal and breast cancer. *Hea lth.*1999;2:266-76.

34. Tversky A, Kahneman D. Loss aversion in riskless choice: a reference-dependent model. *Q J Econ.* 1991;106(4):1039-61.

35. Koszegi B. Health, anxiety and patient behavior. *J Health Econ.* 2003;22(6):1073-84.

36. Volpp KG, Troxel AB, Pauly MV, et al. A randomized, controlled trial of financial incentives for smoking cessation. *N Engl J Med.* 2009;360:699-709.

37. Pai A. Two Blues discuss health behavior change rewards, loss aversion, and regret theory. Mobihealthnews. 2013. http://mobihealthnews.com/24129/two-blues-discuss-healthy-behavior-change-rewards-loss-aversion-and-regret-theory/. Accessed October 4, 2014.

38. Employer investments in improving employee health. National Business Group on Health and Fidelity Investments. 2014. http://www.businessgrouphealth.org/pub/58aad383-782b-cb6e-2763-7baeda20697a. Accessed October 4, 2014.

39. Reducing the risk of heart disease and stroke: a six-step guide for employers. Centers for Disease Control and Prevention. 2003. http://www.cdc.gov/dhdsp/pubs/docs/six_step_guide.pdf. Accessed October 4, 2014.

40. Loewenstein G, Brennan T, Volpp KG. Asymmetric paternalism to improve health behaviors. *JAMA.* 2007;298(20):2415-7.

41. Anderson D, Grossmeier J, Seaverson E, et al. The role of financial incentives in driving employee engagement in health management. *ACSM's Health & Fitness Journal.* 2008;12(4):18-22.

42. Mattke S, Liu H, Caloyeras JP, et al. Workplace wellness programs study: final report. *RAND Corporation.* 2013;1-170.

43. Osterberg L, Blaschke T. Adherence to medication. *N Engl J Med.* 2005;353(5):487-97.

44. DiMatteo MR. Variations in patients' adherence to medical recommendations: a quantitative review of 50 years of research. *Med Care.* 2004;42(3):200-9.

45. DiMatteo MR, Giordani PJ, Lepper HS, et al. Patient adherence and medical treatment outcomes: a meta-analysis. *Med Care.* 2002;40(9):794-811.

46. Molfenter TD, Bhattacharya A, Gustafson DH. The roles of past behavior and health beliefs in predicting medication adherence to a statin regimen. *Patient Prefer Adherence.* 2012;6:643-51.

47. Giuffrida A, Torgerson DJ. Should we pay the patient? Review of financial incentives to enhance patient compliance. *BMJ.* 1997;315:703-7.

48. Mahoney J, Hom D. *Total Value, Total Return: Seven Rules for Optimizing Employee Health Benefits for a Healthier and More Productive Workforce.* GlaxoSmithKline Group; 2006.

49. Maciejewski ML, Wansink D, Lindquist JH, et al. Value-based insurance design program in North Carolina increased medication adherence but was not cost neutral. *Health Aff.* 2014;33(2):300-8.

50. DiClemente RJ, Salazar LF, Crosby RA. *Health behavior theory for public health.* Burlington, MA: Jones & Bartlett Learning; 2013.

51. Dillard AJ, McCaul KD, Klein W. Unrealistic optimism in smokers: implications for smoking myth endorsement and self-protective motivation. *J Health Comm.* 2006;11:93-100.

52. Dillard AJ, Midboe AM, Klein W. The dark side of optimism: unrealistic optimism about problems with alcohol predicts subsequent negative event experiences. *Pers Soc Psychol.* 2009;35:1540.

53. Berheim D, Rangel A. Addiction and cue-triggered decision process. *Am Econ Rev.* 2004;94(5):1558–90.

54. Rolls BJ, Roe LS, Meengs JS. Reducing the energy density and portion size of foods decreases energy intake over two days. *Obes Res.* 2004;12:A5 (abs).

55. Jepson RG, Harris FM, Platt S, et al. The effectiveness of interventions to change six health behaviors: a review of reviews. *BMC Public Health*. 2010;10:538-54.

56. Gruber J, Koszegi B. Is addiction "rational"? Theory and evidence. *Q J Econ*. 2001;116(4):1261-303.

57. Cawley J, Ruhm CJ. The economics of risky health behaviors. 2011; Working Paper 5728, Forschungsinstitut zur Zukunft der Arbeit, Institute for the Study of Labor.

58. Higgins ST, Alessi SM, Dantona RL. Voucher-based incentives: A substance abuse treatment innovation. *Addict Behav*. 2002;27:887-910.

59. Prendergast M, Podus D, Finney J, et al. Contingency management for treatment of substance use disorders: a meta-analysis. *Addiction*. 2006;101:1546-60.

60. Cawley J, Price JA. Outcomes in a program that offers financial rewards for weight loss. In: Grossman M, Mocan N, eds. *Economic Aspects of Obesity*. Chicago: University of Chicago; 2011: 91-126.

61. Bornstein BH, Emler AC. Rationality in medical decision-making: a review of the literature on doctors' decision-making biases. *J Eval Clin Pract*. 2001;7(2):97-107.

62. Van Ryn M, Burke J. The effect of patient race and socioeconomic status on physicians' perceptions of patients. *Soc Sci Med*. 2000;50:813-28.

63. LDI Issue Brief. Leonard Davis Institute of Health Economics-University of Pennsylvania. 2011;17(1):1-8.

64. Cawley J, Ruhm CJ. The economics of risky health behaviors. Working Paper 5728, Forschungsinstitut zur Zukunft der Arbeit, Institute for the Study of Labor; 2011.

65. Loewenstein G, Brennan T, Volpp KG. Asymmetric paternalism to improve health behaviors. *JAMA*. 2007;298(20):2415-7.

66. Thaler RH, Sunstein C. *Nudge: improving decisions about health, wealth, and happiness*. New Haven, CT: Yale University Press; 2008.

HEALTH SYSTEM NAVIGATION: THE ROLE OF HEALTH ADVOCACY AND ASSISTANCE PROGRAMS

ESTHER NASH AND ABBIE LEIBOWITZ

Executive Summary

Health advocates—guiding consumers through a disorganized system.

Health care is confusing and difficult to navigate for the average consumer. When faced with a chronic, serious, or life-threatening illness, even those with a reasonable understanding of how health benefits and care delivery systems work are likely to be overwhelmed. As medical costs have risen, companies offering health benefits have found that they can no longer afford to offer health insurance coverage to as many employees and dependents, or at the same levels of coverage. The result has been a combination of higher premiums, plan designs that provide less coverage and require greater individual participation in the care decision process, and greater cost shifts from employers to employees. Individuals who purchase coverage through the public health insurance exchanges (HIEs) also confront the difficulty of dealing with the healthcare system (many of them doing it for the first time). It is easy to "get lost" in the healthcare system.

An increasingly large share of Americans have ongoing healthcare issues or chronic conditions in their families. Without assistance to maximize their use of health benefits and medical services, they are unlikely to achieve the best possible medical outcomes. In this context health advocacy and navigational assistance are essential.

Since the late 1990s, health advocacy and assistance programs (i.e., programs that support individuals and help them navigate through the healthcare system) have developed as a specialized employee benefit category. Employers have embraced these programs as a means of promoting greater employee responsibility for health, lifestyle, and medical decisions. The desired results are more appropriate utilization, better value for dollars spent on health and wellness programs, reductions in absenteeism and presenteeism due to health issues, and deceleration of the upward healthcare cost trend.[1]

There are several models of member* engagement in advocacy and assistance programs. Opt-in, open-ended programs invite health plan members to contact an advocate whenever they have an issue of any sort related to their health care. Other programs analyze claims and other administrative data to identify various clinical populations and proactively target interventions to a specific group.[1]

Because advocacy programs integrate services across multiple vendors and coordinate care between multiple providers, they can improve the efficiency and effectiveness of the medical system and resolve disputes between insurers or administrators of health benefit programs and members. For large employers, these integration opportunities are a means for making their multivendor health benefits programs more accessible to employees.

Helping users navigate the confusing healthcare environment can both improve clinical outcomes and reduce overall healthcare costs. Although health assistance and navigation programs can relieve stress, increase job productivity, and save money by helping patients more readily access qualified providers to receive appropriate care in a timely manner, their value may not be adequately captured by traditional medical claims–based measures of return on investment. By providing vital navigational assistance and support to individuals at their time of need, advocacy and assistance programs can increase consumer engagement in the healthcare system and in the management of their own and their family's health. The results are a greater likelihood of improved medical outcomes and, typically, lower medical costs.

Learning Objectives

1. Examine the forces driving increased demand for health advocacy.
2. Review the different types and varying challenges of health benefits programs offered in different employer market segments.
3. Appreciate consumers' needs for help in navigating the healthcare system.
4. Assess the total value of advocacy and assistance programs.

Key Terms

carve-out	Patient Protection and Affordable Care Act
consumer-driven health care	pharmacy benefit manager
health advocacy and navigation	preferred provider organizations
health advocate	self-insured
healthcare consumerism	third-party administrators

---

*In this chapter, the term *member* is used to indicate an individual eligible for advocacy assistance. In an employer-sponsored program, this could be the employee, covered dependent, or extended family member.

INTRODUCTION

U.S. health care is technologically sophisticated, costly, and systematically disorganized. Our healthcare system offers seemingly limitless options to those who understand how to access care, have the means to pay for it, and possess the wherewithal to make reasonable decisions regarding treatment options. Unfortunately, very few individuals possess *all* of these skills. When a person faces a serious medical condition, it can become overwhelming to navigate and sort through the health information available online and comply with the requirements and provisions of a health insurance program.

Healthcare leaders and managers approach healthcare issues in terms of "populations" to discern patterns (associations and causations) and design interventions that are appropriate to particular subpopulations. It is possible to categorize individuals into various groups based on their characteristics and personal medical circumstances. Patients with diabetes, glaucoma, asthma, or heart disease are viewed by healthcare providers and payers as members of subpopulations with a common condition. One can further stratify these subpopulations by clinical severity or predicted medical cost, or one can create subsets based on medications utilized or type of employer, insurance plan, or providers seen.

Substituting order for chaos somehow reassures us that we can, in some way, target interventions that meet the needs of those who make up these disparate groups. However, from a health advocacy viewpoint, all individuals exist in one of two large populations: those with a healthcare system–associated problem and those at risk for developing a healthcare system–associated problem. Regardless of the group in which individuals find themselves, help in navigating the healthcare system can prove tremendously useful in accessing the appropriate care at the appropriate time, and in managing risk of future problems.

Health advocates encounter two types of consumers within the group that has a healthcare-system associated problem: those who are able to navigate the healthcare maze for a current issue and those who cannot. Health advocacy and assistance programs help those who are "lost" somewhere in the process of dealing with health benefits and receiving medical services. Without assistance, they are unlikely to reach the best possible medical outcome. And, because they use the medical care system inefficiently, they can incur unnecessary costs. As individual HIEs, consumer-directed high-deductible health plans, and defined contribution premium models gain traction, people are expected to participate in a "self-service" healthcare environment, without sufficient skills or guidance to succeed. The consequences of this predicament affect us all through higher healthcare expenditures and premiums, lost work productivity, and poor satisfaction with the healthcare system.

THE PROFESSIONALIZATION OF HEALTH ADVOCACY AND ITS EMERGENCE AS A COMMERCIAL SERVICE

The idea of helping individuals to effectively use the healthcare system is not new. Both the primary care physician (PCP) as gatekeeper model in managed care and today's patient-centered medical home model are designed to go beyond clinical interactions to coordinate care and support patients outside of the "exam room." In addition, some health insurers have taken steps to make their policies and processes more transparent and have improved their clinical and administrative offerings under the umbrella of "member support."[2]

Since the late 1990s, a new category of health advocates has emerged. These individuals and companies offer assistance to consumers for a fee that is paid directly to the advocate or that is a benefit incorporated into an employer or group's health benefits program. An Internet search reveals no shortage of companies and individuals offering some version of health advocacy to the consumer marketplace. Some programs feature nurses or other health professionals who help people through a clinical situation. Others focus on negotiating medical bills to lower out-of-pocket costs and charge the patient a percentage of the savings.[3–7]

For the purposes of this chapter, we will focus on the model that has gained impressive traction (i.e., private sector advocacy companies providing health assistance and navigational support as an employer benefit). This service sector has established its value as a means of helping people deal with myriad health benefits and access issues.[*,2]

Education in the special skills of health advocacy has become widely available through conferences, university-sponsored certificate programs, a few undergraduate degree programs, and at least one master's degree program in health advocacy. The growing number of health advocates has given rise to several professional organizations that support the professional development and interests of advocates. These include the Alliance of Professional Health Advocates and the National Association of Health Advocacy Consultants.[8]

---

*The focus on private sector advocacy companies is not meant to detract from numerous advocacy groups across the country that work in support of changes in social and health policy to benefit individuals with special health needs or chronic conditions, nor is it intended to overlook the role played by advocates or case managers who coordinate care and provide navigation assistance for individual clients and patients in the community. In many ways, the goals of these groups are aligned with those of commercial advocacy and assistance organizations (i.e., helping consumers in their quest for better health). Ideally, all of these programs work in concert with the patient's physicians to reinforce the provider's treatment plan and enhance the opportunity for the individual to receive the best possible health outcome.

GOALS OF ADVOCACY AND ASSISTANCE PROGRAMS

Advocacy programs share several potentially measurable goals that vary according to the priorities of the sponsor (i.e., the entity paying for the advocacy and assistance services). These include:

- Greater percentage of employees enrolled in lifestyle management programs or condition management programs
- High employee satisfaction with advocacy program or with overall benefits program
- Higher percentage of employees utilizing in-network providers
- Number of identified clinical gaps in care closed
- Reduction in employee days lost from work due to personal or family health issues

The astute reader will recognize that there are measurement challenges with these goals (e.g., they may overlap with goals of other coexisting health management programs, turnover in the population may make continuity difficult, and factors such as provider relationships are not held constant).

Employer sponsors may also have broader objectives such as improving employee engagement or changing employee behavior to be more healthcare consumerist and thus reducing cost. Such qualitative goals are even more difficult to measure over the 12-month plan year, around which company budgets and employee benefits are based.

When health advocates work intensively, one on one, with individuals experiencing a healthcare issue, the immediate goal of advocacy is to find a solution to the problem at hand. A secondary goal of advanced advocacy programs is to equip the member with skills to better navigate the healthcare system in the future, as well as skills to better self-manage her or his health and wellness. Whether or not advocacy programs explicitly set out to change consumer behavior, most participants learn from the experience and can apply this learning to future situations. Ultimately, the key objective of advocacy and assistance programs is simply to help people navigate the health system and cope (Boxes 9-1 and 9-2).

STAKEHOLDER PERSPECTIVES ON HEALTH ADVOCACY

THE EMPLOYERS' PERSPECTIVE

At this time, 45% of Americans age 18 years and older obtain health benefits through their employers, while 37% report receiving coverage from another source.[9,10] Overall, 57% of employers offer health benefits, and 91% of those with 50 or more employees do so.[10,11]

BOX 9-1 FACTORS DRIVING CONSUMER DEMAND FOR HEALTH ADVOCACY

- Healthcare cost increases and increasing consumer out-of-pocket cost responsibility
- The complexity of health insurance benefits programs
- Uncertainty about healthcare coverage and access during implementation of healthcare reform
- Consumers being asked to assume greater self-management of health conditions
- Medical care system disorganization and inefficiencies
- Difficulty accessing care and getting timely appointments
- Increasing medical technology and super specialization, with more providers involved in any episode of care
- Information overload
- Increasing consumer focus on quality of care and patient safety
- The difficulty of managing a parent's health issues—employees as caregivers
- Privacy concerns—reticence to consult employer or health plan
- Nowhere else to turn for help

BOX 9-2 FACTORS DRIVING PURCHASER DEMAND FOR HEALTH ADVOCACY

- Healthcare premium increases and increasing consumer out-of-pocket cost responsibility
- Knowledge that employee health benefits programs have more "hoops to jump through" as cost-containment strategy
- Increasing frequency of changes to benefit plans
- Desire to support employees during insurance market changes related to healthcare reform
- Concern about lost productivity of employees due to time spent trying to navigate healthcare system for themselves or a family member
- Desire to support employees/dependents being asked to assume greater responsibility for self-management of health conditions
- More employee complaints due to encountering disorganized medical care
- Need to improve rates of employee engagement in multiple health management programs
- Reduction in human resources staffing levels to support employees, at same time as increasing regulatory demands and complexity of benefit offerings
- Desire to have a neutral third party helping employee to maintain employee privacy around health issues
- Desire to attract and retain best employees

Regardless of the size of the firm, companies are focused on the cost of health benefits. They seek to buy health benefits within a budgeted allocation, and, to the degree that it can be measured, they want the best value for the price. Employers understand that good health benefits encourage good employee health, reduce absenteeism, increase productivity, and provide an effective tool for attracting new employees and retaining existing ones. However, in a slowing economy and a competitive global business environment, businesses are forced to take a hard look at the health benefits they offer and to take steps to constrain the seemingly relentless increase in costs.[12] The result of these efforts can be a confusing, multilayered array of benefit packages and programs that become difficult for the average employee to understand and use effectively.

According to the Kaiser Family Foundation, the average health insurance premium for family coverage in 2013 reached $16,351,[11] an increase of 80% since 2003. This rate of rise vastly outpaced average wage increases as well as the overall rate of inflation, productivity, and business profitability.[11,13] In response, more employers are using adjustments in the design of their health benefit offerings to encourage certain employee behaviors that they believe will help control the company's healthcare costs.[14]

When discussing advocacy programs purchased by employers, it is helpful to consider employers on the basis of size, because so many benefit decisions are affected by the number of employees for whom they provide health coverage. For the purposes of this discussion, we will define small employers as those with fewer than 100 employees, the middle market as those employers with 100 to 1,500 employees, and large employers as those with more than 1,500 employees.

In the small employer market, health benefit programs tend to be relatively straightforward. The company is usually insured (i.e., it pays a premium to the insurance company for coverage), and the benefits programs it offers follow one of several standard options offered by the health insurer they choose. The employee benefits options tend to be fewer, and there are typically few supports within the employer's environment to answer complicated benefit questions or deal with coverage or access problems. Small companies rarely have a dedicated human resources or benefits administration staff. This employer segment is most likely to decide to shift employees into the public health insurance exchanges created by the **Patient Protection and Affordable Care Act** (ACA). Employers in this segment that continue to offer health benefits depend on health benefits brokers to help them shop for the best available (and typically least expensive) coverage, and to support their needs after the purchase. While some small employers seek advocacy support independently, they are more likely to obtain it through employer coalitions or through their brokers.

The middle market is a bit more complicated. Depending on the cost of health insurance on an insured or premium basis in a particular market, companies with 200 or fewer employees may decide to be **self-insured**. They contract with an administrator, which may be a health insurer or a **third-party administrator**, to administer their health benefits programs and pay claims using the plan's underlying contracts. While largely a broker-driven employer segment, health benefits consultants also compete for the business of servicing these accounts.

With self-insurance comes the ability to craft a benefits program unique to the perceived needs of the company or organization, which may not align with the needs or desires of the employees. Thus, we begin to see the introduction of **carve-outs**—health benefits services that are provided by a separate company from the company's basic health coverage. Pharmacy benefits are commonly provided using this carve-out approach. Employers that carve out their pharmacy benefits typically contract with a **pharmacy benefit manager** to administer the prescription drug coverage program. These programs promote the use of mail-order pharmacies and are structured around a cost-advantaged formulary that encourages the use of less expensive brand and generic drugs. They feature multiple tiers of copays and several layers of step edits and precertification requirements. It is easy to see how customized benefits and carve-outs can complicate simple consumer tasks, such as getting a prescription filled.[15] Employers in the middle market look to health advocacy support for their employees to balance this extra navigational complexity.

Nearly all large employers are self-insured, and their benefits packages typically include an array of programs purchased from multiple unrelated benefits vendors, a so-called "best of breed" approach. In addition to the health plan administrator (more likely to be a health plan than a third-party administrator in the largest end of this market segment), one commonly sees carve-out pharmacy benefit managers, mental health managers, disease management programs, general case managers, cancer case managers, transplant case managers, an employee assistance program, a telephonic nurse triage service, and a wellness program in addition to the expected dental plan, workers' compensation, and short-term and long-term disability management programs. Sometimes these different vendor relationships are managed by the health plan and are presented as the plan's services, but large employer benefits programs can include more than 20 different vendors that provide some aspect of employee health benefits.[16]

In reality, there are many examples of well intentioned benefit designs (i.e., intended to ensure appropriate cost-effective utilization) that create increased hassle and confusion for employees. Consider the following:

- Limited pharmacy formularies encourage the use of preferred brands and generic drugs, which offer lower cost and equivalent efficacy to branded products but introduce complexity into the simple process of getting a prescription filled.
- Mail-order drug programs reduce costs but require physicians to write a prescription for a 90-day supply and place the responsibility on the consumer for reordering the medication before the supply runs out and therapy is interrupted.
- Mental health provider networks may get more people into care by facilitating appointments with less highly trained and less expensive professionals, but may also make access to traditional psychiatric care more difficult for those who need it.

- Disease management and case management programs help individuals with chronic conditions focus on strategies to improve their health, but may be disconnected from the patients' relationship with their treating physician.
- In their quest to get an injured worker back to work as soon as possible, disability management and workers' compensation programs may paradoxically increase the likelihood that injured workers receive surgery and other aggressive therapies rather than allowing time for conservative treatment to work.[17–20]

Despite the ability of sophisticated large employers and their consultants to select the best employee benefit programs, they are commonly frustrated by low rates of employee utilization of these valuable programs. Because advocates are aware of all the programs, they proactively guide employees and their dependents to the appropriate program for their needs. Adding an advocacy and assistance program helps employers to get value out of all the other benefit programs.

It is little wonder that advocacy and assistance programs have gained popularity among employers of all sizes to assist as a means of helping employees to navigate the healthcare system. Employers see advocacy programs as supplementing their constrained internal resources while they manage complex benefits that often change on an annual basis.

THE CONSUMER'S PERSPECTIVE—CONSUMER-DRIVEN HEALTHCARE

While many employers offer a choice of plans, **preferred provider organization** (PPO) plans that include in- and out-of-network options continue to be the dominant choice of employees, holding a steady proportion of 50% to 60% of covered workers since 2010.[11] Compared to an HMO model, with only an in-network benefit, or a traditional indemnity plan with broadly inclusive provider coverage, PPO benefit designs introduce an increased level of complexity. More narrow networks within networks are increasingly the norm, and individuals are left to deal with unpredictable charges and balance billing from partially or completely out-of-network providers. Even for care delivered in network, health benefit programs are increasingly shifting costs to the consumer in the form of higher payroll contributions, larger deductibles, greater coinsurance responsibilities, and benefit limitations and exclusions. This trend is shown by the fact that average monthly premium contributions for employer-sponsored family coverage have increased over 250% from 1999 to 2013 and the majority of plans today, including those offered in the public HIEs, include sizeable annual deductibles for both individuals and families.[11]

Health plan designs with a high annual deductible paired with savings arrangements (i.e., health reimbursement arrangements or health savings accounts) have been dubbed **consumer-driven health care**, with the hope that consumers' increased financial contribution will encourage them to take a greater role in making healthcare decisions and managing their own health. The lever is the higher out-of-pocket cost for the consumer. The belief is that if people have to spend more of their own money on health care they will spend it more wisely.[14,21] Many emphasize the potential of these programs to motivate individuals to be more conscious of their health and the impact of lifestyle choices, believing that consumers will take better care of themselves to avoid preventable health expenses in the future.[22] Compared to the past, when insured consumers were completely insulated from the costs of healthcare services they received, there is now a reason to care about prices and another reason to consult an advocate.

As yet, the long-term population health impacts of high-deductible health plans are unknown. Regardless of the health outcomes, shifting costs to employees and requiring them to be more engaged in managing their own health is an approach that continues to gain traction. In fact, as of 2013, 23% of all firms offering health benefits included one of these consumer-directed models as an option, and 20% of covered workers were enrolled in them.[11]

Along with a greater role in managing their own healthcare spending, consumers are expected to be more actively involved in healthcare decision making. Consumers are being encouraged to seek out multiple opinions on treatment, and, gradually, a greater acceptance of the consumer's role in comparing the cost, quality, and safety of healthcare providers is emerging. However, the availability and utility of tools to help consumers function as informed users of the healthcare system (so-called transparency tools) is fairly limited. Quality comparisons between facilities and individual physicians are often restricted to certain diagnoses or procedures, or use data that no longer reflect current practice. Cost transparency tools may be difficult to use or lack features relevant to a consumer's actual health insurance coverage. One would have to conclude that today's healthcare system is far from transparent.

Finding quality provider information applicable to one's needs, discussing billing issues with a hospital, appealing a denial of coverage, finding qualified physicians, getting appointments with specialists, understanding what is said at a doctor's visit, and evaluating the validity of information from the Internet are daunting tasks, and dealing with them creates great consumer frustration. Advocacy and assistance programs are a good fit in all of these situations, providing support to help individuals organize information, interpret policies, and navigate care delivery and payment systems. For example, when a patient receives conflicting advice, an independent advocate can coach the patient on the right questions to learn the rationale for different approaches and support the individual through the decision process.

THE PHYSICIAN'S PERSPECTIVE

U.S. healthcare provider training has an intense focus on clinical information and generally overlooks the more practical aspects of health care (e.g., office practice management, insurance benefit design), leaving most physicians unprepared to deal with their patients' health benefit issues. As healthcare practices join multiple insurance provider networks with differing administrative rules, physicians must add staff (e.g., to handle billing, precertification approvals, and various treatment protocols), thus increasing their overhead.

Although most physicians are willing to help their patients deal with administrative issues, they have neither the time nor the expertise to do so, and, typically, healthcare reimbursement does not reward providers for time spent on these activities. Even physicians who are willing to make a reasonable effort to assist patients with a formulary exception or to obtain coverage for medical equipment tend to drop out of the process when the problem becomes too time intensive, leaving patients to deal with it on their own. As a consequence, physicians have become supporters of health advocacy and assistance programs. They recognize that these programs support the medical home concept and reinforce the patient–physician relationship.

Many specific activities of advocates support coordination of care and help patients follow the provider's treatment plan. For example:

- Collecting the patient's prior treatment records and reports
- Locating primary care physicians in the health plan network for patients without one
- Locating appropriate specialists in the health plan network for specific clinical issues
- Guiding the patient to the most cost-effective source of prescription medication prescribed by the provider
- Interpreting and reinforcing the physician's treatment plan
- Assisting the patient in resolving coverage issues with the insurer and returning the patient's focus to treatment and removing stress
- Helping the patient enroll in disease management and wellness programs

Although some physicians assume that every instruction given to a patient in the exam room will be remembered and followed, astute physicians realize that the limited face-to-face encounter with the patient is insufficient to address all the barriers (behavioral and administrative) to patient adherence. Thus, doctors understand the value of the help and support offered by advocacy and assistance companies because it is similar to what they would do for a patient if time permitted.

THE PERSPECTIVE OF HEALTH PLANS AND ADMINISTRATORS

While all health plans have customer or member service departments, several commercial health plans have added their own advocacy programs. These programs primarily focus on issues involving the plan's network, benefits, and programs. As enhancements to their member assistance and clinical management services, they may provide a competitive market advantage by positioning the insurer or third-party administrator as a high-touch health plan of choice. A few health plans have added advocacy to select segments of their businesses to attract and retain customers. In the Medicare Advantage arena, several plans have incorporated advocacy to help seniors—who may be new to managed care—to navigate and access care. Under the present Medicare Stars reimbursement model, this assistance can accrue to the plan's benefit by increasing compliance with recommended care, improving plan performance, and increasing government payments.

Advocacy provided by a health plan faces two major challenges. First, consumers generally mistrust health plans. In the Kaiser Family Foundation's April 2004 health poll, two-thirds of consumers said that they were "very worried" or "somewhat worried" that their health plan was more concerned about saving money than providing the right treatment for its members.[23] In an earlier study, almost half of the adult health plan members surveyed reported having a problem with their health plan in the previous year.[24] If the advocacy program is perceived as working for the health plan, and therefore part of the problem, the member may be reluctant to utilize the program or to provide complete information to the advocate.

Second, to be effective, advocates must interface with multiple providers, health plans, and other health support programs objectively, on the member's behalf. An experienced advocate understands the member's array of benefits and services and the specific employer policies, and can quickly get to the root of the problem. Thus, health plans sponsoring advocacy programs may choose to position the program as a separate entity (e.g., using a different phone number or different branding). In this way, member interactions are typically free of the acrimony that might exist if the members contacted the plan directly, and the advocacy staff members can spend their interaction time dealing with the members' navigation issues rather than handling their dissatisfaction with the health plan. Although the advocate's answer is frequently the same one the member would receive from the health plan, it is more likely to be well received, trusted, and acted upon when it has come from a source perceived to be working on the member's behalf.

ENGAGEMENT MODELS IN COMMERCIAL HEALTH ADVOCACY SERVICES

There is no shortage of individuals and organizations offering health advocacy–related services. Depending on your search engine and Internet speed, typing "health advocate" into the search engine yields between 1 million and 27 million hits in English in under 0.40 second![25] However, the commercial **health advocacy and navigation** marketplace is dominated by a handful of companies that sell their services, primarily to employers and health plans to help employees and family members navigate the healthcare system. Several reasons for the limited number of commercially successful healthcare advocacy firms include:

- The need for broad availability to consumers at any time for a huge array of healthcare needs
- The extensive ongoing investment in expert staff hiring, training, and development; information systems; and communications

Advocacy programs must be available to individuals in their time of need, regardless of the circumstances. Opt-in advocacy and assistance programs encourage those eligible to reach out to the advocate for help at any time they face a health issue. There is only partial ability to predict when such needs will arise and who will have them, so the availability of health advocacy support must be repeatedly communicated throughout the year to increase the likelihood that the employee, plan member, or consumer will remember to contact the advocate when she or he has an issue. A broad message of "We'll help with anything," encourages consumer participation.

Increasingly, advocacy programs are developing predictive models based on administrative data (e.g., medical and pharmacy claims, laboratory result values, self-reported health risk assessments) to anticipate member needs. One use of this information is to target outbound communications to those members most likely to benefit from health navigation and to tailor the type of outreach and support. While predictive models have more often been associated with disease management programs, advocacy programs that work across large populations can also benefit from this approach to develop customized outbound communications.

In addition, medical history and health risk information about members can be made available to advocates at the time of a member's inbound call through prepopulating software platforms used by advocates. This allows the advocate to opportunistically offer additional support (e.g., disease management, wellness, preventive services, referral to employee assistance program) that matches with the member's clinical situation. Even if the initial contact was for an unrelated issue, the ability to provide a broader degree of support and clinical integration and close identified gaps in care extends the impact of advocacy interactions and is more likely to get to the root of the problem that inspired the call to the advocacy program.

Outbound engagement models encounter problems familiar to other population health programs using healthcare claims data (i.e., the information typically reflects past events, and its ability to predict future needs is imperfect at best). In addition, sending any outbound communication—whether by phone, e-mail, postal mail, or text—to a consumer who is not "activated" or motivated to respond has repeatedly proven costly and inefficient.

Ultimately, effective health navigation and advocacy combine both inbound and outbound engagement approaches, but round-the-clock inbound availability of broad and deep advocate expertise is the tested model of independent advocacy services.

A MATTER OF TRUST

Trust is an important component of any population health intervention. With trust, healthcare consumers are more likely to engage and to change suboptimal behaviors. As mentioned previously, a key advantage of health advocacy and assistance programs that are not associated with health plans is their independence. They can be viewed as a trusted party by patients and family members. Information provided to advocacy programs must be strictly protected in accordance with the Health Insurance Portability and Accountability Act (HIPAA) requirements.[26] Users typically sign a release allowing the advocate to represent them in dealing with physicians, hospitals, and health plans. Moreover, none of the individual's protected health information is ever shared with the health plan or the employer without the individual's explicit permission.

Advocacy programs create personal relationships between users and advocates. This bond is founded on trust and instills confidence that the advocate's only motive is to get the right answer for the user. In many cases, there is a difference between the correct answer and what the consumer may have wanted to hear. It is not surprising that people often want services that are not covered by their health plans or want to pay less out of their own pockets than their benefits program requires. The advocate is often called upon to explain that the issue is not one of medical necessity but one of medical coverage, or that the problem is not the plan's failure to pay a claim properly but the member's responsibility for paying a deductible or copayment.

Health advocates try to help members find the most appropriate provider for a required service. Advocates can explore the level of experience a provider has with a particular clinical condition, or the cost of treatment, by asking questions that a prospective patient is uncomfortable asking. Advocates can research and assist members to access community resources or compassionate care programs for needed services or medications that are not covered under the consumer's health benefits. Taking these extra steps is an important part of being the individual's true advocate.

WHAT HELP DO HEALTHCARE CONSUMERS NEED?—LESSONS FROM ADVOCACY DATA

Most people who have access to a health advocacy and navigation service do not use these assistance programs when measured over the course of a year as a stand-alone program. In fact, 17% of adults do not have contact with any healthcare professional in a given year.[27] For the vast majority of those who do, the health system works as intended, or if a medical or billing issue arises, they can either resolve it on their own or accept a certain level of dissatisfaction. Despite increasing criticism about the non-patient-centric nature of our healthcare system, most consumers choose to address issues on their own.

So, who does choose to use the help of an advocate and what type of help do they need? Utilization varies significantly across employers and is greatly influenced by communications promoting the service as well as changes occurring in benefit plans. In general, advocacy programs serve about 6% to 10% of the families in large companies and 10% to 15% in small companies.[28] This reflects that the fact that larger companies often have more staff in their internal benefits departments to assist employees. Overall, the reasons consumers use advocacy programs reflect changes in an employer's benefit design and circumstances in the local medical delivery system. When companies change health insurers, requests for help finding new in-network providers increase. When plan designs are altered, benefit questions spike. When specialized care is unavailable locally, members are more likely to ask for help finding qualified experts elsewhere. The rate of member utilization of advocacy can also be influenced by the positioning of advocacy services in the overall employer benefit design. For example, channeling calls for multiple employee services through a single point of access dramatically increases engagement rates. Many employers offer employee incentives to participate in wellness programs or chronic condition support services that can be accessed by calling the all-purpose advocacy/navigation service, thus driving additional employee engagement.

From a population health standpoint, meaningful insights can be gained from reviewing the reasons consumers contact an advocate for assistance. Approximately 60% of all initial reasons given by consumers for contacting advocacy programs today are related to an administrative issue. This is partly driven by the accelerated pace of changes in benefit designs over the past several years, which has increased the complexity of dealing with health benefits.

Administrative issues include questions about or problems with a bill, a benefit, a denial of coverage, an appeal, a grievance, or a referral. (See Figures 9-1 through 9-3.) Any of these can get in the way of people dealing health issues, and contact with an advocate typically occurs during treatment or after the individual has received care.

The remaining first calls are driven by direct health needs (e.g., the need for health information, problems accessing care, finding a new doctor, identifying an appropriate specialist, arranging second opinions). Questions about physician interactions and the need to locate community-based resources are also included in this group. Help dealing with senior care issues is a common need. Interestingly, considering the greater share of healthcare costs coming out of pocket from the consumer, requests for information about the price of medical care that has not already been delivered represent a relatively small fraction of the calls. As pricing transparency tools become more prevalent, it remains to be seen whether they will meet consumers' needs or generate more assistance requests to advocates.

As advocacy services have developed, it has become apparent that focusing narrowly on the reason for the patient's initial call results in many missed opportunities to help with underlying medical issues and influence consumer health behavior. For example, employees may call after receiving a bill for a service that they believe was processed incorrectly. Typically, the advocate assesses the bill from the standpoint of the service provided, how it was billed, how it was adjudicated, and how the adjudication was applied to the provisions of the individual's benefits policy. In the case of an error, the advocate

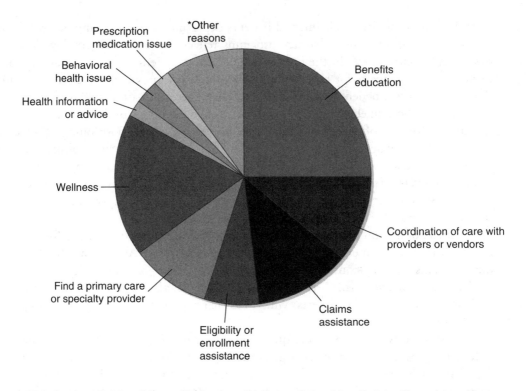

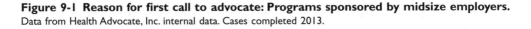

*"Other" category includes: Eldercare, Genitourinary, Respiratory, Serious Injury, Podiatry, Rheumatology, Allergy, Plastic/Reconstructive, Rheumatology, Sleep Disorders

Figure 9-1 Reason for first call to advocate: Programs sponsored by midsize employers.
Data from Health Advocate, Inc. internal data. Cases completed 2013.

attempts to facilitate correction of the problem. But, resolving the billing issue will not address the health problem that led to the healthcare transaction.

Other people inquire about a benefit and usually do so because they either have used or anticipate using the benefit in the near future. Using their experience and listening skills, health advocates can anticipate other needs the member may have. For example, a woman calling about the company's maternity benefit is probably pregnant, contemplating getting pregnant, or has recently delivered a child. During the benefit discussion, there is a teachable moment to talk about selecting an in-network obstetrician or a pediatrician, address any outstanding questions about pregnancy and child care, and guide the woman into a prenatal care program. Similarly, an inquiry about a bill for emergency room care for asthma is an opportunity for the advocate to confirm that the member has a physician helping her or him to manage the asthma and to offer help with scheduling follow-up appointments, coordinating more affordable

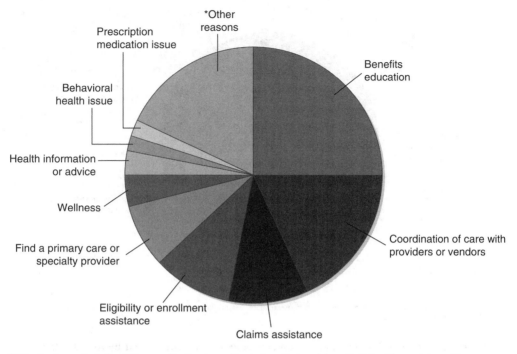

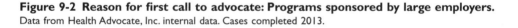

*"Other" category includes: Eldercare, Genitourinary, Respiratory, Serious Injury, Podiatry, Rheumatology, Allergy, Plastic/Reconstructive, Rheumatology, Sleep Disorders

Figure 9-2 Reason for first call to advocate: Programs sponsored by large employers.
Data from Health Advocate, Inc. internal data. Cases completed 2013.

prescriptions, and referring the patient for additional support (e.g., an asthma disease management program).

Data and information systems can facilitate these broader encounters by analyzing past medical claims, use of medications, lab results, and self-reported health information to develop a personal profile of the individual. This information helps in identifying ongoing needs and gaps in care in a manner that encourages a discussion of additional issues at the time of engagement. Using data in this way allows for the potential to convert every consumer–advocate contact into a broader discussion of a health issue and add value to the role of health advocacy.

In some cases, the reasons for health-related calls involve relatively simple problems (e.g., acute care services that will likely have no further consequences). However, as demonstrated in Figure 9-4, many reasons are related to chronic conditions or other ongoing needs, and the opportunity to intervene can have a dramatic effect on the future care of the individual.

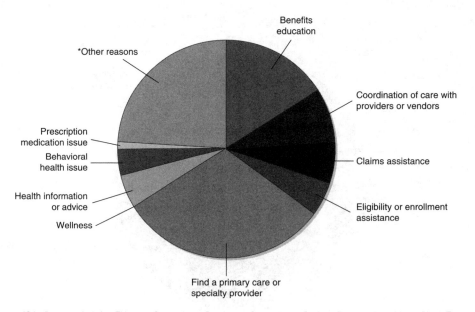

*"Other" category includes: Eldercare, Genitourinary, Respiratory, Serious Injury, Podiatry, Rheumatology, Allergy, Plastic/Reconstructive, Rheumatology, Sleep Disorders

Figure 9-3 Reason for first call to advocate: Programs sponsored by health plans.
Data from Health Advocate, Inc. internal data. Cases completed 2013.

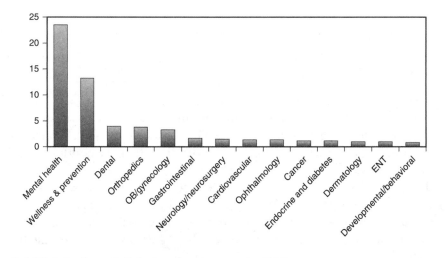

Figure 9-4 Distribution of clinical support requests, 2013.
Data from Health Advocate, Inc. internal data. Cases completed 2013.

ADVOCACY AND ACCESS TO QUALITY HEALTH CARE

One of the most common requests for assistance is help with finding a doctor. Ensuring that consumers have a relationship with a primary care medical home is foundational to improving population health, and advocates play a key role in promoting access to primary care. Although most consumers have difficulty communicating the attributes of what they consider to be a good doctor, studies have shown that consumers judge the value of the medical care they receive based on the provider's communication style, interpersonal skills, and availability.[29]

Many health plans now make some provider quality and cost information available, and federal and state agencies are beginning to report comparative quality data. In the present form, the data are not very useful to the average consumer.[30] Most published information pertains to facilities, with relatively little pertaining to individual physicians. Consumers may wrongly assume that a lower-cost provider is a lower-quality provider.[31] Limited health literacy and comfort with healthcare statistics may challenge consumers who are trying to interpret provider performance numbers. Thus, the personal interaction found in advocacy programs can be key to helping consumers understand what information is relevant to their conditions and important when choosing a physician or hospital.

The most frequent requests for help with finding a physician involve finding "common" physicians. It is more difficult to find and apply quality criteria to discriminate among the many providers of common care than it is to locate highly specialized providers. One can start by checking the doctor's credentials, training, society memberships, and years of experience. The fact that a physician is in a health plan's network can be taken as a sign that he or she has passed the plan's credentialing review, and public databases can be searched for sanctions.

Beyond checking these characteristics, the advocate can identify what members want and what characteristics they are looking for in a doctor (e.g., man or woman, group practice or solo practice, evening hours, languages spoken, hospital preference). These objective criteria can be used to define the member's view of a desirable doctor. Similar criteria may be useful in finding the best provider match for a specialist with availability that meets the member's health needs. A match is made against the member's criteria, and several options are developed and presented to the member. Depending on the member's preference, appointments are scheduled, records transferred, and referrals and authorizations facilitated.

The process is similar when identifying specialists who deal with unusual clinical conditions. Although the conditions presented may be of greater urgency and compel the advocate to complete the search quickly, the advocate can seek out information about the proficiency of specific physicians and hospitals in the context of a particular medical condition. Advocates are adept at researching comparative provider information from health plans or in the public domain to identify experts in the particular field in different locations.

COORDINATION OF CARE ACROSS THE SPECTRUM—PROVIDERS AND BENEFIT PROGRAMS

Health advocates are skilled at making connections across multiple benefit programs. To illustrate this point, consider the case of a parent who called for assistance because she received a balance bill from an out-of-network emergency room physician who treated her 5-year-old son for an asthma attack at an in-network hospital. After obtaining a HIPAA-compliant release, the health advocate examined the physician's bill, the employer's health benefit documents, and how the plan paid the claim. In this case, the emergency room physician's services should have been processed at an in-network level of benefit because the employer's plan design stated that the participation status of the hospital would govern how bills from out-of-network physicians would be adjudicated. Correcting the mistake reduced the member's payment from $350 to $50, the amount of her emergency room copay, and ostensibly satisfied the parent's reason for calling.

But what about the child's underlying clinical needs? There was an opportunity to explore the poorly controlled asthma that sent the child to the emergency room in the first place. Building on the trust developed by resolving the billing issue, the advocate was able to confirm that the member had an in-network provider and to enroll the child in the asthma management program offered by the health plan. If no asthma program had been available, the clinical advocate could have provided the family with educational information about asthma, discussed common management strategies and proper use of medications, obtained an expedited appointment with the child's physician, and prepared the parent for the discussion with the doctor. The advocate might even have contacted the doctor's office in advance to alert the physician of the child's impending visit and his history and needs and coordinated any required lab tests or x-rays before the visit to make the physician encounter more useful.

There are many opportunities to save dollars through the entry point of navigational assistance and advocacy support. Even in seemingly straightforward claims or administrative issues, recognizing clinical opportunities increases the opportunity for advocacy services to save future medical costs. Addressing these otherwise hidden clinical opportunities allows employers to maximize the value of their benefit programs, increase the effectiveness of other care management programs, and improve medical outcomes.

Realizing the pivotal care coordination role of advocates, many large employers with benefits programs involving multiple vendors now position health advocacy programs as a gateway to all of the employee benefits programs and services offered. The obvious advantage of this "800-Call-Advocate" model is that employees need to remember only one phone number. After discussing the case with the employee, the health advocate links him or her to the correct service provider. In this personal, single-point-of-contact model, the advocate functions as a case coordinator, helping individuals navigate both the health system and the benefit environment.

Using the previous case illustration, an advocate could connect the 5-year-old asthma patient to an in-network allergist for evaluation. After the visit, the advocate may coordinate services with the health plan's case managers, speak to the plan-affiliated durable medical equipment supplier, and enroll the child in an asthma disease management program. If the child's illness resulted in the mother's missing work, the advocate can contact the employer to help ensure coverage could make arrangements under the Family and Medical Leave Act (FMLA).

It is easy to see how intertwined the system is and how difficult it can be for a patient who is struggling with a health issue. This single, seemingly straightforward and common case could involve the child and his family, an emergency room physician, the hospital that operates the emergency room, the pediatrician, an allergist, a disease management nurse, the case manager at the health plan, a durable medical equipment provider, the company's benefits administrator for FMLA approvals, the carve-out pharmacy benefits administrator, and a query of the health plan's claims system. A serious or complex illness—or having both private and public insurance—could magnify the complexity many times. Is it any wonder that people find the healthcare system difficult to navigate?

HEALTHCARE CONSUMERISM AND HEALTH ADVOCACY

The implied hope of consumer-driven health plans (i.e., high-deductible benefit designs) is that consumer behavior can be changed in ways that will lower costs and improve the quality of care.[32] These models embrace the belief that consumers who bear a greater share of healthcare costs and spending can be motivated to assume greater responsibility for managing their own care. If the hope is realized, consumers will make smarter and more informed decisions about the care they receive and the professionals and hospitals from whom they receive it.

The RAND studies of the 1970s offer good documentation that consumers who are asked to pay more money out of pocket get less care.[33] There is also evidence that consumers do not discriminate well between care they need and care that is unnecessary when making these decisions.[34] New studies reveal that activated or engaged patients have improved health outcomes and that some may also have lower healthcare costs.[35] But after decades of insulating consumers from healthcare costs and market forces, simply shifting cost to the consumer will not automatically create activated, smarter healthcare consumers, nor does it make the system more transparent or easier to navigate.

Consumers who function well in a consumer-driven model and who embrace self-management tools differ from the overall consumer population. They appear to be more motivated or activated from the start and are innately better prepared to manage their own health.[22] Advocates can play an important role in helping the remainder of the population function better in a consumer-driven environment—by helping them find and use information for comparing provider cost, quality, and safety, and by coaching them to be active questioners of their providers. (See box 9-3.) As **healthcare consumerism** becomes the norm, advocacy and assistance programs can provide timely support to those who need help with navigating the healthcare system.

BOX 9-3 HOW HEALTH ADVOCATES PROMOTE HEALTHCARE CONSUMERISM

- Help individuals find and interpret medical information about their condition
- Prepare individuals for provider encounters
- Help individuals find and use comparative quality and safety information about providers
- Assist individuals to find the most cost-effective source of treatment
- Obtain cost information and negotiate price of services

THE PATIENT PROTECTION AND AFFORDABLE CARE ACT—IMPLICATIONS FOR THE FUTURE OF HEALTH ADVOCACY

The ACA includes several provisions that support the concept of health advocacy. In particular, the law provided funding to expand upon existing state programs that assist consumers with private health insurance. One stated goal was to foster nationwide support to consumers in navigating issues of coverage, eligibility, enrollment in health plans, and appeals of claims or coverage denials. Another goal was to study the outcomes of this assistance program. The appropriation was modest—$30 million in the first round of funding in 2010–2011—and only state agencies were permitted to apply. Ultimately, 33 states utilized this initial funding. Experience showed that slightly more than one third (36%) of the people utilizing these state-run programs received "information or referral," whereas the remainder received advocacy support.[36]

The shift of health plan purchasing responsibility to consumers created a greater consumer need for assistance in accessing coverage on state and federal HIEs. Recognizing this, the ACA authorized funding for "navigators," unrelated to insurers, who would be trained to promote availability of insurance exchanges and premium tax credits to consumers and facilitate their enrollment in qualified health plans. These navigators specifically do not have a role in resolving issues for consumers already enrolled in a health plan or for consumers having a specific health issue.[37] Although the ACA greatly raised general awareness of the term "navigator," it narrowed the definition in comparison with health advocacy–type navigators in the private realm.

The rollout of HIEs in late 2013 was marred by technical issues and, more importantly, by ineffective communication to affected populations. Looking ahead, subject to the political landscape, the individual mandate should become more effective, and a greater proportion of individuals will seek coverage through the HIEs. Driven by the ACA, this movement may be a cultural tipping point for health advocacy in that personal responsibility to seek and evaluate benefits annually will become the norm for more

Americans. As choices proliferate, so will complexity, and consumers will need neutral counsel and assistance to navigate the process. As more consumers utilize and become satisfied customers of advocacy and assistance services, they may share their experiences and drive additional demand.

The patient-centered medical home (PCMH) movement also got a boost with the funding of several medical home pilot programs of the ACA. It is fair to say that if all individuals were cared for by mature medical home practices adhering to all the of PCMH principles (i.e., whole-person orientation, patient centeredness, coordination of care, focus on quality and safety, enhanced patient access), there would be less need for external health advocate support. However, the medical home movement is not the dominant care model at present, and it does not include a heavy focus on navigating the administrative issues facing patients.

Accountable care organizations (ACOs) are increasingly common healthcare delivery models. Supported by the ACA for Medicare members and by commercial health plans more widely, there were almost 400 (commercial and Medicare) such practice organizations as of 2014. Each ACO is accountable for the financial and clinical outcomes of its population through complex contracts with payers. To be effective, ACOs face a long list of clinical integration tasks, including cultural transformation, data integration, and focus on overall long-term population health. Eventually, ACOs will, by necessity, have to incorporate aspects of navigation and advocacy assistance to ensure that patients access the right care at the right time, and no more or less. Although some early interest exists, it is too soon to say whether and when ACOs will become sponsors of health advocacy programs—and whether they will help consumers with the many issues and healthcare interactions individuals face beyond the limits of their ACO provider networks.

CONCLUSION

As the United States embarks on a multiyear journey of incremental reforms to its healthcare delivery and payment system, certain needs remain obvious. Employers will continue to struggle with their role in providing health benefits to employees until some way of constraining the explosive increases in healthcare costs is found. Companies that choose to continue offering health insurance benefits will have no option but to increase the share that employees must pay for their health coverage and to increasingly tie health behaviors to this coverage through incentive programs and other strategies. As a result, individuals will increasingly be required to assume greater responsibility for managing their own health. Health advocacy and assistance programs provide support to these individuals in navigating the healthcare environment. By providing help at the consumer's moment of need, these programs are optimally placed to help people make better healthcare choices. The efforts of advocates support healthcare consumerism. Their interactions with individuals provide a framework for educating participants to make wiser medical and lifestyle decisions, leading to better medical outcomes and value for the consumer and the payer.

STUDY AND DISCUSSION QUESTIONS

1. What considerations are driving increased consumer and employer demand for advocacy support?
2. How does a company's size influence its use of advocacy and assistance in its overall employee benefits program?
3. Compare the advantages and disadvantages of data-driven versus opt-in advocacy programs.
4. What can we learn from patterns of health advocacy program utilization?
5. How will the ACA impact navigation and advocacy?

SUGGESTED READINGS AND WEBSITES

READINGS

Herzlinger RE, ed. *Consumer Driven Health Care: Implications for Providers, Payers, and Policymakers.* Hoboken, NJ: John Wiley & Sons; 2004.

WEBSITES

American Medical Association. White paper on patient navigators. https://www.ama-assn.org/ama/pub/advocacy/topics/health-insurance-market-reforms.page. Accessed October 7, 2014.

Health Advocate website: www.healthadvocate.com. Accessed October 7, 2014.

Kaiser Family Foundation. 2013 Employer Health Benefits Survey. http://kff.org/private-insurance/report/2013-employer-health-benefits/. Accessed October 7, 2014.

Kaiser Family Foundation. Healthcare Costs. http://kff.org/health-costs/ Accessed January 21, 2015.

The Center for Health Affairs. The Emerging Field of Patient Navigation. http://www.chanet.org/TheCenterForHealthAffairs/MediaCenter/NewsReleases/~/media/A92355F0A6E140F1A13493BC3C349CAB.ashx. Accessed October 7, 2014.

REFERENCES

1. Leibowitz A. The role of health advocacy in disease management. *Dis Manag.* 2005:8:141-3.
2. Cigna Newsroom. Cigna introduces new service model that pairs individuals with a personal health advocate; making it easier to be healthy. http://newsroom.cigna.com/article_display.cfm?article_id=933&. Accessed October 7, 2014.
3. The Karis Group. http://www.thekarisgroup.com/index.html. Accessed October 7, 2014.
4. My Medical Negotiator. https://www.mymedicalnegotiator.com. Accessed October 7, 2014.
5. Alderman A. After a diagnosis, someone to help point the way. *New York Times*, September 11, 2009. http://www.nytimes.com/2009/09/12/health/12patient

.html?_r=1&scp=1&sq=patient%20advocates&st=cse. Accessed October 7, 2014.

6. Gerencher, K. Advocates can help. *Wall Street Journal*, April 17, 2011. http://online.wsj.com/news/articles/SB100014240527487044879045762675033361027560. Accessed October 7, 2014.

7. Tergesen, A. Help navigating health-care system. *Wall Street Journal*, August 15, 2012. http://online.wsj.com/news/articles/SB10000872396390444443504577603140897758680. Accessed October 7, 2014.

8. The Alliance of Professional Health Advocates. http://www.healthadvocateprograms.com/index.htm. National Association of Healthcare Advocacy Consultants. http://nahac.memberlodge.com/. Both accessed October 7, 2014.

9. Kaiser Family Foundation. Health care costs, a primer. http://kff.org/healthcosts/report/health-care-costs-a-primer. Accessed October 7, 2014.

10. Fewer Americans getting health insurance from employer. *Gallup Well-Being*, February 22, 2013. http://www.gallup.com/poll/160676/fewer-americans-getting-health-insurance-employer.aspx. Accessed October 7, 2014.

11. Kaiser Family Foundation and Health Research and Educational Trust. Employer Health Benefits 2013 Annual Survey. http://kaiserfamilyfoundation.files.wordpress.com/2013/08/8465-employer-health-benefits-20132.pdf. Accessed October 7, 2014.

12. Haynes VS. A premium sucker punch. *The Washington Post*, January 25, 2009: F1. http://www.washingtonpost.com/wp-dyn/content/article/2009/01/24/AR2009012400181.html. Accessed October 7, 2014.

13. Arnst C. CEOs secretly want health-care reform. *BusinessWeek*, May 6, 2009: 23. http://www.businessweek.com/stories/2009-05-06/ceos-secretly-want-health-care-reform. Accessed October 7, 2014.

14. Bloche MG. Consumer-directed health care. *N Engl J Med*. 2006;355(17):1756-9.

15. California Healthcare Foundation. Navigating the pharmacy benefits marketplace. January 2003. http://www.chcf.org/publications/2003/02/navigating-the-pharmacy-benefits-marketplace. Accessed October 7, 2014.

16. Blumenthal D. Employer-sponsored health insurance in the United States: origins and implications. *N Engl J Med*. 2006;355:82-8.

17. Ray WA, Daugherty JR, Meador K. Effect of a mental health "carve-out" program on the continuity of antipsychotic therapy. *N Engl J Med*. 2003; 348:1885-94.

18. Goldman HH, Frank RG, Burnam MA. Behavioral health insurance parity for federal employees. *N Eng J Med*. 2006;354:1378-86.

19. Stano M. Carve outs: comments on the workshop. *Am J Manag Care*. 1998;4:sp23-6.

20. Blumenthal D, Buntin MB. Carve outs: definition, experience, and choice among candidate conditions. *Am J Manag Care*. 1998;4:sp45-57.

21. Rosenthal MB. What works in a market-oriented health policy? *N Engl J Med*. 2009;360(21): 2157-60.

22. Hibbard JH, Greene J, Tusler M. Plan design and active involvement of consumers in their own healthcare. *Am J Manag Care*. 2008;14(11):729-36.

23. The Kaiser Family Foundation/Harvard School of Public Health. National survey on consumer experiences with and attitudes toward health plans. https://kaiserfamilyfoundation.files.wordpress.com/2013/01/national-survey-on-consumer-experiences-with-health-care-plans-chartpack.pdf. Accessed October 7, 2014.

24. Kaiser Family Foundation. Health poll survey, March/April 2004. http://kaiserfamilyfoundation.files.wordpress.com/2013/01/march-april-2004-kaiser-health-poll-report-survey-selected-findings-on-the-knowledge-and-understanding-of-the-new-medicare-rx-drug-program-toplines.pdf. Accessed October 28, 2014.

25. Google. Available at https://www.google.com/#q=health+advocate. Accessed October 28, 2014.

26. U.S. Department of Health and Human Services. The Health Insurance Portability and Accountability Act (HIPAA). http://www.hhs.gov/ocr/privacy/. Accessed October 7, 2014.

27. Centers for Disease Control and Prevention. Ambulatory care use and physician visits. http://www.cdc.gov/nchs/fastats/physician-visits.htm. Accessed October 28, 2014.

28. Health Advocate Book of Business Internal Analysis, 2013.

29. Robert Wood Johnson Foundation. Consumer beliefs and use of information about health care cost, resource use, and value. October, 2012. http://forces4quality.org/consumer-beliefs-and-use-information-about-health-care-cost-resource-use-and-value-findings-consumer. Accessed October 7, 2014.

30. Sinaiko A, Eastman D, Rosenthal M. How report cards on physicians, physician groups, and hospitals can have greater impact on consumer choices. *Health Aff.* 2012;31(3):602-11.

31. Hibbard JH, Greene J, Sofaer S, et al. An experiment shows that a well-designed report on costs and quality can help consumers choose high-value health care. *Health Aff.* 2012;3:560-8.

32. Dixon A, Greene J, Hibbard J. Do consumer-directed health plans drive change in enrollees' health care behavior? *Health Aff.* 2008;27(4):1120-31.

33. Chernew ME, Newhouse JP. What does the RAND health insurance experiment tell us about the impact of patient cost sharing on health outcomes? *Am J Manag Care.* 2008;14(7):412-14.

34. Reed, M. High-deductible health insurance plans: efforts to sharpen a blunt instrument. *Health Aff.* 2009;28(4):1145-54.

35. Hibbard J, Greene J, Overton V. Patients with lower activation associated with higher costs; delivery systems should know their patients' 'scores.' *Health Aff.* 2013;32(2):216-22.

36. Grob R, Schlesinger M, Davis S, et al. The Affordable Care Act's plan for consumer assistance with insurance moves states forward but remains a work in progress. *Health Aff.* 2013;32(2):347-56.

37. Patient Protection and Affordable Care Act; Exchange Functions: Standards for Navigators and Non-Navigator Assistance Personnel; Consumer Assistance Tools and Programs of an Exchange and Certified Application Counselors-Final Rule. *Federal Register* 78 FR 42823-42862. July 17, 2013. http://www.gpo.gov/fdsys/pkg/FR-2013-07-17/pdf/2013-17125.pdf. Accessed October 7, 2014.

Chapter 10

TRANSITIONS OF CARE

JASON LEE AND BONNIE ZELL

Executive Summary

Connecting the components across the continuum is critical to supporting each patient's journey to maximize his or her health over time.

Population health provides a framework for understanding much that is wrong with the U.S. healthcare system, including difficulties in transitions of care. Its "big picture" perspective derives from integrating ideas about changing how the practice of medicine is organized and how the industry is managed. The extent to which these ideas are resisted is due more to inertia and not wanting to buck the status quo than to lack of evidence that their implementation would, in practice, improve quality and/or reduce costs without diminishing quality. Two (probably related) megatrends run against currents of modern practice and management. First is the fact that 20% of the population accounts for 80% of the costs of health care in any given year. Second is the transformation of the U.S. healthcare system from one that provides acute "sick" care to one that promotes prevention and provides chronic care services with the intent of keeping people out of the hospital. As the chapter unfolds, it will become increasingly apparent that a population health perspective with a focus on chronic care provides key lessons on the need to improve care transitions. Considered along with a patient-centric approach and one that utilizes information technology (IT) connectivity and interoperability, the implications for health reform are both numerous and important for quality and costs.

Learning Objectives

1. Understand the shift from acute care to chronic care management, the associated costs, and the need to address the continuum of care, especially care transitions from home to health care and back to home.
2. Synthesize knowledge of how context and circumstances of the individual and community influence health outcomes and associated medical and societal costs of chronic care.
3. Describe emerging models of chronic care management and delivery of primary care, including new financial models.

Key Terms

accountable care organization

acute care

care transitions

chronic care

hot spotting

models of care delivery

Pareto principle

patient centeredness

population health

patient-centered medical home

self-determination theory

INTRODUCTION

"The **Pareto principle** states that, for many events, roughly 80 percent of the effects come from 20 percent of the causes."[1] This is true for land ownership (i.e., the wealthiest 20% own 80% of the land) and for the distribution of peas in a crop of peapods (i.e., 80% of peas are found in 20% of peapods). But what does this have to do with health care? A great deal, it turns out. The Pareto principle says that in any given year, 20% of the U.S. population will account for about 80% of national healthcare expenditures—and this is true. Even more striking is that a mere 5% of the population accounted for almost 50% of national healthcare expenditures (in 2009, the most recent year for which reliable data are available).[2]

The 80–20 rule has two major implications for how we think about the way healthcare is organized, structured, and financed in the United States. First, if only a small fraction of people use a large amount of healthcare resources, we should strive to know everything we can about each of them to manage their health and control their costs. Second, because relatively little of the healthcare pie is left for the majority of the U.S. population, we should do everything we can to keep people healthy so that they don't require expensive healthcare services. These are two of the key lessons learned from adopting a **population health** perspective.

In 2003, David Kindig and Greg Stoddart described the now widely adopted population health conceptual framework (see Figure 10-1) made up of three pillars: health outcomes, health determinants, and policies and procedures.[3] One of the most striking

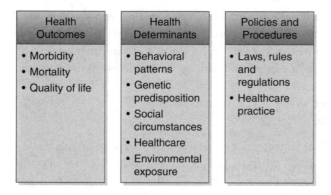

Figure 10-1 Population health conceptual framework.
Data from Kindig, David and Greg Stoddart, "What is Population Health," *Am J Public Health*, v.93(3); Mar 2003, accessed at http://www.ncbi.nlm.nih.gov/pmc/articles/PMC1447747/, March 19, 2014.

observations incorporated in this framework is that of the five health determinants, health care accounts for only 10% of health outcomes.[4]

This framework (and its associated causal model, which holds that health outcomes are directly affected by health determinants and that policies and procedures directly affect health determinants and indirectly affect health outcomes through their effects on health determinants) provides many points of traction for addressing problems with the ailing healthcare system.[5] In addition to the 80–20 rule and its implications, we must recognize that there has been a significant shift in clinical focus. Fifty years ago, the primary activity of doctors was diagnosing and treating acute illnesses; today, the primary activity is managing chronic disease. A distinct but closely overlapping phenomenon with respect to the 80–20 rule is that 75% of healthcare resources are consumed by the care for and consequences of the five major chronic diseases (heart disease, cancer, trauma, mental disorders, pulmonary disorders). Despite this, we continue to deliver health care in a manner that is essentially unchanged from the mid-20th century. We charge separately for each diagnostic test and are reimbursed for pills prescribed and procedures delivered. We perpetuate a system designed to generate profit from illness—a business model that would surely fail if patients were kept healthy.

Many factors perpetuate this outdated model of delivering health care. The underlying premise is one that casts the clinician as the most important actor in the healthcare experience, and the consequences include difficulty in scheduling appointments at times convenient for the average person, challenges in accessing one's personal health information, and a continual fount of mixed messages coming from multiple providers.

Because the transformation of the U.S. healthcare system from one that provides acute sick care to one that provides prevention and **chronic care** management (keeping people out of the hospital) is so radical a change, with implications for change throughout the system, this chapter will examine the transition closely in the context of the population health framework elaborated in this introduction. As the chapter unfolds, it will become increasingly apparent that a population health perspective with a focus on chronic care provides key lessons on the need to improve care transitions. Taken together, the implications for health reform are both numerous and important.[6]

CHRONIC CARE

In the United States, an estimated 125 million people have at least one chronic condition, and half of these people have multiple chronic conditions.[7] This number is expected to rise to 157 million by 2020.[7] The prevalence of chronic disease increases with age; 82% of Medicare beneficiaries have one or more chronic conditions, and 25% have four or more conditions.[8–10] Seventy percent of all deaths are attributable to chronic illnesses. Medicare beneficiaries with four or more chronic conditions are 99% more likely to be hospitalized,[11] and they receive services from 14 different physicians (on average).[7]

Chronic conditions are generally classified as those illnesses and diseases that are expected to persist beyond 1 year and may lead to functional limitations, disability, and the need for long-term medical care. One quarter of persons with chronic disease are limited in their ability to perform basic activities of daily living (ADLs), including bathing, dressing, self-feeding, and toileting. Many more people with chronic conditions struggle to perform those activities classified as instrumental ADLs (IADLs), such as preparing meals; performing household tasks (doing laundry, cleaning, paying bills); using technology, such as telephones, televisions, and computers; shopping; and adhering to medication and treatment schedules.[12] Data from the Medical Expenditure Panel Survey (MEPS) indicate that people with chronic medical conditions require more inpatient hospital care, emergency department visits, and prescription medications, and they utilize more outpatient, community, and home health services than those without chronic conditions.[12]

The effects of chronic illness are experienced at both individual and societal levels in terms of productivity, quality of life, morbidity and mortality, and healthcare costs. Chronic medical conditions typically progress to disability and additional comorbidities. For example, many individuals with advanced diabetes will experience chronic renal failure and partial or complete amputation of an extremity. Among Medicare-eligible patients, management of chronic conditions constitutes a disproportionate level of spending compared to the number of people affected. For example, 14% of Medicare patients suffer from heart failure, yet 43% of all Medicare funding is spent on providing care to heart failure patients. Diabetes is another chronic condition in which a relatively small proportion of Medicare patients (18%) utilize a disproportionate share of spending (32%).[13]

CHRONIC CARE MANAGEMENT, CARE TRANSITIONS, AND COORDINATION OF CARE

It is not surprising that the need for improved chronic care management is one of the major challenges facing the U.S. healthcare system. As the longevity of Americans increases, so does the prevalence of people living with chronic disease. The lifestyle factors of tobacco use, physical inactivity, and weight gain also play a role in the recent increase in the development of chronic conditions at younger ages. Some people with chronic conditions do not receive any health care or receive inadequate care; both result in poor disease control and unnecessary complications and disease morbidity. Improving the coordination of care and services is a critical challenge and a goal in many reform efforts.

Patients without access to, or dissatisfied with, primary care services have drifted toward specialty care. The resultant multiplicity of providers increases the complexity and fragmentation of health care, which, in turn, increases the cost of care without sufficient evidence of improved disease status. While evidence of better outcomes is apparent when a specialist is consulted for an acute problem, the same has not proven true for chronic conditions.[14-16] Chronic care involves transitions among and between multiple care settings, creating management challenges and bottlenecks that impede the smooth flow of information. Combined, these issues may increase the risk of harm to the patient and often result in preventable rehospitalizations.

For years, hospital readmissions within 30 days of discharge have been used as a marker of quality of care as well as an indicator of financial burden for hospital administrators and health plans. Yet, these outcomes have proven resistant to change.[17] Readmissions occur as a result of a number of factors including lack of effective healthcare services and lack of effective discharge planning. Readmissions cost the healthcare system a substantial amount of money, and the recently instituted Centers for Medicare and Medicaid Services (CMS) rules that eliminate payment for preventable readmissions occurring within 30 days of discharge are forcing hospitals to become accountable for transitions of care. These financial consequences are encouraging better in-hospital discharge planning and, more generally, a more thorough and realistic understanding of the life/situational context and personal circumstances of the individuals they care for. Until recently, most of the research on the causes of relatively high 30-day readmission rates has focused on practices and procedures that occur solely in the hospital.[18,19] Because most care transitions happen in the broader community, with the hospital being just one component, new efforts conceptualize readmissions as part of a broader social/environmental complex. Hospitals and providers now must understand what resources are needed to support a discharged individual (e.g., a connection to their primary care physician, home support services, transportation to appointments, access to medications, ability to pay for medications and services, social support).

REIMAGINING CONTINUITY OF CARE

Despite health care's newfound enthusiasm for **patient centeredness**, patients must still overcome many organizational and logistic hurdles to access needed services. Beneath this is the assumption that face-to-face time with providers is irreplaceable and that accessing such services is so critical and valuable that patients will endure any inconvenience to maintain the status quo.

In a world where health information was not widely available and a majority of disease required **acute care**, this may have been true. However, the current social, political, and technological landscape is shifting around a fundamentally stagnant medical system. Chronic disease, which requires more interaction rather than less, and inaccessible, over-burdened primary care systems are combining to create pent-up demand—in business terms, a *market inefficiency*—for health care and health information. Frustration is rampant. As a result, new ways are emerging for patients to access health information and health care that were not available 15, 10, or even 5 years ago. These new models of care circumvent the traditional medical system, responding to increasingly unmet needs and helping to fill health care's market inefficiencies. Many of these new models of care are significantly more patient centered than those that are prevalent today.

REDEFINING CONTINUITY

In fits and starts, health care is becoming *continuity* focused, but it is doing so in a way that remains largely provider centered. In a world dominated by chronic disease, a majority of health activities do not involve doctors, nurses, or hospitals. They occur in the context of patients' daily lives: in their homes, their communities, and their neighborhood grocery stores and at their children's schools. The few moments spent by a patient in a clinic are relatively insignificant in comparison. Yet, for many clinicians, the world outside the clinic doors is an abstraction. Granted, it is where patients adhere or fail to adhere to "orders," but too often there is too little connection between what happens in the clinic and what happens outside of the clinic.

Continuity of care should become less about ensuring that a patient's records are sent to a primary care provider or that they are able to schedule an appointment with a specialist after their hospital course and more about focusing broadly on the interaction between a patient's daily life and the healthcare system. In their brief face-to-face interactions, the standard method of delivering health care, clinicians have struggled to meaningfully shape their patients' adherence with lifestyle modifications and medication usage. New models of care must start with the patients' daily life activities as the epicenter of the healthcare experience, and under that assumption, clinicians must consider how they can participate in their patients' lives rather than expect patients to blindly follow their orders.

The State Action on Avoidable Rehospitalizations (STAAR) Initiative, led by the Institute for Healthcare Improvement in collaboration with four states, found that teams formed by representatives in each of the agencies that may be used by a patient along the continuum of care may be the ideal solution.[20] They propose that these teams be built on mutual trust to improve communication and care transition by following a four-point model of change. Their change model consists of the following points:

1. Enhanced assessment of posthospital needs
2. Effective teaching to facilitate learning by the patient and family caregivers
3. Posthospital care follow-up, including medical and social services
4. Boundaryless transfer of critical information as the patient transitions to the next clinician or healthcare organization or home[20]

Another successful program is Dr. Eric Coleman's Care Transitions Program, which focuses on four key dimensions:

1. Medication self-management
2. Use of a dynamic patient-centered record, the personal health record, that has patient-related clinically relevant information in an easy-to-comprehend format
3. Timely primary care/specialty care follow-up based on empirical research
4. Knowledge of signs or "red flags" that indicate a worsening in condition and how to respond

The program consists of patients and their caregivers working with a "transitions coach," who teaches them self-management skills and provides them with specific tools to ensure that their needs are met during the transition from a healthcare setting to their home setting. It is a low-cost, 4-week program that includes one home visit and three phone calls. Research has shown this program to be instrumental in "reducing rehospitalization, helping to contain costs for complex patients, and improving hospital bed capacity for patients admitted with more favorable DRG (Diagnostic Related Groups). The program is self-sustaining, consistent with both Medicare Advantage and Medicare fee-for-service financial incentives, and promotes better performance on new Joint Commission initiatives aimed at post-hospital care."[21]

RECENTERING CARE

Patients often receive care in multiple settings (e.g., hospital, skilled nursing facility, rehabilitation facility) during a single episode of illness. Too often, this results in fragmented care and poorly coordinated care transitions. Even when a patient is transferred from one setting to another within the same hospital, information from the previous site often is not transmitted effectively to providers at the receiving end. The negative consequences of fragmented care include medication errors, patient and caregiver distress, duplication of services, preventable and unnecessary emergency room visits, and inappropriate or conflicting care recommendations.

People with chronic conditions and those with complex healthcare needs often require repeated services from several entities (e.g., surgeons, hospitalists, hospital nurses, physicians at skilled nursing facilities, physical therapists, primary and specialty care hospitals, and, most important of all, caregivers in the patient's home). Patients in these situations are usually in a vulnerable condition, and their caretakers are often overwhelmed by a complex set of responsibilities (e.g., keeping track of discharge and medication information from one site, coordinating and arranging for postacute care). Although the task of coordinating services following a hospital discharge typically falls to the patients' caregivers (often family members), in the absence of appropriate information regarding the medical needs of the patient from medical and support staff, caregivers may feel ill prepared to make appropriate arrangements.

The patient in the context of his or her daily life—*not the patient–provider interaction*—is the fundamental unit of health creation. This truth stems from the fact that individual behavior accounts for the largest share of health outcomes, as revealed in the population health model discussed at the start of this chapter.

Self-determination theory is a thoroughly researched and well supported set of postulates about the fundamental motivators of human behavior that successfully predict, even in clinical trials, that *autonomy, confidence*, and *relatedness* are the key drivers of human behavior that affect positive health outcomes, from broad (e.g., smoking behavior, dietary patterns, exercise habits) to specific actions (e.g., medication adherence).[22] Autonomy is supported by many factors, but a controlling healthcare environment that treats patients as subjects rather than as self-directed actors in their own lives hinders it. Confidence is strengthened by successful interactions with healthcare providers. When they leave the clinician's office, too many patients feel that they were shuffled through a process, that they were not heard, that they did not understand what just happened, and that the suggested interventions are not in line with their preferred lifestyle, cultural preferences, and circumstances. Relatedness is the feeling that one is connected to one's providers and one's plan for health maintenance. It is also a function of external social supports at all levels.

EMERGING MODELS OF CARE

Providers, payers, regulators, patients, and other stakeholders in the healthcare system know that chronic disease is on the rise, and many understand the added burden this trend places on a system already stressed to the breaking point. In theory at least, today's emerging models of care acknowledge that disease management requires different strategies and skills than diagnosis and treatment of acute illness. However, acknowledging a problem in need of a solution is one thing; solving it is another. A common theme among mainstream and emerging chronic disease management models is a continued focus on the interaction between the patient and provider, and on coordination among providers. Because the emerging models of care perpetuate the traditional, provider-centered model of care, the struggle to meaningfully alter health outcomes (by failing to motivate human behavior) continues.

With the advent of **accountable care organizations** (ACOs), hospitals now face the challenge of improving the patient's experience of care, improving the health of populations, reducing per capita costs of health care, and distributing payment to providers based on their contribution to positive patient outcomes over an episode of care. **Patient-centered medical homes** (PCMHs), best known in the recent past as primary care medical centers, have traditionally focused their efforts on preventing illnesses and managing chronic conditions in communities. Increasingly, they are developing and testing ways to collaborate with community-based organizations, including schools, churches, and businesses. ACOs and PCMHs are emerging **models of care delivery** that can incorporate new principles of care that focus on chronic disease and population health.

ACCOUNTABLE CARE ORGANIZATIONS

An ACO is Medicare's shared savings program. According to the CMS, ACOs:

> are groups of doctors, hospitals, and other health care providers, who come together voluntarily to give coordinated high quality care to their Medicare patients. The goal of coordinated care is to ensure that patients, especially the chronically ill, get the right care at the right time, while avoiding unnecessary duplication of services and preventing medical errors. When an ACO succeeds in both delivering high-quality care and spending health care dollars more wisely, it will share in the savings it achieves for the Medicare program.[23]

Irrespective of the definition, the burden of serving patients remains on hospital-, office-, and clinic-based providers despite the reality that most patients require well integrated collateral services (e.g., home and/or outpatient coaching, counseling, medication management assistance).

PATIENT-CENTERED MEDICAL HOMES

The National Committee for Quality Assurance describes PCMHs as:

> a healthcare setting that facilitates partnerships between individual patients and their personal physicians and office teams, and when appropriate, the patient's family. Care is facilitated by registries, information technology, health information exchange and other means to assure that patients get the indicated care when and where they need and want it in a culturally and linguistically appropriate manner.[24]

Other organizations define a PCMH more arbitrarily, selecting specific service elements and omitting others.[25]

The current healthcare reform environment—encompassing the prevailing models discussed earlier—provides a platform fertile for testing integrated systems of care to better serve populations in general and patients' needs in particular. To meet these challenges we must broaden the evaluation metrics for effective care to include public health-oriented indicators of successful outcomes as well as clinical measures.[26] In short, the practice of health care must shift from being responsible for a section of the population (e.g., Medicare beneficiaries affiliated with a specific organization) to include entire geographic areas in order to harness community resources to optimize and sustain population-based services.

PRINCIPLES OF NEW MODELS OF CARE

One of the most radically disruptive new models of primary care uses a subpopulation "**hot spotting**" approach that focuses on the chronically ill and highest-cost patients. As described in Gawande's profiles of actual programs created in Camden, New Jersey and Atlantic City, New Jersey, the key to the success of hot spotters is creating innovative ways of providing intensive outpatient care to the most at-risk chronically ill patients, who account for a disproportionately high percentage of medical expenditures. Gawande observes that "the critical flaw in our health-care system . . . is that it was never designed for the kind of patients who incur the highest costs."[27] Doctor's offices are perfect for "a thirty-year old with a fever" for whom a "twenty minute visit . . . may be just the thing" and for a "pedestrian hit by a minivan there's nowhere better than an emergency room," but, he observes, "these institutions are vastly inadequate for people with complex problems."[27] For the chronically ill, high-utilizer patient, a high-touch, less intense approach has resulted in substantially higher quality care at an unprecedented lower cost. Many of the essential components of this approach—from workforce issues to technology to communication strategies to reimbursement methodology—are captured in a set of principles of new models of care. It is the multitude of innovative ways in which these principles can be put into practice that is our focus here rather than any specific approach that incorporates them.

A NEW HEALTHCARE PARADIGM FOR THE PRACTICE OF MEDICINE

Because chronic disease is more prevalent than acute disease, healthcare services are now more management driven relative to diagnosis. In addition to connecting health-related sites through transitions, we must begin to think and act beyond the walls of health care to reverse the perspective of the historical model. A good place to start is with the premise that health and wellness start at home and that a patient's life does not revolve around his or her interactions with healthcare providers.

HEALTH STARTS AT HOME

Interactions with the healthcare system are a small portion of a patient's life. Furthermore, medically modifiable etiologies of disease are a small minority of all disease, and an even smaller component of chronic disease. In a modern environment, the physician's office or clinic doesn't matter as much as it did in the past. Care providers should be equipped and financially motivated to take into consideration a patient's home situation, and the healthcare system should be available to the patient when he or she is home. Changes in the workforce and mobile technologies are key to enabling change of this kind.

COMPLEXITY

Although it is easier to reduce causality to a linear model, more often it is a web of inter-relationships. True problems are diffuse and interwoven with many facets of life, and patient outcomes are rarely determined by a single determinant. Solutions must respond to this complexity with comprehensiveness. Among the multiple factors that influence health outcomes are various service-related events (e.g., availability and competency of caregivers; information provided to postacute care facilities; procedures and practices of home health agencies, physicians, allied health professionals, pharmacies, and public health and social services agencies).[28,29]

FINANCIALLY RATIONAL

We must recognize that financial incentives play into the institutional will of most health-care entities, and providers are known to be sensitive to financial incentives as well. It follows that any sustainable solution must be financially rational for all involved. Sometimes one person's loss is another person's gain; thus, we recognize that what is rational may not be always realistic.

COMMUNITY COORDINATED

We must establish and activate strategic relationships with other community resources, local governments, schools, religious organizations, and others to find ways of diffusing the cost burden of intensive, at home, interventions.

UPSTREAM

We must address root causes; an ounce of prevention . . .

INDIVIDUALIZED CARE

We should customize care both on the clinical and contextual spectrum. Creating a spectrum of "touch" allows us to more closely match resources to patient needs, resulting in efficient and patient-centered healthcare provision.

DATA INTEGRATED

Medicine and health care stand to learn a great deal from the way other industries exploit data to further their aims and goals. The opportunities for medicine are great, largely because the industry is so far behind virtually every other industry. Data should be granular, immediate, usable, and freely transferrable among contexts. Sharing data, using common standards, protecting privacy, reducing redundancy, avoiding errors, employing algorithms to improve care, and using big data analytic techniques to practice smarter and more efficiently at micro and macro levels are some of the ways data can be better integrated and used to improve healthcare delivery.

TECHNOLOGY SAVVY

Trends in mobile technology carry great promise for moving healthcare data collection and delivery into a patient's home, increasing information flow, enabling a high-touch approach for those with chronic conditions, avoiding rehospitalization, and increasing motivation. Increasingly, we are able to provide services through tele-health connections, e-mail, and online questionnaires that do not require any face-to-face visits but rather utilize evidence-based algorithms to direct interventions.

CONTEXT AS A VITAL SIGN

As an extension of a person, a community should be considered in the management and promotion of health. A person's preferences, social situation, home and neighborhood environment, and access to needed support services influence his or her outcomes and functional capability. Arguably, these realities have more impact on an individual's health than does her or his access to healthcare services alone. Therefore, the healthcare system must have knowledge about this context for each individual.

COMMUNICATION AND COMMUNICATIONS TECHNOLOGY

Medicine has been conspicuously insulated from the radical transformation of communication technology. The use of e-mail to communicate with a physician, a fairly recent phenomenon, is being adopted cautiously by a small subset of providers. Mobile technology, cloud-based information systems, and algorithm-based decision making have transformed other industries and yet are largely unharnessed by medicine.

More broadly, clinicians should consider how the words and language they use are "heard" by patients and consumers. Ross and colleagues conducted a focus group that highlights the importance of the patient–physician relationship and identifies opportunities to use this bond to communicate more clearly by avoiding technical jargon and terms that may be laden with unintended values and meanings for consumers.[30]

RESHAPING THE CARE INTERACTION

Disease management requires high-frequency, low-touch interactions as opposed to low-frequency, high-touch, face-to-face interactions in our traditional way.

PATIENT RESPONSIVE

In modern America, patient centeredness has more to do with provider coordination and integration than it does with directly responding to the needs of a patient. Patient-centered models still expect patients to come to the provider, to wait, to miss work, and to coordinate future appointments. PCMHs have all of the same shortcomings of other clinics; they just seek to reduce those shortcomings in some way.

Patient responsiveness is an acknowledgment that, in the future, physicians may not have the monopoly on providing healthcare information. Patients can turn, alternatively, to disease management forums, self-diagnostic apps, video chat (e.g., Skype) appointments, and online meetings. A patient may eventually be able to seek care without ever leaving home.

EVIDENCE BASED

As we gather reliable data on basic disease processes, management of uncomplicated disease becomes algorithmic. The challenge of managing simple disease with a well established foundation of research is shifting away from diagnostic complexity or clinical nuance and toward consistency, efficiency, and safety.

BARRIERS AND CHALLENGES

FINANCIAL

The fee-for-service payment model encourages excess intervention and fragmentation over coordination. Payment reform is an essential component of any strategy to shift the provider perspective away from illness treatment and toward wellness promotion.

LEGAL

Disruptive models of care will inevitably infringe on domains of certain physicians' practices. As a new workforce emerges and forms of high-access, low-touch health care gain a foothold, traditional physician roles will eventually be challenged and produce a legal backlash to preserve the status quo.

POLITICAL

By expanding insurance, healthcare reform will increase the traffic of patients in an already overburdened system. The bottleneck for basic healthcare services will only worsen, providing fertile ground for other models of care.

HISTORICAL

Medical culture is, by and large, risk averse. Even evidence-based findings can be surprisingly slow to permeate into the daily practice of physicians. Additionally, current models of care are deeply rooted and designed to thrive on the current methods of reimbursement.

CONCLUSION

Chronic disease is the new world of medicine, yet, in many ways, our system is unchanged. Even the more progressive models of today are extensions of historical systems and thus unsuited to face the challenges of ongoing disease management and prevention. We must replace the physician as the central point in the healthcare experience with the patient's community and life circumstances for better health management. Treatment of chronic disease requires continuity of care and management of **care transitions** that maintain an ongoing connection with patients as they live their lives. To do this in a way that is financially feasible, models of care must be fundamentally restructured. We must trend away from high-resource, low-frequency interaction toward frequent, low-intensity interactions. This could be accomplished via telephonics, the freer flow of connected information, and the integration of patient-centered health information available with increased frequency through mobile health devices.

STUDY AND DISCUSSION QUESTIONS

1. Discuss the risk factors and circumstances that lead to the development of chronic diseases.
2. Compare and contrast the impact and incentives of financial models for prevention and chronic care management, including ACOs, bundled payments, and fee-for-service. Compare and contrast the effect of new models of care. What are their relative strengths and weaknesses?
3. What information do healthcare providers need to solicit from patients and families to better understand their context, circumstances, and cultural and personal preferences?
4. Consider what metrics are needed to assess progress in incorporating patient and family perspectives and preferences, as well as social and home needs.

SUGGESTED READINGS AND WEBSITES

READINGS

Berwick DM, Nolan TW, Whittington J. The Triple Aim: care, health and cost. *Health Aff.* 2008;27(3):759-69.

Gawande A. The hot spotters. *The New Yorker.* 2011;(January 24):41-51.

Jencks SF, Williams MV, Coleman EA. Rehospitalization among patients in the Medicare fee-for-service program. *N Engl J Med.* 2009;360(14):1418-28.

Kindig D, Stoddart G. What is population health? *Am J Public Health.* 2003;93(3):380-3. http://www.ncbi.nlm.nih.gov/pmc/articles/PMC1447747/. Accessed October 27, 2014.

Schroeder S. We can do better—improving the health of the American people. *N Engl J Med.* 2007;357(12):1221-8. http://www.nejm.org/toc/nejm/357/12/. Accessed October 27, 2014.

WEBSITES

The Care Transitions Program: http://www.caretransitions.org/

Health Affairs Blog, David Kindig, Beyond the Triple Aim: Integrating the Nonmedical Sector: http://healthaffairs.org/blog/2008/05/19/beyond-the-triple-aim-integrating-the-nonmedical-sectors/. Accessed October 27, 2014.

Improving Population Health, David A. Kindig, MD, PhD, editor: http://www.improvingpopulationhealth.org/blog/about-this-blog.html. Accessed November 2, 2014.

Institute for Healthcare Improvement, State Action on Avoidable Rehospitalizations (STARR) Initiative: http://www.ihi.org/engage/Initiatives/completed/STAAR/Pages/default.aspx. Accessed October 27, 2014.

REFERENCES

1. Pareto principle: http://en.wikipedia.org/wiki/Pareto_principle. Accessed October 27, 2014.
2. Health Spending: Trends and Impact: http://kff.org/slideshow/health-spending-trends-and-impact/. Accessed October 27, 2014.
3. Kindig D, Stoddart G. What is population health? *Am J Public Health.* 2003;93(3):380-3. http://www.ncbi.nlm.nih.gov/pmc/articles/PMC1447747/. Accessed October 27, 2014.
4. Schroeder S. We can do better—improving the health of the American people. *N Engl J Med.* 2007;357(12):1221-8. http://www.nejm.org/toc/nejm/357/12/. Accessed October 27, 2014.
5. Nash D. Managing the Health of the Nation, July 17, 2103. http://new.livestream.com/opengroup/Nash-philly13. Accessed October 27, 2014.
6. Nash D, Reifsynder J, Fabius R, Pracilio V. *Population Health: Creating a Culture of Wellness.* Sudbury, MA: Jones & Bartlett; 2011.
7. Mollica RL, Gillespie J. Care coordination for people with chronic conditions, January 2003. http://www.partnershipforsolutions.org/DMS/files/Care_coordination.pdf. Accessed October 27, 2014.
8. Machlin SR. Trends in health care expenditures for the elderly age 65 and over: 2006 versus 1996, August 2009. http://www.meps.ahrq.gov/mepsweb/data_files/publications/st256/stat256.pdf. Accessed October 27, 2014.
9. Hoffman C, Rice D, Sung HY. Persons with chronic conditions, their prevalence and costs. *JAMA.* 1996;276(18):1473-9.
10. Wagner EH. Meeting the needs of chronically ill people. *BMJ.* 2001;323(7319):945-6.
11. Wolff JL, Starfield B, Anderson G. Prevalence, expenditures, and complications of multiple chronic conditions in the elderly. *Arch Intern Med.* 2002;162(20):2269-76.
12. Administration on Aging. A Profile of Older Americans: 2008. Washington, DC: US Department of Health and Human Services. http://www.mowaa.org/Document.Doc?id=69. Accessed October 27, 2014.
13. Linden A, Adler-Milstein J. Medicare disease management in policy context. *Health Care Finance Rev.* 2008;29(3):1-11.
14. Harrold LR, Field TS, Gurwitz JH. Knowledge, patterns of care, and outcomes of care for generalists and specialists. *J Gen Intern Med.* 1999;14(8):499-511.
15. Greenfield S, Rogers W, Mangotich M, Carney MF, Tarlov AR. Outcomes of patients with hypertension and non-insulin dependent diabetes

mellitus treated by different systems and specialists: results from the medical outcomes study. *JAMA*. 1995;274(18):1436-44.

16. Greenfield S, Kaplan SH, Kahn R, Ninomiya J, Griffith JL. Profiling care provided by different groups of physicians: effects of patient case-mix (bias) and physician-level clustering on quality assessment results. *Ann Intern Med*. 2002;136(2):111-21.

17. Jencks SF, Williams MV, Coleman EA. Rehospitalization among patients in the Medicare fee-for-service program. *N Engl J Med*. 2009;360(14): 1418-28.

18. McCarthy D, Johnson MB, Audet AM. Recasting readmissions by placing the hospital role in community context. *JAMA*. 2013;309(4):351-2.

19. Oddone EZ, Weinberger M. Hospital readmission rates: are we measuring the right thing? *Ann Intern Med*. 2012;157(12):910-1.

20. Institute for Healthcare Improvement, State Action on Avoidable Rehospitalizations (STARR) Initiative. http://www.ihi.org/engage/Initiatives/completed/STAAR/Pages/default.aspx. Accessed October 27, 2014.

21. The Care Transitions Program. http://www.caretransitions.org/overview.asp. Accessed October 27, 2014.

22. Ryan R, Patrick H, Deci E, Williams G. Facilitating health behaviour change and its maintenance: interventions based on self-determination theory. *The European Health Psychologist*. 2008;10(3):2-5.

http://www.selfdeterminationtheory.org/SDT/documents/2008_RyanPatrickDeciWilliams_EHP.pdf. Accessed October 27, 2014.

23. Centers for Medicaid and Medicare Services, Accountable Care Organizations. http://www.cms.gov/Medicare/Medicare-Fee-for-Service-Payment/ACO/index.html?redirect=/ACO/. Accessed October 27, 2014.

24. Mitka M. Patient-Centered Medical Homes offer a model for better, cheaper healthcare. *JAMA*. 2012;307(8):769-72.

25. Vest JR, Bolin JN, Miller TR, et al. Medical homes: where you stand on definitions depends on where you sit. *Med Care Res Rev*. 2010;67(4): 393-411.

26. Gourevich MN, Cannel T, Boufford JI, Summers C. The challenge of attribution: responsibility for population health in the context of accountable care. *Am J Public Health*. 2012;102(Suppl 3):S322–S4.

27. Gawande A. The hot spotters. *The New Yorker* 2011;(January 24):41-51.

28. Kocher RP, Adashi EY. Hospital readmissions and the Affordable Care Act: paying for coordinated quality care. *JAMA*. 2011;306(16):1794-5.

29. Kangovi S, Grande D. Hospital readmissions—not just a measure of quality. *JAMA*. 2011;306(16):1796-7.

30. Ross M, Igus T, Gomez S. From our lips to whose ears? Consumer reaction to our current health care dialect. *Perm J*. 13(1):8-16.

HEALTHCARE QUALITY AND SAFETY ACROSS THE CARE CONTINUUM

BETTINA BERMAN, VALERIE P. PRACILIO, AND
JANICE L. CLARKE

Executive Summary

Improving healthcare quality and safety requires a coordinated effort among all stakeholders.

Quality and safety are central to the healthcare reforms underway in the United States. The collective effect of quality initiatives will be positive if the goals, strategies, and payment models are aligned and all stakeholders are considered. The Patient Protection and Affordable Care Act (ACA) aims to make quality health care accessible and affordable via programs wherein the patient is central to the delivery of care, the provider is compensated based on quality rather than quantity, and health benefits purchasing is value based. The metrics used to evaluate these programs—especially those that address chronic or costly conditions and provide some context for good quality—are useful tools for population health management. With greater provider accountability, better coordination of care, and more emphasis on quality and safety, health reform is likely to have a positive effect on population health. This chapter discusses quality and safety in the context of the changing U.S. healthcare environment across a broad range of healthcare settings.

Learning Objectives

1. Understand the evolution of the healthcare quality and safety movement in the United States.
2. List and describe the roles of key U.S. quality organizations.
3. Explain how quality is measured.
4. Describe governmental and private payer strategies for quality and safety.
5. Identify strategies to improve quality across healthcare sectors.
6. Understand the implications of the ACA for healthcare quality and safety.

Key Terms

CMS quality initiatives

Healthcare Effectiveness Data and
  Information Set (HEDIS)

hospital quality improvement

National Quality Forum

National Quality Strategy

patient safety organizations

retail clinic

INTRODUCTION

Central to all efforts aimed at improving population health is the goal of delivering better quality and safer care. This is evident even in the definition of population health, which places a strong emphasis on health outcomes.[1-3] We have learned a great deal since the Institute of Medicine's (IOM's) seminal report, *To Err Is Human,*[4] which focused a national spotlight on the health system's shortcomings in 1999: We've recognized that systems are the issue rather than people, that we can't improve what we don't measure, and that coordination is integral to quality care. We are gaining valuable experience in setting aims, taking action, measuring change, and coordinating care. Moreover, we've come to understand that quality health care, delivered in a system that can keep patients safe, is essential to advance population health. Although a number of successful programs have been implemented, it will take commitment and cooperation from a broad range of stakeholders to transform the system.

Quality of care affects a population's overall health. It is complex and broad in scope, making it difficult to measure. Beyond the clinical sphere, healthcare quality encompasses the health of a community and access to care. The four factors that affect health are clinical care, health behaviors, social and economic factors, and the physical environment. A healthy population requires that all four factors be considered in combination; this chapter focuses specifically on the quality of care and how it can be evaluated and improved.[5]

As defined by the IOM, quality is "the degree to which health services for individuals and populations increase the likelihood of desired health outcomes and are consistent with current professional knowledge."[4] Advancing quality, and ultimately population health, requires improving the current system, wherein measuring quality and safety at the population level remains a challenge.[1] Measurement systems have evolved and become more robust since the early 2000s, but many opportunities for improvement remain, in particular, the timeliness of data for review and appropriate action.

Similar opportunities exist for improving measurement of patient safety (i.e., freedom from accidental injury). In general, quality and safety gain attention reactively—in other words, once an incident occurs or when the data are available—but measurement systems must also support proactive quality and safety evaluation and improvement to prevent incidents before they occur.

Quality measurement is not a new concept. As early as the 1960s, Dr. Avedis Donabedian recognized the reciprocal influence of healthcare quality on the community and vice versa.[6–8] Resources available in a community and the processes used to allocate those resources affect outcomes of care. The healthcare industry can be described as a set of inputs (e.g., health behaviors, social and economic factors, the physical environment) and outputs (e.g., outcomes such as quality of care). Differences among communities in terms of structural and process-based inputs (e.g., available resources, insurance coverage, cultural values) help explain the large variations in practice patterns and patient outcomes across the United States.[6]

Positive changes are underway to ensure that care delivery is based on evidence and is of the highest quality. As organizations engage in federally funded programs that incentivize providers to meet quality targets, they create strategic alliances to address their population's needs and begin to form larger organizations through partnerships, mergers, and affiliations, thereby strengthening their positions in the community. Underscoring these changes is a reliance on quality data to guide decisions and align strategies to better serve their patients.

Over the past few decades, researchers, analysts, and healthcare consortia have compiled evidence demonstrating the magnitude of quality and safety challenges. In response, leading organizations such as the **National Quality Forum** (NQF), the Agency for Healthcare Research and Quality (AHRQ), the Institute for Healthcare Improvement (IHI), and the National Patient Safety Foundation (NPSF) have devised strategies to address these needs. Immediately following the publication of *To Err Is Human*, these and other organizations began to develop metrics for evaluating quality and safety. The NQF established a process for validating and endorsing sound and reliable metrics. The process entails bringing together stakeholders from various healthcare sectors to evaluate and validate a measure based on four criteria: The measure must be (1) important to measure (i.e., there is sufficient evidence to indicate that it can affect quality), (2) scientifically acceptable to produce valid and reliable results, and (3) usable in quality improvement and decision making, and what is being measured must be (4) feasible to collect.[9] For each measure, the NQF assembles a committee to assess its merits, invites the public to comment, and reaches a consensus on whether to endorse the measure. Once endorsed, the measure becomes publicly available for use.[10] NQF-endorsed measures are available in a searchable database maintained by the NQF. Another source of measures is the National Quality Measures Clearinghouse maintained by the AHRQ.[11] Not all measures in this resource are endorsed by the NQF; however, this database provides detailed information related to the use and application of and evidence to support the measures, along with tutorials, technical assistance videos, and other resources. The clearinghouse also categorizes measures by domain, thus enabling healthcare organizations to search defined measures by topic. Included are four "Population Health Quality" measure domains related to structure, process, outcome, access, and experience.[12]

In similar fashion, the IHI and NPSF have brought together key thought leaders to devise strategies to effect quality and safety. The IHI gained recognition for its campaigns aimed at reducing morbidity and mortality. Today, its Triple Aim seeks to improve patients' experience of care, improve the health of populations, and reduce costs.[13] More than 100 teams that have committed to pursuing the Triple Aim in the United States and internationally are well on their way to improving population health. The NPSF's focus is on reducing harm through a variety of educational initiatives and collaboratives.[14] Both of these organizations offer a wide range of resources to evaluate, measure, and improve quality and safety.

Although efforts to date have all yielded positive results and led to progress, a significant opportunity exists in advancing measurement beyond today's retrospective evaluation systems to achieve real-time quality and safety monitoring systems. Current IHI and NPSF initiatives will lead to improvement over time, but the tools for measurement are not fully matured. Increasing technology adoption by healthcare systems will undoubtedly enable more rapid feedback to providers at the point of care. With the benefit of access to real-time data, a population approach to quality and safety improvement will become more targeted, and resources will be used more efficiently to provide quality care. Such an approach will go a long way toward advancing population health.

The following sections trace the evolution of healthcare quality and safety, from groundbreaking work in the private sector, to the Centers for Medicare and Medicaid Services (CMS) programs and initiatives, to the ACA and its substantial impact on healthcare providers and patients.

GOVERNMENT AND PRIVATE SECTOR CONTRIBUTIONS TO HEALTHCARE QUALITY AND SAFETY

EARLY ADOPTERS OF QUALITY AND SAFETY MEASURES

In 1989, the National Committee for Quality Assurance (NCQA) established the Health Maintenance Employer Data Set, which in 2007, was renamed the Healthcare Effectiveness Data and Information Set (HEDIS). HEDIS was developed to enable consumers to compare a health plan's performance with other health plans and with national and regional benchmarks. The most widely reported set of performance measures used to evaluate and rank the performance of health plans and providers, the HEDIS measures are developed with input from all stakeholders, including the public. The measure development cycle can be as long as 12 to 24 months.[15]

There are two types of HEDIS measures: (1) Process measures evaluate the process of care (e.g., Is the diabetic patient receiving eye exams at the recommended intervals? Is the patient's blood pressure being measured and controlled with the appropriate medications?), and (2) outcomes measures evaluate the end point of care (e.g., Is the patient's hemoglobin A1c [a measure of how well diabetes is controlled] within the recommended parameters? Is the patient's blood pressure controlled?).[16]

HEDIS measures address a broad range of quality and safety concerns, from recommended screenings to appropriate medical management of chronic conditions to access to important services (e.g., dental care, drug and alcohol dependence treatment, pre- and postnatal care, mental health services). Measures are added, deleted, and revised annually. The data are collected by means of surveys, chart reviews, and health insurance claims (e.g., hospitalizations, procedures, office visits). Aggregate data and analyses are reported by the NCQA in its annual State of Health Care Quality Report.[17]

HEDIS measures are used by the NCQA as part of its health plan accreditation process and by employers to help select high-performing health plans that will provide the highest value of care for their employees. NCQA's Quality Compass is a tool that enables employers to generate custom reports to compare select health plans on the basis of quality improvement and benchmarks. Performance measures also play an increasing role in the evaluation of health plans and service providers. Although more than 90% of U.S. health plans use HEDIS to measure their performance,[18] there is considerable variability in how the measures are used (e.g., some organizations use "HEDIS-like" measures), which complicates how providers are evaluated. Many health plans tie physician incentives and reimbursement to performance on HEDIS metrics, and performance metrics play an integral part in today's healthcare environment.

Another early adopter of performance metrics, the Joint Commission (JC), developed and tested several sets of hospital performance measures in 1986. This led to the development of the 1998 JC initiative, ORYX.[19] Today, the ORYX hospital-based performance measures are used by the JC in the hospital accreditation process and are publicly reported on the JC website.

CMS QUALITY INITIATIVES

In an effort to hold hospitals accountable for the quality of care they deliver, the CMS initiated a program to financially penalize hospitals that failed to report the ORYX measures to the CMS. Later, the CMS began to report ORYX results publicly on its Hospital Compare website. With increased public reporting, hospitals began to invest significant resources to improve their performance on the metrics.[20] Since the early 2000s, **CMS quality initiatives** have been implemented incrementally and with increased sophistication. Although the CMS has been especially successful in standardizing processes for reporting, there remains a need for greater coordination of measurements across a broad range of programs, which is discussed later in this chapter.

THE PATIENT PROTECTION AND AFFORDABLE CARE ACT

The focus on healthcare quality was brought to the forefront with the 2010 passage of the ACA, which effectively increased the scope of performance measurement and strengthened the existing CMS performance measurement programs. The central objective of the law is to improve healthcare quality and access to care while lowering healthcare costs.[21]

The ACA mandates that metrics be used to evaluate quality of care, that quality metrics be publicly reported, and that hospital and provider payments be tied to performance.[22] The law also established the not-for-profit Patient-Centered Outcomes Research Institute (PCORI) to conduct comparative effectiveness research. PCORI's mission is to identify national priorities for healthcare research to "help people make informed health care decisions, and improve health care delivery and outcomes, by producing and promoting high-integrity, evidence-based information that comes from research guided by patients, caregivers, and the broader health care community."[23]

VALUE-BASED PURCHASING

The two greatest needs in U.S. health care today are to decrease cost and improve quality. These two needs are the foundation on which the ACA was built, and they are the basis for one of its key concepts—value-based purchasing (VBP). VBP programs vary in their design, but they share a common goal and two components to help achieve it: (1) defined performance goals for select quality metrics and (2) financial incentives for the hospital or the individual provider.[24,25] Although reported results of VBP "pay-for-performance" (P4P) programs have been mixed and questions remain on their ability to create sustainable value and affect health outcomes, federal and commercial programs continue to proliferate.[24] VBP aligns a portion of Medicare payments with provider performance on quality metrics and shifts the current volume-based fee-for-service (FFS) model to a methodology that pays for value of care. The VBP programs established by the ACA will affect providers in multiple healthcare settings.

CMS HOSPITAL READMISSIONS REDUCTION PROGRAM

The ACA includes provisions to reduce hospital payments for certain readmissions that are deemed preventable. Under the CMS Hospital Readmissions Reduction Program (HRRP), hospitals are subject to rate reductions if they have high readmission rates for certain conditions (e.g., heart attacks, heart failure, pneumonia). The goal is to encourage hospitals and providers to improve care transitions. Insufficient attention to patient hand-offs to the primary care provider poses a high risk for error and inadequate provider communication and follow-up. These, in turn, can lead to costly readmissions through the emergency department.[26]

PATIENT-CENTERED MEDICAL HOME

The ACA incorporated and authorized funding for the patient-centered medical home (PCMH) model. The PCMH is modeled on an enhanced, multidisciplinary team-care concept with a primary care physician coordinating care between different specialty providers and practice sites. Access to providers is enhanced through extended hours of operations and greater patient communication, and the payment structure is designed to reward providers for rendering enhanced services. The PCMH strategy charges the primary care provider (PCP) with leading the care team and coordinating care for patients, with a focus on prevention of illness and optimal treatment of the whole person. The ultimate goal is to equip a comprehensive team of providers with the information needed to coordinate patient care.[19] PCMH patients have the opportunity to become actively engaged in their care, and studies have shown that PCMHs enhance the experience of and satisfaction with care for clinically complex patients.[27]

ACCOUNTABLE CARE ORGANIZATIONS

Fragmentation of care and waste in the healthcare system led to the establishment of care delivery reform proposals under the ACA. Accountable care organizations (ACOs) are affiliations of healthcare providers (hospitals, physicians, and others involved in patient care) that together are accountable for the health care of a defined population and its associated costs. An ACO is defined as a patient-centered organization in which the patients and the providers are partners in the decision-making process surrounding care decisions.

The Medicare Shared Savings Program (MSSP) for ACOs is a voluntary program aimed at improving patient care and meeting the **National Quality Strategy**'s (NQS's) three aims: (1) better care, (2) healthy people and healthy communities, and (3) affordable care.[28] To receive the shared savings reward from Medicare, ACOs must meet quality standards in the following areas: (1) patient and caregiver care experiences, (2) care coordination, (3) patient safety, (4) preventive health, and (5) at-risk population and frail elderly health.[29] ACOs will be held accountable for multiple quality metrics (e.g., preventive care screenings, blood pressure control, diabetes control), and the results will be available for public review. For satisfactory performance on quality measures, ACOs must reach out to their patients and address needs for preventive care and chronic disease management.[30]

ROLE OF HEALTH INFORMATION TECHNOLOGY

The American Recovery and Reinvestment Act (ARRA) of 2009 established financial incentives for hospitals and eligible providers to invest in and utilize health information technology (HIT) under the Electronic Health Record (EHR) Incentive Program, also called the Meaningful Use (MU) Program, which stipulates that providers demonstrate performance on certain CMS-defined core and menu measures for their EHR systems. The goal of the program is to build a national HIT infrastructure that, ultimately, could be leveraged to improve population health, patient engagement, and access to care.[31]

HIT has the potential to enhance the clinical care process and improve patient outcomes in several ways:

- HIT systems afford providers access to up-to-date clinical care guidelines by means of clinical decision support tools.
- Prescribing clinicians can be alerted to patient allergies and potentially harmful drug interactions via alerts generated by computerized provider order entry (CPOE) systems.
- Providers can use EHR systems for medical management of their patient populations (e.g., by creating alerts and outreach messages for preventive care, by focusing practice resources on complex medical patients).
- The EHR infrastructure allows providers to track their performance on quality measures and to report clinical quality measures to the CMS as part of the EHR incentive program.

In theory, and used optimally, EHR systems have the potential to improve population health. To date, the literature on HIT as it relates to quality and safety of patient care is inconclusive.[32]

PATIENT SAFETY ORGANIZATIONS

With heightened awareness of healthcare safety issues, a new framework for reporting and addressing medical errors and adverse events became a national priority. The Patient Safety and Quality Improvement Act of 2005 encouraged reporting and the establishment of **Patient Safety Organizations** (PSOs). PSOs are neutral external parties that support quality and safety improvement in a secure environment in which providers and organizations can collect, aggregate, and analyze data.[33] What distinguishes PSOs from peer-review processes is that information reported to a PSO is protected from legal liability or professional sanctions. This important distinction serves to allay fears and encourage reporting and review to promote improvement.

As the lead federal agency for patient safety research, the Agency for Healthcare Research and Quality (AHRQ) was granted authority by Congress to designate PSOs in accordance with the patient safety rule. An organization can seek PSO status if its primary activity is to "improve patient safety and the quality of health care delivery" and it meets 15 statutory requirements.[34] A complete list of PSOs can be found at http://www.pso.ahrq.gov/pso-list.

ENSURING QUALITY AND SAFETY ACROSS THE POPULATION HEALTHCARE CONTINUUM

INPATIENT HOSPITAL QUALITY IMPROVEMENT

For more than a decade, the CMS has tested programs aimed at providing high-quality and cost-effective care. The Premier Hospital Quality Incentive Demonstration project, implemented as a pilot program in 2003, was aimed at measuring performance in several disease domains (e.g., acute myocardial infarction, congestive heart failure, pneumonia, coronary artery bypass graft surgery, hip and knee replacement surgery, management of surgical patients).[19] VBP metrics are related to each of these disease types, and achieving performance goals earns participating hospitals a financial incentive. Population health improvement relies on understanding population needs, and VBP metrics are useful to providers in managing care for populations of patients.

Financial incentives were a fundamental component of early VBP programs. However, as efforts to integrate related processes and strategies into standard practice increase, the trend has shifted to financial penalties. For example, under the Deficit Reduction Act (2005), hospitals no longer receive additional payments for hospital-acquired conditions (HACs) (e.g., bloodstream infections, urinary tract infections, falls, and pressure ulcers that were not present on admission). HACs resulting from medical errors are a leading cause of mortality and a financial burden on the healthcare system. The belief is that these cases can be reduced or eliminated through the consistent use of evidence-based guidelines.[20] Accountability for **hospital quality** is increasing as well. Since 2005, the CMS Hospital Compare website has been making the public aware of hospital performance data on process and outcomes measures, spending, and resource utilization.[19] Clearly, the shift from incentives to penalties reflects a drive toward improving the standard of care.

A multitude of quality programs have been launched by the CMS in an effort to transform our system from one that is volume based to one that is value based in terms of purchasing healthcare services. In concert with the three aims of the NQS, the goals of quality reporting programs are to improve care and control costs.[21] Beginning in October 2012, the ACA[22] mandated the establishment of a VBP program for all acute care hospitals—the most comprehensive of the quality initiatives implemented by the CMS. Under this program, payments to hospitals are based on performance measured in six domains:

- Safety
- Patient- and caregiver-centered experience and outcomes
- Care coordination
- Clinical care
- Population or community health
- Efficiency and cost reduction

The quality measures for the fiscal year 2014 VBP program include 17 measures in the areas of clinical care, patient experience, and patient outcomes (Table 11-1). Additional outcomes measures (e.g., bloodstream infections, patient safety measures) will be added in 2015 along with an efficiency (cost) measure.[20]

The HCAHPS survey tool, developed by the CMS and the AHRQ, is composed of 18 questions in 10 domains related to the hospital experience.

As VBP programs evolve, they have shifted from mere reporting to performance by incorporating outcomes measures. These programs are also increasing provider accountability for the patient experience by including metrics related to the HCAHPS, a standardized tool used by all hospitals to assess and compare patient experience.[23] Since 2006, hospitals have voluntarily submitted HCAHPS data to the CMS, which initiated public reporting of results on the CMS Hospital Compare website in 2008. Although submission is voluntary, hospitals must provide the data to the CMS to receive their full annual payment update.[23,24]

Table 11-1   Measure Domains for the 2014 VBP Program

Clinical Processes of Care Measures
Acute myocardial infarction
Heart failure
Pneumonia
Healthcare-associated infections
Surgery indicators

Patient Experience of Care Measures
Hospital Consumer Assessment of Healthcare Providers and Systems (HCAHPS) Survey

Outcomes Measures
Mortality rates for acute myocardial infarction, heart failure, and pneumonia

Efficiency Measures (2015)
Medicare spending per beneficiary

AMBULATORY CARE QUALITY IMPROVEMENT

Historically, ambulatory care quality initiatives have lagged behind those in the inpatient setting. This changed in 2007 when the CMS implemented the Physician Quality Reporting System (PQRS) program, a voluntary, pay-for-reporting program for Medicare providers. This is the first CMS program to tie performance on quality metrics to incentives and penalties.[25] In 2014, eligible providers could report on 284 quality measures including smoking cessation counseling, measurement of body mass index (BMI), and laboratory values (e.g., cholesterol and hemoglobin A1c levels for diabetes patients). Multistakeholder groups develop the CMS quality measures, and, as a result, discussions regarding ambulatory quality have expanded. However, some question the ability to relate performance on the measures to quality improvement.[26] Although measurement is an essential step to raise awareness, it is the actions taken in response to results that lead to quality improvement.

Programs such as the PQRS and improved transparency via websites such as Physician Compare are increasing accountability for ambulatory care providers. Established by the ACA and launched in December 2010, the Physician Compare website serves a two-fold purpose: to provide patients with information to make informed healthcare decisions and to provide physicians with an incentive to improve quality of care.[27] Currently, Physician Compare includes basic demographics and information on providers' participation in the PQRS and CMS Meaningful Use incentive programs. PQRS measure data for large group practices, and ACOs are also available on the website. Soon, Physician Compare may include ambulatory patient experience data as reported through the Clinician Group Consumer Assessment of Healthcare Providers and Systems (CGCAHPS) survey. The goal of the CGCAHPS is to improve the quality of patient care through assessments of patient experience as well as access to healthcare providers.

Federal VBP programs are becoming a mainstay in efforts to improve quality and reduce cost. Each program takes a slightly different approach, but all of them hold a mirror to the stakeholders involved—from government policy makers to physicians and patients—in meaningful ways. Although these programs place a substantial reporting and financial burden on the nation's hospitals and ambulatory practices, the hope is that the associated incentives and penalties will be an impetus for positive change. Observers have already seen an increase in demand for hospital and provider accountability that might lead to better quality of care for covered populations.

QUALITY AND PATIENT SAFETY IN ALTERNATE CARE SETTINGS

RETAIL CLINICS

Conveniently located in pharmacies and "big box" stores across the country, **retail clinics** staffed by nurse practitioners (NPs) and physician assistants (PAs) provide basic preventive care and select primary care to a growing segment of the population. Recently, the Center for Studying Health System Change reported that an estimated 4.1 million families visited a retail clinic in 2010—a nearly threefold increase from 2007.[35]

Most retail care clinics are members of the Convenient Care Association (CCA), a professional organization representing various companies and health systems that provide care in a retail setting. Since its inception in 2006, the CCA has fostered a culture of quality and safety throughout the retail industry by requiring member clinics to demonstrate compliance with a comprehensive set of quality standards. The organization retains a third-party reviewer to certify that member clinics conform with or exceed these standards.

The initial certification process assures that a clinic's policies and procedures are consistent with CCA quality standards. Performance is assessed on elements such as provider credentialing, ongoing quality monitoring, coordination of care with primary care and other providers, health promotion and preventive screening information, compliance with regulatory standards (e.g., Health Insurance Portability and Accountability Act, Occupational Safety and Health Administration, and Centers for Disease Control and Prevention guidelines), use of an EHR, peer and collaborating physician chart review, maintenance of a safe environment, and mechanisms to empower patients to make informed choices.[36] Once any deficiencies have been fully addressed, a 2-year initial certification is issued.

The recertification process is designed to review a clinic's performance, identify opportunities for improvement, and discuss new strategies. Evidence of ongoing quality improvement submitted by a clinic may include quality initiatives undertaken since the initial certification, minutes from quality improvement committee meetings, and quality reports generated by the clinic (e.g., waiting time reports, patient satisfaction surveys, appropriateness of care based on a chart review). Action plans to address deficiencies must also be submitted. To be recertified, a clinic must demonstrate how it uses EHRs in a "meaningful" way (e.g., how the EHR interfaces with other providers' systems, how the EHR provides alerts for potential drug interactions, how the EHR is utilized to track quality data).

The Joint Commission also identifies elements of performance for retail clinics and makes them available as part of its *Comprehensive Accreditation Manual for Ambulatory Care.*

There is substantial evidence of the high quality of care provided in retail clinics. One study compared the cost and quality of care provided for three common conditions (otitis media, urinary tract infections, pharyngitis) and preventive care in a retail clinic with care provided in physician offices, urgent care centers, and emergency rooms. Overall costs were significantly lower in the retail clinics, and although not statistically different from physician offices or urgent care centers, aggregate data on quality metrics were best for retail clinics. In comparison with emergency departments, retail clinics demonstrated statistically superior quality. A second study found that NPs and PAs in the retail setting adhered to guidelines more than 99% of the time for testing and treatment of pharyngitis.[37] After studying data from visits to one CCA member's clinics (Take Care Clinic®) over a 2-year period, another group of researchers found that appropriate treatment was rendered for children with upper respiratory infections in 88% of visits, and for pharyngitis in 93% of visits. Both results surpassed leading ambulatory care benchmarks (i.e., HEDIS).[38]

URGENT CARE CENTERS

Driven by a disturbing decrease in the number and availability of primary care physicians, long wait times in emergency rooms for nonemergent care, and the public demand for immediate access to medical care, the urgent care (UC) industry has experienced considerable growth since its inception in the mid-1990s, with more than 9,000 facilities operating in 2014.[39]

The American Academy of Urgent Care Medicine (AAUCM) is a national organization dedicated to elevating standards, improving education and training, and encouraging scientific and medical research in the field of UC medicine and, by doing so, improving the overall quality of medical care.[38] The AAUCM offers an accreditation program for UCs, a voluntary process by which these organizations can measure the quality of the services they deliver and compare their performance against nationally recognized standards.[40] The Urgent Care Center Accreditation (UCCA) program sets quality standards, measures performance, and provides consultation and education as needed. Accreditation of a UC practice is based on a reasonable assessment of the practice's compliance with applicable standards and its adherence to the policies and procedures of the UCCA program. Accreditation standards encompass rights of patients, governance, administration, quality of care provided, quality management and improvement, facilities and environment, immediate/urgent care services, pathology and medical laboratory services, diagnostic imaging services, employee and occupational health services, and health education and wellness.[40]

The NQF has endorsed ambulatory care measures for assessing the quality of care in a wide variety of clinical settings including UC centers. However, implementation of the measures in the UC setting is challenging because urgent care is, by definition, episodic and most measures focus on providing longitudinal care to a panel of patients.[41] A survey conducted by Weinick and colleagues suggests that UC compares favorably with other practice settings on select quality indicators including integration with the healthcare system, postvisit follow-up, quality of care, and patient satisfaction.[41]

LONG-TERM CARE

In recent years, the concept of long-term care has evolved to encompass a multitude of settings and forms based on a patient's needs and wishes. However, nursing home care remains a key component of long-term care (LTC) and the quality of LTC remains a concern for many stakeholders. As the largest payer for nursing home care of the disabled and elderly populations, the federal government has an obvious interest in providing high-value care for its beneficiaries. In 2002, the CMS initiated the Nursing Home Quality Initiative (NHQI), and today nursing home quality is assessed using a mix of process and outcome metrics. The current nursing home quality measures are endorsed by the NQF and publicly reported on the CMS Nursing Home Compare website,[42] thus enabling consumers to compare quality of care information on more than 15,000 Medicare and Medicaid certified nursing homes across the country. The website includes information on Five-Star Quality Ratings of overall and individual performance on health inspections and quality measures and hours of care provided per resident by staff performing nursing care tasks.[43]

The goals of the CMS nursing home quality measures are to assist consumers in evaluating nursing home care quality and to provide the nursing homes with data that can be used to improve quality. Current quality measures for nursing home stays over 100 days are related to the following:

- Falls with major injury
- Self-report of moderate to severe pain
- Pressure ulcers
- Influenza and pneumococcal vaccine administration
- Urinary tract infections
- Loss of control of bowel or bladder
- Bladder catheters
- Physical restraints
- Increased need for help with daily activities
- Excessive weight loss
- Depressive symptoms
- Antipsychotic medications[44]

In the future, the CMS quality metrics may be tied to payment for long-term care, and a VBP demonstration project has been implemented in several states to evaluate the participants' performance on an array of metrics.

Under Medicare, LTC hospitals are certified as short-term acute care hospitals. LTC hospitals treat patients with multiple conditions requiring long-stay (average length of stay 25 days), hospital-level care. Per reporting requirements established by the ACA, beginning in 2012, LTC hospitals must submit data to the CMS on three quality measures endorsed by the NQF:

- NQF #0138—National Health Safety Network (NHSN) Catheter-Associated Urinary Tract Infection Outcome Measure
- NQF #0139—NHSN Central Line–Associated Bloodstream Infection Outcome Measure
- NQF #0678—Percent of Residents with Pressure Ulcers That Are New or Worsened (Short-Stay)

Beginning in 2014, a financial penalty will be assessed for failure to submit data on these measures. In January 2014, two measures were added, with financial penalties for failure to report commencing in 2016:

- NQF #0680—Percent of Nursing Home Residents Who Were Assessed and Appropriately Given the Influenza Vaccine (Short-Stay)
- NQF #0431—Influenza Vaccination Coverage Among Healthcare Personnel[45]

The Joint Commission offers a Medicare/Medicaid LTC certification based on a facility's success in meeting five National Patient Safety Goals: (1) identify residents correctly, using at least two ways (e.g., name and date of birth) to ensure that each resident receives the appropriate medication and treatment; (2) use medicine safely by taking extra care with patients receiving anticoagulants, keeping careful records, communicating changes in prescriptions and dosages, and updating medication lists following physician visits; (3) prevent infections by using nationally recognized hand-washing guidelines and setting goals to improve adherence and by using proven guidelines to prevent bloodstream infections from forming in central lines; (4) prevent residents from falling by identifying those at greatest risk and taking appropriate action; and (5) prevent bed sores by identifying residents at greatest risk and taking preventive measures.[46] Nursing homes that are not certified under this program may be licensed by individual state survey agencies.

HOME HEALTH CARE

Home health, a covered service under Medicare, consists of part-time, medically necessary skilled care (i.e., nursing, physical therapy, occupational therapy, and speech-language therapy) ordered by a physician. In 2010, a total of 10,800 Medicare-certified home health agencies made 122,578,603 visits to patients throughout the United States.[47] Three types of CMS Home Health Quality Measures—process, outcome, and potentially avoidable event measures—have been reported since 2011. The tool used to collect and report home health agency performance data is the Outcome and Assessment Information Set (OASIS). Since 1999, the CMS has required Medicare-certified home health agencies to collect and transmit OASIS data for all adult patients whose care is reimbursed by Medicare or Medicaid (with the exception of patients receiving pre- or postnatal services only).[48] OASIS data are used to calculate quality reports that are provided to agencies as a guide for quality and performance improvement efforts. Effective in 2010, agencies are required to collect data items supporting measurement of rates for use of specific evidence-based processes. The CMS anticipates that these process measures will promote the use of best practices across the home health industry.

Beginning in the fall of 2003, the CMS has posted a subset of OASIS-based quality performance information on the Medicare.gov Home Health Compare website. These publicly reported data include outcome measures that indicate how well agencies assist their patients in regaining or maintaining their ability to function and process measures that evaluate the rate of the agency's use of specific evidence-based processes of care. The home healthcare quality measures currently reported on Home Health Compare are related to (1) managing daily activities; (2) managing pain and treating symptoms, such as symptoms of worsening heart failure or trouble breathing; (3) treating wounds and preventing pressure ulcers; (4) preventing harm, such as education on medications; and (5) preventing unplanned hospital care (e.g., how often the person was treated in the emergency department or admitted to the hospital).[49]

The CMS plans to introduce additional depression screening and pressure ulcer measures in 2015.[50] Home Health Compare also includes results of the Home Health Care (HHC) Consumer Assessment of Healthcare Provider Survey (CAHPS).

CONSUMER PERSPECTIVE

One of the six goals of the CMS Quality and Safety Strategy for 2013 and Beyond is to "strengthen person and family engagement as partners in their care."[51] The IOM defines patient-centered care as "providing care that is respectful of and responsive to individual patient preferences, needs and values, and ensures that patient values guide all clinical decisions."[52] The ACA directs the CMS to promote a focus on patient experience, self-management, and shared decision making. Because patients have limited data with which to make informed decisions as they relate to their care in the current provider-oriented system, the CMS intends to alter the healthcare landscape by encouraging and incentivizing providers to actively engage patients in their care. The consensus is that informed, engaged consumers will select high-quality care providers and share in the healthcare decision-making process.[52]

The AHRQ promotes patient-centered care through its family of patient experience surveys. Initially developed to evaluate the quality of health plans, the CAHPS program now includes a multitude of patient experience surveys for a variety of patient care settings. The goals of the CAHPS programs are to (1) develop standardized surveys that organizations can use to collect comparable information on patients' experience with care and (2) generate tools and resources to support the dissemination and use of comparative survey results to inform the public and improve healthcare quality.[53] The HCAHPS survey is a standardized tool used by all hospitals to compare patient experience.[23] Developed by the CMS and the AHRQ, the HCAHPS survey tool is composed of 18 questions in 10 domains related to the hospital experience:

- Nurse communication
- Doctor communication
- Responsiveness of hospital staff
- Pain management
- Communication about medicines
- Discharge information
- Cleanliness of hospital environment
- Quietness of hospital environment
- Overall rating of hospital
- Willingness to recommend hospital

The AHRQ has a variety of different CGCAHPS surveys to capture patient experience in ambulatory settings.[54] Common quality measures on the surveys include the following:

- Getting timely appointments, care, and information
- How well providers (or doctors) communicate with patients

- Helpful, courteous, and respectful office staff
- Patients' rating of the provider (or doctor)

The Home Health CAHPS survey includes questions related to provider professionalism, communication, and discussions about medication safety and pain management. Beneficiaries are also asked to rank the agency and whether they would recommend its services to friends and family.[54]

Since 2006, hospitals have voluntarily submitted HCAHPS data to the CMS, which started public reporting of results on the Hospital Compare website in 2008. Although submission is voluntary, hospitals must provide the data to the CMS to receive their full annual payment update.[23,24] For providers in the outpatient setting, the CMS will start to tie performance on the CGCAHPS to the Physician Value-Based Payment Modifier and provide payment to physicians based on the quality of care compared to cost. The Home Health CAHPS survey was developed by the AHRQ in 2008 and received NQF endorsement in 2009. In 2012 the CMS started reporting the results from the HHCAHPS surveys on Home Health Compare to provide consumers with comparative data on patients' perspectives, to improve transparency, and to create incentives for home health agencies to improve the care provided to CMS beneficiaries.[55] Using the same strategy of financial penalties in the home care setting as those used in other provider settings, the CMS stipulates that home health agencies must contract with a certified survey vendor and submit the CAHPS data to the CMS to receive the annual payment update.

CONCLUSION

Improving healthcare quality and safety requires change, and such change will rely on a coordinated effort among all stakeholders—government policy makers, clinicians, healthcare organizations, and patients alike. Building on existing initiatives, the ACA set in motion ACOs, PCMHs, and VBP programs to improve care coordination and increase provider accountability. Although the full value of these approaches will take time to realize, advances toward better quality and lower cost are likely to be achieved in the process. Embracing current and future changes will require a shift in thinking, a shift in culture, and advances in technology.[28]

STUDY AND DISCUSSION QUESTIONS

1. What elements of the ACA have the potential to improve quality?
2. How can a PCMH support population health management?
3. What are the core components of the CMS VBP programs?
4. How will public reporting of quality measures improve quality of care?

SUGGESTED READINGS AND WEBSITES

READINGS

Institute of Medicine. *To Err Is Human: Building a Safer Health System*. Washington, DC: National Academy Press; 2000.

Nash DB, Clarke J, Skoufalos A, Horowitz M. *Health Care Quality: The Clinician's Primer*. Tampa, FL: American College of Physician Executives; 2012.

WEBSITES

Centers for Medicare and Medicaid Services. Hospital Value-Based Purchasing: http://www.cms.gov/Medicare/Quality-Initiatives-Patient-Assessment-Instruments/hospital-value-based-purchasing/index.html?redirect=/hospital-value-based-purchasing/ and http://www.cms.gov/Outreach-and-Education/Medicare-Learning-Network-MLN/MLNProducts/downloads/Hospital_VBPurchasing_Fact_Sheet_ICN907664.pdf. Accessed November 2, 2014.

Health Affairs. Health Policy Brief. Pay-for-Performance: http://healthaffairs.org/healthpolicybriefs/brief_pdfs/healthpolicybrief_78.pdf. Accessed November 2, 2014.

Medicare Hospital Compare: http://www.cms.gov/Medicare/Quality-Initiatives-Patient-Assessment-Instruments/HospitalQualityInits/HospitalCompare.html. Accessed November 2, 2014.

Medicare Physician Compare: http://www.cms.gov/Medicare/Quality-Initiatives-Patient-Assessment-Instruments/physician-compare-initiative/Physician-Compare-Overview.html. Accessed November 17, 2014.

National Committee for Quality Assurance (NCQA). HEDIS and Performance Measurement: http://www.ncqa.org/HEDISQualityMeasurement.aspx. Accessed November 2, 2014.

National Quality Forum (NQF). http://www.qualityforum.org/Home.aspx. Accessed November 10, 2014.

REFERENCES

1. Pracilio VP, Reifsnyder J, Nash D, Fabius R. The population health mandate. In: Nash D, Reifsnyder J, Fabius R, Pracilio VP, eds. *Population Health: Creating a Culture of Wellness*. Sudbury, MA: Jones & Bartlett; 2011:xxxv-lii.

2. Kindig DA. Understanding population health terminology. *Milbank Q*. 2007;85:139-61.

3. Kindig D, Stoddart G. What is population health? *Am J Public Health*. 2003;93:380-3.

4. Institute of Medicine. *To Err Is Human: Building a Safer Health System*. Washington, DC: National Academy Press; 2000.

5. County Health Rankings and Roadmaps. A Robert Wood Johnson Foundation Program. http://www.countyhealthrankings.org/our-approach. Accessed October 28, 2014.

6. DesHarnais S, Pracilio VP. Population health quality and safety. In: Nash D, Reifsnyder J,

Fabius R, Pracilio VP, eds. *Population Health: Creating a Culture of Wellness*. Sudbury, MA: Jones & Bartlett; 2011:89-104.

7. Donabedian A. Evaluating the quality of medical care. *Milbank Mem Fund Q*. 1966;44(Suppl):166-206.

8. The Dartmouth Atlas of Health Care. Understanding of the Efficiency and Effectiveness of the Health Care System. http://www.dartmouthatlas.org/index.shtm. Accessed October 28, 2014.

9. National Quality Forum. What NQF Endorsement Means. http://www.qualityforum.org/Measuring_Performance/ABCs/What_NQF_Endorsement_Means.aspx. Accessed October 28, 2014.

10. National Quality Forum. How Endorsement Happens. http://www.qualityforum.org/Measuring_Performance/ABCs/How_Endorsement_Happens.aspx. Accessed October 28, 2014.

11. Agency for Healthcare Research and Quality (AHRQ). National Quality Measures Clearinghouse. http://www.qualitymeasures.ahrq.gov/about/. Accessed November 17, 2014.

12. National Quality Measures Clearinghouse. Template of Measure Attributes. http://www.qualitymeasures.ahrq.gov/about/template-of-attributes.aspx. Accessed October 28, 2014.

13. Institute for Healthcare Improvement. IHI Triple Aim Initiative. http://www.ihi.org/Engage/Initiatives/TripleAim/Pages/default.aspx. Accessed October 28, 2014.

14. National Patient Safety Foundation. NPSF at a Glance. http://www.npsf.org/?page=npsfataglance. Accessed December 31, 2014.

15. National Committee for Quality Assurance (NCQA). HEDIS Life Cycle. http://www.ncqa.org/tabid/425/Default.aspx. Accessed October 28, 2014.

16. National Committee for Quality Assurance (NCQA). The Essential Guide to Health Care Quality. http://www.ncqa.org/Portals/0/Publications/Resource Library/NCQA_Primer_web.pdf. Accessed October 28, 2014.

17. National Committee for Quality Assurance (NCQA). Focus on Obesity and on Medicare Plan Improvement. The State of Health Care Quality 2012. http://www.ncqa.org/Portals/0/State%20of%20Health%20Care/2012/SOHC_Report_Web.pdf. Accessed October 28, 2014.

18. National Committee for Quality Assurance (NCQA). What Is HEDIS? HEDIS and Quality Compass. http://www.ncqa.org/HEDISQualityMeasurement/WhatisHEDIS.aspx. Accessed October 28, 2014.

19. Goodrich K, Garcia E, Conway, P. A history of and a vision for CMS quality measurement programs. *Jt Comm J Qual Patient Saf*. 2012;38(10):465-70.

20. Chassin MR, O'Kane ME. History of the quality improvement movement. In: Burns SD, Kott A, eds. *Toward Improving the Outcome of Pregnancy III*; 2010:1-8. http://www.marchofdimes.com/materials/toward-improving-the-outcome-of-pregnancy-iii.pdf. Accessed October 28, 2014.

21. Marjoua Y, Bozic KJ. Brief history of quality movement in US healthcare. *Current Rev Musculoskelet Med*. 2012;5:265-73.

22. Millenson ML, Macri J. Will the Affordable Care Act Move Patient-Centeredness to Center Stage? Robert Wood Johnson Foundation. http://www.rwjf.org/en/research-publications/find-rwjf-research/2012/03/will-the-affordable-care-act-move-patient-centeredness-to-center.html. Accessed October 28, 2014.

23. Washington E, Lipstein SH. The patient-centered outcomes research institute—promoting better information, decisions, and health. *N Engl J Med*. 2011;365(15):e31.

24. Benzer JK, Young GJ, Burgess JF, et al. Sustainability of quality improvement following removal of pay-for-performance incentives. *J Gen Intern Med*. 2014;29(1):127-32.

25. Blumenthal D, Jena AB. Hospital value-based purchasing. *J Hosp Med*. 2013;8(5):271-7.

26. North Carolina Institute of Medicine. Examining the Impact of the Patient Protection and Affordable Care Act in North Carolina. Chapter 7: Quality. January 2013. http://www.nciom.org/wp-content/uploads/2013/01/FULL-REPORT-2-13-2013.pdf. Accessed October 28, 2014.

27. Wang QC, Chawla R, Colombo CM, et al. Patient-centered medical home impact on health plan members with diabetes. *J Public Health Manag Pract*. 2014;20(5):E12-20.

28. Berwick DM. Launching Accountable Care Organizations—the proposed rule for the Medicare

Shared Savings Program. *N Engl J Med.* 2011; 364(16):e32.

29. Health reform implementation time line. http://kff.org/interactive/implementation-timeline/. Updated 2013. Accessed October 28, 2014.

30. American College of Physicians. Accountable Care Organizations (ACOs) Summary. http://www.acponline.org/advocacy/where_we_stand/assets/aco.pdf. Accessed October 28, 2014.

31. Moore R, Rachman FD, Lardiere MR. Using Health Information Technology to Improve Quality. National Association of Commnity Health Centers. June 2010. http://iweb.nachc.com/downloads/products/HCCN_15_10.pdf. Accessed October 28, 2014.

32. Institute of Medicine. Health IT and Patient Safety. Building Safer Systems for Better Care. November 8,2011.http://www.iom.edu/Reports/2011/Health-IT-and-Patient-Safety-Building-Safer-Systems-for-Better-Care.aspx. Accessed October 28, 2014.

33. Agency for Healthcare Research and Quality. Frequently Asked Questions. What is a PSO? https://www.pso.ahrq.gov/faq#WhatisaPSO. Accessed December 31, 2014.

34. Agency for Healthcare Research and Quality. Frequently Asked Questions. Who can seek listing as a PSO? http://www.pso.ahrq.gov/faq#whocanseeklisting. Accessed December 31, 2014.

35. Tu HT, Boukus ER. Despite rapid growth, retail clinic use remains modest. Health System Change Research Brief No. 29. http://www.hschange.org/CONTENT/1392/. Accessed October 28, 2014.

36. Miller JM, Nash DB. Quality metrics and initiatives in the clinic setting. In: Riff J, Ryan SF, Hansen-Turton T, eds. *Convenient Care Clinics: The Essential Guide to Retail Clinics for Clinicians, Managers, and Educators.* New York: Springer Publishing Company; 2013.

37. Mehrotra A, Liu H, Adams JL, et al. Comparing costs and quality of care at retail clinics with that of other medical settings for 3 common illnesses. *Ann Intern Med.* 2009;151:321-8.

38. Woodburn JD, Smith KL, Nelson GD. Quality of care in the retail health care setting using national clinical guidelines for acute pharyngitis. *Am J Med Qual.* 2007;22(6):457-62.

39. American Academy of Urgent Care Medicine. Future of Urgent Care. http://aaucm.org/about/future/default.aspx. Accessed October 28, 2014.

40. American Academy of Urgent Care Medicine. Urgent Care Center Accreditation. https://aaucm.org/professionals/accreditation/default.aspx. Accessed October 28, 2014.

41. Weinick RM, Bristol SJ, DesRoches CM. Urgent care update: the quality of care at urgent care centers. *JUCM.* February 2009. http://jucm.com/pdf/The_Quality_of_Care_at_Urgent_Care_Centers.pdf. Accessed October 28, 2014.

42. Centers for Medicare and Medicaid Services. Nursing Home Compare. https://www.medicare.gov/nursinghomecompare/?AspxAutoDetectCookieSupport=1. Accessed October 28, 2014.

43. Centers for Medicare and Medicaid Services. What is Nursing Home Compare? http://www.medicare.gov/nursinghomecompare/About/What-Is-NHC.html. Accessed October 28, 2014.

44. Centers for Medicare and Medicaid Services. Nursing Home Quality Initiative. Quality Measures. What's New? http://www.cms.gov/Medicare/Quality-Initiatives-Patient-Assessment-Instruments/NursingHomeQualityInits/NHQIQualityMeasures.html. Accessed October 28, 2014.

45. Centers for Medicare and Medicaid Services. Long term care hospital prospective payment system: news. http://www.cms.gov/Outreach-and-Education/Medicare-Learning-Network-MLN/MLNProducts/downloads/ltch-news.pdf. Accessed October 28, 2014.

46. The Joint Commission Accreditation. Long Term Care Medicare/Medicaid Certification-based Option. National Patient Safety Goals, 2014. http://www.jointcommission.org/assets/1/6/2014_LTC2_NPSG_E.pdf. Accessed October 28, 2014.

47. Centers for Medicare and Medicaid. Home Health Quality Initiative. Quality Measures Used in the Home Health Quality Reporting Program. http://cms.gov/Medicare/Quality-Initiatives-Patient-Assessment-Instruments/HomeHealthQualityInits/HHQIQualityMeasures.html. Accessed October 28, 2014.

48. Scharpf TP, Madigan EA. Functional status outcome measures in home health care patients with heart failure. *Home Health Care Serv Q.* 2010;29(4):155-70.

49. Centers for Medicare and Medicaid Services. Home Health Compare. http://www.medicare.gov/homehealthcompare/search.html. Accessed October 28, 2014.

50. Centers for Medicare and Medicaid Services. Upcoming Changes to Home Health Quality Reporting. March 19, 2014. http://www.nahc.org/assets/1/7/MoW14-101.pdf. Accessed October 28, 2014.

51. Centers for Medicare and Medicaid Services. CMS Quality Strategy 2013–Beyond. November 18, 2013. https://www.cms.gov/Medicare/Quality-Initiatives-Patient-Assessment-Instruments/QualityInitiativesGenInfo/Downloads/CMS-Quality-Strategy.pdf. Accessed October 28, 2014.

52. Institute of Medicine. Crossing the Quality Chasm: A New Health System for the 21st Century. March 2001. http://www.iom.edu/~/media/Files/Report%20Files/2001/Crossing-the-Quality-Chasm/Quality%20Chasm%202001%20%20report%20brief.pdf. Accessed October 28, 2014.

53. Agency for Healthcare Research and Quality (AHRQ). CAHPS: Assessing Health Care Quality From the Patient's Perspective. https://cahps.ahrq.gov/about-cahps/cahps-program/14-p004_cahps.pdf. Accessed October 28, 2014.

54. Agency for Healthcare Research and Quality (AHRQ). Clinician and Group Surveys. https://cahps.ahrq.gov/surveys-guidance/cg/index.html. Accessed October 28, 2014.

55. Centers for Medicare and Medicaid Services. Home Health Care CAHPS Survey. https://homehealthcahps.org/GeneralInformation/AboutHomeHealthCareCAHPSSurvey.aspx. Accessed October 28, 2014.

Chapter 12

INFORMATION TECHNOLOGY

JOHN K. CUDDEBACK AND DONALD W. FISHER

Executive Summary

Good data are the cornerstone of population health management.

Health information technology sits at the intersection of two very dynamic fields, health care and information technology (IT). Healthcare providers are finally recognizing the importance of managing population health, which is possible only by using IT at multiple levels. At the same time, health IT is moving beyond traditional, provider-focused systems. Providers and payers are collaborating to integrate data to better understand the populations they serve. Many individuals are assuming greater accountability by using mobile apps to measure and manage their own health, proactively, outside the boundaries of the traditional healthcare system. And many provider organizations are broadening their focus to encompass health promotion and wellness, although few are yet able to integrate data from mobile apps into their systems.

This evolution will be the focus of this chapter, but we should also mention that health care is on the threshold of another dramatic change enabled by IT. The cost of genetic testing is rapidly declining, which will make it more widely available. That will create larger pools of genetic information, and new analytic methods will enrich our understanding of the genetic correlates of health and disease, particularly for conditions associated with multiple genetic factors.[1] Over the next decade or two, this will promote a highly personalized approach to preventing, diagnosing, and treating a variety of health conditions.

Learning Objectives

1. Become familiar with the benefits of capturing clinical data in structured form in an electronic health record (EHR).
2. Understand the relationship between point-of-care systems (e.g., EHRs), surveillance and tracking systems (e.g., patient registries), and retrospective analytic systems (e.g., data warehouses).
3. Explain some of the challenges of integrating data collected by a patient's mobile apps into a provider organization's EHR.
4. Evaluate the strengths and weaknesses of clinical and administrative data for health services research.
5. Become familiar with ways in which provider organizations can use population-level analyses for performance improvement.
6. Understand the potential of cognitive systems in assisting healthcare providers in "keeping up with the literature" and applying new findings in caring for their patients.
7. Recognize critical success factors for EHR implementation and unintended consequences of inserting information technology into healthcare workflows.

Key Terms

administrative data
alert fatigue
Blue Button initiative
care coordinator
case management
claims data
clinical data
clinical decision support
clinical guidelines
computable data
computerized physician order entry
controlled vocabulary
cost accounting
data warehouse
diagnosis-related groups
discrete field
disease registry
electronic health record
enterprise master patient index
episode of illness
evidence-based guidelines
gaps in care
genomic profile

grouper
health information exchange
Health Insurance Portability and
    Accountability Act of 1996
Health Level Seven
health services research
longitudinal patient record
meaningful use (of health information
    technology)
national provider identifier
natural language processing
Office of the National Coordinator for
    Health Information Technology
ontology
outlier
patient attribution
patient portal
patient registration
patient registry
pharmacovigilance
population management systems
practice management system
predictive models

process redesign
prospective payment
protected health information
revenue cycle
risk adjustment

semantic interoperability
structured data
transaction systems
transparency

IT FOUNDATIONS FOR POPULATION HEALTH: FROM PAPER MEDICAL RECORDS TO EHR, PATIENT REGISTRY, AND DECISION SUPPORT

Traditional paper medical records have many shortcomings, including illegible handwriting and a lack of templates to guide clinicians in documenting critical clinical information. Paper records can be used in only one place at a time and can be misplaced or lost. They cannot provide **clinical decision support**—alerts and reminders driven by **evidence-based guidelines**, plus context-sensitive reference material to assist clinicians in caring for individual patients. For population health, the critical shortcoming of paper records is that patient-level data cannot be aggregated to create a picture of the population, their care, and the outcomes of that care. Moving from paper to an **electronic health record** (EHR) is essential for managing population health.

An EHR is much more than a record. At the patient level, it is a dynamic tool that enables a new approach to clinical workflow, evidence-based decision making, and team-based care. At the population level, it enables both care and learning—*care* in the sense of identifying patients who may be at risk for poor outcomes because they have not received care, which is indicated according to current evidence, and *learning* in the sense of using aggregate data to refine and expand the evidence base, to enhance our understanding of what interventions are most effective, and cost-effective, for certain subsets of patients within a population.

Healthcare has lagged far behind other information-intensive industries in its use of IT. Broad adoption and "meaningful use" of interoperable EHRs with clinical decision support is recognized as essential for substantially improving quality and reducing overall cost. Promoting effective use of IT has become a key area of focus for U.S. health policy and healthcare reform. Although healthcare providers have used information technology for decades, IT was initially used for administrative functions, such as patient registration, billing, and financial management. Ironically, the extreme fragmentation and complexity of healthcare payment in the United States has forced providers to continue investing in administrative systems to protect their financial stability, deferring implementation of clinical systems that could actually improve the quality, safety, and efficiency of the core business—promoting health and providing care to patients. Early EHRs focused on transcribed dictation, which addressed the problem of lost or illegible records and made patient information available to multiple users at once. But prescriptions for medications were still written on paper, so these systems could not alert physicians to potential drug-to-drug interactions. Many hospitals installed computerized order communication systems on nursing units, but these systems simply replaced slips of paper sent to the laboratory or the radiology department. They did not assist physicians in deciding what to order.

These early clinical systems lacked three things that are essential for improving patient care and supporting population health: (1) entry of key data elements in structured form, (2) decision support for physicians and other clinicians, and (3) support for workflow and communication among members of the care team within an organization and interoperability with other providers. The value of EHRs and the data they capture can best be understood in terms of a twofold problem in evidence-based medicine: the non-application of relevant existing evidence in the care of individual patients and the lack of evidence germane to common clinical situations.[2] Two classic studies illustrate these problems. First, McGlynn and colleagues found that U.S. adults received only 55% of recommended preventive care, acute care, and care for chronic conditions such as hypertension (high blood pressure) and diabetes.[3] EHRs can address this gap at the patient level by ensuring that a patient's chronic conditions are addressed and that appropriate preventive care is provided on every visit, even if the visit is for a minor acute condition. Provider organizations can address this gap at the population level by using a **patient registry**, a database of all the provider's patients who have certain chronic conditions or need periodic screening or preventive care. It enables the organization to identify patients who need care but are not scheduled for, or have missed, an appointment. These are often referred to as "**gaps in care**." A registry is typically used by a **care coordinator**, who contacts patients who need care but are not receiving it. Information about outreach efforts should be sent back to the EHR, giving clinicians a complete view of all interactions with the patient. Second, Boyd and colleagues reviewed current **clinical guidelines** for common chronic diseases and found that they generally fail to account for multiple comorbid conditions.[4] The strict application of existing guidelines to a hypothetical elderly patient with five common chronic conditions yielded a medication regimen so complex it would be unmanageable. In practice, physicians often make thoughtful compromises when treating complex patients. Capturing data from these "natural experiments" allows us to develop optimized protocols for specific patient populations by aggregating the data for those patients and then studying the relationships between the actual process of care and the resulting outcomes.

IMPORTANCE OF STRUCTURED DATA

To improve the care of individual patients through clinical decision support, data must be captured in structured form. For example, the EHR should contain a problem list with the patient's symptoms and diagnoses coded so the software can apply guidelines that recognize and adjust for specific comorbid conditions. The patient's allergies and intolerances should also be coded so the EHR's decision support logic can recognize, for example, that the first-line therapy for a new diagnosis is a drug in the same class as one to which the patient has had an allergic reaction in the past. The EHR could then suggest using an alternative drug that is not likely to cause an allergic reaction. This type of decision support requires that information about the patient's allergies be selected from a pulldown list of drugs and drug classes rather than entered as error-prone free text.

There are two key aspects of **structured data**: (1) a **discrete field**, or data element, for each concept and (2) a standard set of codes, or a **controlled vocabulary**, for expressing the content of each field. Because they can be used directly by computerized clinical decision support algorithms, structured data are referred to as **computable data**. For example, current hypertension guidelines recommend treatment for patients age 60 years or older whose blood pressure is 150/90 mm Hg or higher, unless the patient has diabetes or chronic kidney disease, in which case blood pressure should be controlled to 140/90 or lower.[5] If an EHR contains a structured problem list, medication list, and blood pressure readings over time, it can provide very precise clinical decision support. It can alert clinicians during a visit (1) if the patient's blood pressure exceeds the applicable threshold, depending on age and comorbid conditions; (2) if the patient's blood pressure is trending upward over time, despite prescribed therapy; and (3) in an e-prescribing system that receives updates from pharmacies, whether the patient is refilling his or her prescriptions for antihypertensive medications on schedule or perhaps is continuing to refill a prescription that the physician had meant to discontinue.

At the population level, structured data are required to assemble patient registries that show the current status of all patients who have certain chronic conditions. This involves aggregating data for all patients who have a particular diagnosis on their problem list in the EHR, and it requires that data for all patients be expressed using common code sets. Structured data are also essential for comparative effectiveness research, which requires information on the health and health care of many patients, over time and across providers. Capturing data in structured form imposes a greater burden on the person who enters the data, but it yields downstream benefits—in the care of individual patients, in managing population health, and in developing new knowledge to expand the evidence base with specific guidance for real-world clinical situations.

An important concept related to structured data is **semantic interoperability** between two computer systems. *Semantics* is the study of meaning, and the term is similar to the concept of computable data. If two systems exchange a scanned image of a narrative progress note, written legibly by hand, they would enable their human users to gain a common understanding of the patient's status. But an e-prescribing system receiving only the scanned image cannot use it to warn the prescriber that the patient is allergic to the medication that is about to be prescribed. Two systems exchanging a scanned note are interoperable, but they are not semantically interoperable. If they exchanged a coded allergy list using a common coding system, they would be.

Commonly used code sets include ICD-9-CM and ICD-10-CM (International Classification of Diseases, 9th or 10th Revision, Clinical Modification), used for patient diagnoses on insurance claims, and CPT-4 (Current Procedural Terminology, 4th Edition) and HCPCS (Healthcare Common Procedure Coding System), used for coding professional services like physician office visits, consultations, and surgical procedures.[6] Medicare and most commercial insurance plans pay hospitals a fixed amount for each admission, dependent on the patient's diagnoses and surgical procedure(s) performed. This is called **prospective payment**. Each hospital admission is classified into one of about 750 categories, called **diagnosis-related groups** (DRGs), and a fixed payment rate is established for every patient in a given DRG, with some adjustments for very costly cases, called **outliers**. The software that assigns cases to DRGs is called a **grouper**. DRGs are convenient, but dividing the entire spectrum of hospital care into just 750 categories yields relatively coarse groupings, particularly for pediatrics and other low-volume populations, so the patients and the care provided within these DRGs may be quite heterogeneous. It is also important to remember that DRGs were designed for payment, so they group patients by overall cost of hospital resources consumed (excluding professional fees), which may not be correlated with risk of mortality or other clinical outcomes.

ADMINISTRATIVE DATA VS. CLINICAL DATA

The **Health Insurance Portability and Accountability Act** (HIPAA) of 1996 established privacy and security requirements for individually identifiable health information, commonly known as **protected health information**, and it also established standard formats and coding systems for billing and for payment of insurance claims—the administrative simplification provisions of the act. The series of bills or insurance claims for each patient, typically called **administrative data** or **claims data**, provide a useful view of the care process. It is a stylized view, filtered through billing rules that depend on the way providers are organized and the nature and continuity of a patient's insurance coverage. The diagnosis information may be incomplete, especially for ambulatory care, and claims indicate only that a lab test or diagnostic procedure was done, not the result. Claims data are blind to noncovered services, for which no claim is generated, and patient outcomes must be inferred from subsequent care (e.g., for a complication) or the lack of it. Physician office visits are typically reflected in claims data, but activities such as care coordination, visit planning, patient outreach, patient education, and health coaching are not. These are often critical to achieving good outcomes, yet they are seldom reflected in claims data because they are seldom reimbursed. Medications are often a crucial part of therapy, so pharmacy claims can provide important information. Because they reflect drugs actually dispensed, they indicate whether patients are refilling their prescriptions on schedule. Yet claims data reflect only prescription medications for which patients used their pharmacy benefit, so they may exclude over-the-counter medications, nutraceuticals, and prescriptions filled through low-cost generic programs. Claims data also suffer discontinuities when the patient changes health plans, which often happens with a change in employment.

Despite some blind spots, administrative data have the advantage of being structured, with discrete fields and common code sets for the patient's diagnoses, services provided, and procedures performed. They reflect all covered services that a patient received, from any provider, and the sequence of billable events constitutes a standardized framework for a longitudinal patient record. **Clinical data** are much richer but were historically recorded in unstructured form. EHRs permit key data—from allergies and smoking status to physical findings, pain scales, and functional assessments—to be recorded in structured form. Lab results, clinical observations like height, weight, and blood pressure, and key results of diagnostic tests are typically available as structured data. Providers are increasingly using patient portals, not just to allow patients to access their lab results but also to obtain patient-reported outcomes and health risk factors. However, unless a patient receives essentially all her or his care from a single provider organization, or providers are sharing data via a health information exchange (described later in this chapter), clinical data may mirror the fragmentation of the delivery system, with each provider's record providing a rich but narrow view.

INCENTIVES FOR EHR ADOPTION

Large, multispecialty medical groups have been using EHRs and disease registries, and e-prescribing for more than a decade, as has the Veterans Health Administration. But few small practices have had the time or money to undertake a disruptive IT implementation, and the EHR market for smaller practices has been relatively fluid, making vendor selection challenging. With few clinical support staff, small practices also have limited potential to gain efficiencies through workflow redesign. Fortunately, EHRs and **practice management systems** are becoming available as cloud-based systems, which simplifies technical support, and configuration of clinical decision support and workflow features is getting easier. These factors, combined with federal incentive payments, are accelerating EHR adoption by small and medium-size practices, as well as implementation of **computerized physician order entry** (CPOE) and structured documentation systems in hospitals. As part of the economic stimulus legislation passed in 2009, Congress authorized the Centers for Medicare and Medicaid Services (CMS) to provide financial incentives up to $44,000 per physician for practices and hospitals who achieve **meaningful use** of EHRs. The systems must meet certain standards for capture of structured data, interoperability with other providers, and reporting population-based quality measures. Rewarding meaningful use recognizes that improved health and health care do not result simply from adoption of IT but rather from using the technology to inform clinical decisions; enhance efficiency and patient safety by ensuring that relevant information is not forgotten or overlooked; engage patients and families; monitor and improve quality, safety, and cost efficiency; and reduce health disparities among minorities and disadvantaged populations. The meaningful use criteria mirror the themes of this chapter and address population health explicitly. Incentive payments began in 2012, with the first of three stages of requirements. Later stages require that patients actually use Web portals and that providers report quality measures in order to receive the full incentive payment. By April 2014, 53% of physicians had received at least one incentive payment.[7] This is a dramatic increase in EHR adoption, up from an estimated 11% in 2006.[8] Not all of these EHRs meet the full, later-stage meaningful use criteria, and many aspects of EHR software can still be improved. But most experts believe federal incentives have brought us to a tipping point in adoption and use of EHRs and e-prescribing.

USING POPULATION-LEVEL ANALYTICS FOR IMPROVEMENT

We have discussed the use of existing evidence, generally in the form of clinical guidelines, to ensure that patients receive the appropriate care: (1) individualized alerts and reminders, delivered via an EHR at the point of care when a patient is being seen, and (2) the surveillance function of a patient registry, which entails looking across a patient population to determine who is overdue for screening, periodic testing, or follow-up care to facilitate outreach by a care coordinator. Both involve comparing what is known about patients (in the form of structured data) to established guidelines or care protocols, at the patient level and at the population level. We have also mentioned the use of aggregate data from multiple provider organizations for comparative effectiveness research, which contributes to periodic national or international efforts by expert panels to update established guidelines.

Provider organizations can use analyses of population-level data in two important ways. Figure 12-1 shows a hypothetical distribution of patients—say, a population of patients with diabetes—by overall cost of care, over a period of time. As with most distributions of patients, it is skewed to the right. The majority of patients have relatively low overall cost, but a few incur high cost, perhaps because they develop a complication that requires them to be admitted to a hospital or because they have several other conditions that also require treatment. One use of data like these is for **process redesign**, with the goal of improving care for the typical patient—in this case reducing overall cost while maintaining or improving quality. An important principle of quality improvement is that doing something consistently enables continual learning by using data to stimulate conversation about ways to enhance the consistency and reliability of care and to discover where small variations lead to better outcomes. Reducing case-to-case variation is a key goal of care coordination, to ensure that all patients receive consistent, complete, and timely care. For example, there is often wide variation in the medications used by different physicians for the same condition or in how heavily primary care physicians rely on specialist referrals for patients with multiple chronic conditions. These situations may represent opportunities for improvement by developing evidence-based care protocols, which is one form of process redesign.[9]

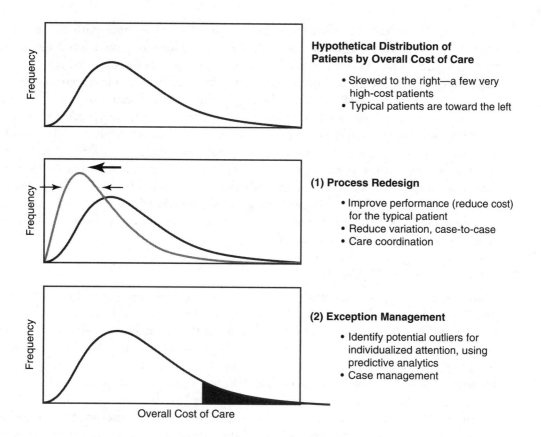

Figure 12-1 Two components of performance improvement.

Key to managing population health is the Pareto principle, commonly called the "80–20 rule." The 80–20 figure is actually quite accurate for the noninstitutionalized U.S. civilian population: 20% of the people consume 80% of the total medical costs. Within that group, however, there is even more extreme concentration: just 5% of people consume 50% of costs.[10] Some of these high utilizers are already sick and are relatively easy to identify. But others can be identified through **predictive models**, which use large databases to determine factors that identify patients at risk for future illness and consequent utilization. Not all of this utilization can be averted, but the patients at highest risk should be considered for intervention. Unlike care coordination, which is focused on ensuring that mainstream patients reliably receive routine care, the **case management** function is broader and tailored to the individual needs of complex patients. It could involve using telehealth to monitor daily weights in a patient with congestive heart failure or helping the patient deal with social issues that affect compliance with treatment or present barriers to receiving care. Health plans (insurers) have long done broad risk stratification, based on past utilization as reflected in claims data, but newer predictive models based on clinical data extracted from EHRs perform much better. One current model can identify 15% of patients with chronic obstructive pulmonary disease who make up more than half of the patients who will, absent intervention, have an emergency department (ED) visit or inpatient admission over the next 6 months.[11] Such models can help provider organizations focus limited case management resources on the patients for whom they are likely to be most effective. An important theme in managing population health is using data to identify people who have needs—whether for routine care or screening in people who are generally healthy (using registries) or for individualized support in complex patients at high risk (using predictive models)—and then reaching out proactively to these people to ensure that their needs are met.

MOBILE HEALTH AND SOCIAL MEDIA

Most of the core applications used by healthcare providers were designed long before the first iPhone was introduced in 2007. These applications have seen incremental improvements in software functionality, new population health and analytics modules, and better end-user devices, but their core architecture remains provider centric. Meanwhile, mobile computing and social media have fundamentally changed the way most Americans interact with information and with each other. We now expect a level of **transparency** and convenience in business transactions that could barely have been imagined in 2007. Why has online healthcare lagged so far behind online banking and the purchase of airline tickets? There are obvious differences in the nature and circumstances of the interactions: Healthcare providers deal with people at their most vulnerable, as they address matters of life and death; family members and other caregivers are usually involved; and health care has a spiritual dimension that is seldom associated with banking. In the discussion about structured data, we got a glimpse of the depth and complexity of the data needed to describe health and health care, plus the challenges of expressing these data in standardized form. In banking, a person has opened an account in advance and carries a standardized ATM card, and everything is expressed in terms of dollars. In health care, there is no standard for identifying individuals (who sometimes want to conceal their identity), and data about health and health care are far more complex and nuanced.

Mobile health apps are evolving rapidly, enabling patients to track and manage aspects of their health "in the white space between office visits" and promoting patient engagement and accountability. New sensor technologies will make it practical for patients to measure a variety of clinical parameters, and mobile apps can also facilitate access to an expert. Telemedicine is rapidly becoming mainstream. There will be a growing demand for home care as baby boomers age, and mobile technology promises to empower teams of caregivers, just as EHRs have done within medical practices. Patients are increasingly using **patient portals** offered by providers and connected to the provider's EHR. Indeed, later stages of the Meaningful Use incentives require providers to use secure electronic messaging to communicate with a portion of their patients. Portals can help patients' family members, such as adult children of elderly patients, to participate in their care. However, apps not obtained from the provider organization can present significant challenges. Protocols for responding to patient messages on a portal can be relatively straightforward, but clarifying expectations and liability for a provider organization to monitor and take action on unsolicited physiologic data, such as home blood pressure readings, is far more difficult. Few provider-sponsored portals accept data directly from mobile apps such as electronic scales or blood pressure cuffs. Third-party services are available to transfer data between patient devices and provider EHRs, but they are seeing only limited use.[12]

SYSTEMS FOR PROVIDER ORGANIZATIONS

The IT systems within a typical healthcare provider organization can be grouped into three major categories: (1) transaction systems, (2) population management systems, and (3) data warehouses and analytics. These categories are distinguished by the business functions they support and the level of data aggregation, from individual patients to broad populations. Figure 12-2 shows major "logical" systems within each category (i.e., functions that must be performed, whether by discrete software systems or by modules within a larger system, as well as some typical data types). As noted at the top of the figure, transaction and population management systems are used concurrently to support operations, and data warehouses are generally retrospective. But as shown at the bottom of the figure, care protocols developed through retrospective analysis are implemented in the concurrent systems. Transaction systems are generally focused at the level of an individual patient, while population management and data warehouses aggregate data from all patients within a provider organization's population.

PATIENT- AND POPULATION-LEVEL OPERATIONAL SYSTEMS

Systems that support granular business or clinical processes are considered **transaction systems**. An EHR focuses on a series of patient care events, one patient at a time. A patient scheduling system arranges individual appointments. These systems provide some natural data aggregation, such as patient problem lists and medication lists in an EHR, or a scheduling system view showing all patient appointments with a given provider on a given day. But these systems aggregate limited types of data for a particular purpose. EHRs typically support care planning, order entry and management, communication among the care team, and documentation of care, from progress notes to medication administration. Provider organizations may also have specialized systems for certain

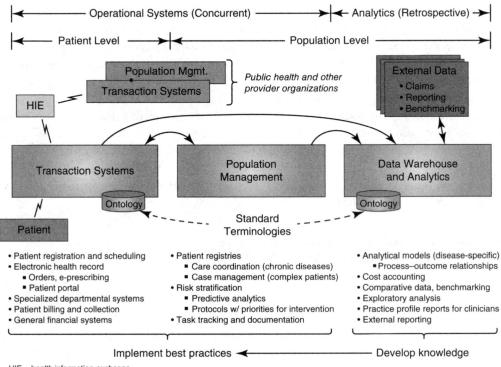

Figure 12-2 Systems used by provider organizations.

departments and functions. A surgical system schedules the rooms, equipment, personnel, and supplies necessary for each procedure and also tracks implants. Laboratory, blood banking, pharmacy, and radiology systems manage both clinical data and departmental workflow. Medical imaging requires dedicated systems for picture archiving and communication (PACS). These may be modules of a comprehensive hospital information system (HIS), or they may be dedicated departmental systems that are interfaced via a messaging protocol called **Health Level Seven** (HL7). As health care becomes more specialized and sophisticated, information demands escalate, and the need for precise coordination among an expanding team of direct care providers and essential support services continues to grow.

A core system within every provider organization is **patient registration**, which maintains a record of every patient who receives care and cross-references the way each patient is identified in the organization's systems. If an organization has older ("legacy") systems with different ways of identifying patients, an **enterprise master patient index** (EMPI or MPI) may be used to translate among the patient identifiers used in different systems. Identifying patients can be quite complex because a person's name may change over time, as with marriage or adoption, and other data, including address, phone number, driver's license number, and insurance coverage, change frequently. Patients may provide inconsistent information, and data may be entered incorrectly. These practical challenges of patient identification should be kept in mind when using datasets obtained from provider organizations. Patient registration is viewed as the front end of a "**revenue cycle**" that culminates in sending bills to patients and claims to third-party payers and managing collections. These patient financial systems are distinguished from general financial systems, which mirror the management systems used in any business: general ledger, human resources, payroll, and materials management. These systems support operational processes within the organization, rather than the care of individual patients, but they are often specialized for health care. Materials management systems may have modules for pharmaceuticals, surgical supplies, and custom orthopedic implants. General financial systems hold a wealth of data about processes that support care delivery, but they generally do not contain information on the care of individual patients.

Most of the systems in Figure 12-2 are designed to support providers and provider organizations in delivering care and third-party payers in paying for care. There is a single box for the **patient portal**, representing a window into provider systems. But organizations that succeed in achieving broader synergy between their systems and the mobile apps used by patients will have an advantage in managing population health.

At the other end of the spectrum from transaction systems, a **data warehouse** assimilates data from multiple transaction systems. It facilitates analysis across an entire patient population and offers diverse ways to drill down to specific subsets of patients, clinical services, or parts of an organization. Patient billing systems and EHRs can summarize all services for a given patient over time, but they generally cannot identify all patients who received a given service. That requires a different slice through the data. For example, no single transaction system allows us to analyze the use of advanced imaging in patients with an initial episode of low back pain. The radiology system has information about patients who had imaging studies, but for this analysis, we also need to know about similar patients who did not have imaging studies. We need longitudinal records to distinguish the initial episode of low back pain, and we need to understand the full picture for both groups of patients—their other diagnoses, medications, and other services provided, before and after the imaging. This question illustrates the importance of collecting data from multiple transaction systems in a data warehouse.

Population management systems are a hybrid, used concurrently for operations but providing a population-level view. A patient registry collects data about all patients in a defined population, such as those with particular chronic conditions (sometimes called a **disease registry**). It is a fundamental tool of population management, enabling surveillance (case finding) and risk stratification, based on historical utilization or predictive analytics, across a broad population. Registries typically help to manage care coordination workflow, with task tracking and documentation of outreach contacts and interventions. Most EHR vendors now offer a registry module, and physicians may access a registry at the point of care. Logically, however, an EHR remains a transaction system, designed mainly for caring for individual patients, while registries and data warehouses are designed for a population view.[13]

CREATING DATA WAREHOUSES

Data warehouses enable organizations to create additional value from the data that accumulate as a by-product of using EHRs and other systems that support patient care and operations. Data warehouses may be created at multiple levels, within an organization or across organizations. The term may be applied to any database that aggregates and organizes data from multiple source systems that has a defined process for keeping it current and offers the ability to query the system in ways that were not (fully) anticipated when the warehouse was designed. A data warehouse may be optimized for certain types of queries, but all warehouses should permit some degree of exploratory analysis. Data warehouses often bring in external data. For example, each patient's home address may be combined with census data to impute an education level based on the median education level within the area. These imputed variables are not specific to an individual patient, but they can be useful in population-level analyses to inform decisions about where to locate programs to improve health literacy, for example.

A terminology system that provides names for concepts within a certain domain and defines relationships among the concepts is called an **ontology**. Most ontologies specify hierarchical relationships, mapping detailed terms to one or more higher-level classes. For example, the U.S. Food and Drug Administration (FDA) assigns a unique National Drug Code (NDC) to each drug (or combination), dosage form, and strength, from each manufacturer. This code serves as a universal product identifier, and supply chain systems track NDCs and even lot numbers. But this is too much detail for an e-prescribing system. There, the generic name of the drug and the available dosage forms and strengths are useful, but not the manufacturer or the lot number. Consider a retrospective analysis to determine whether certain patients received a beta blocker upon discharge from the hospital. It would be unwieldy to construct a query that names every drug in this class, let alone every dosage form, strength, and manufacturer. Rather, data about drugs are loaded into a data warehouse at multiple levels of granularity: the NDC and lot number that was dispensed by the pharmacy for a particular patient at a particular time, all forms of a given drug (e.g., a certain beta blocker), and all medications that fall into a given class (e.g., all beta blockers). Medications are often grouped into therapeutic classes, although the classes are not strictly hierarchical, because some drugs are used for multiple purposes and thus fall into multiple classes.

There are three ways to describe the costs associated with an episode of care. The least accurate is to add up the charges for all the billable services involved. Prices charged by provider organizations are often highly artificial, because third-party payers typically negotiate deep discounts or pay according to a fee schedule, regardless of what the provider charges. The second approach, especially useful for comparing cost of care for different providers, is to assign a standardized cost to each billable service and add up the standard-ized costs.[14] This is essentially a cost-weighted measure of utilization. The third approach, which is most useful for managing a provider organization, involves a **cost accounting** system, a retrospective analysis in which all of the organization's expenses, represented in its general financial systems, are allocated across its billable services, which are represented in its patient financial system. This may be done at varying levels of precision, distinguish-ing direct and indirect, fixed and variable components of cost for each service. Cost accounting is standard practice in other industries, and its use is growing in health care. But not all provider organizations have a clear understanding of the actual cost of provid-ing care. For population health, it is important to consider costs beyond those strictly related to the provision of care, such as the lost productivity of an employee who is unable to work or absent because of visits to care providers. From this perspective, using IT to provide care via patient portals and "virtual visits," or "e-visits," becomes even more com-pelling, taking on an economic dimension in addition to patient convenience.

We have discussed aggregating data from multiple patients to create a population view. At the patient level, there is also a need to assemble data from a series of encounters to create a **longitudinal patient record** reflecting the patient's health and health care over time. Occasionally, we may need only a cross-sectional view to study a particular service provided to patients during a hospital stay, but we are usually interested in care processes and patient outcomes that evolve over time, which requires a longitudinal record. Accu-mulating diagnoses over time is often the only way to gain a complete picture of a patient's chronic conditions. The diagnosis codes on the claim for an individual encounter do not necessarily reflect all of the patient's diagnoses, only those that were treated or that affected treatment during the corresponding encounter. Consider a patient with diabetes, hyper-tension, and congestive heart failure. Owing to limited time, the physician may document only the principal condition addressed during each office visit, perhaps diabetes during one visit and heart failure during another. Even with a longitudinal record, some impor-tant conditions may never be coded. Up to 20% of adults with clear clinical evidence of diabetes may lack a code for diabetes in their claims data, or even on their problem list in the EHR.[15] Algorithms have been developed to identify **episodes of illness**, using longitudinal claims data to distinguish acute episodes from ongoing care for one or more chronic conditions. To understand the cost of care for a patient's chronic illness, we need to distinguish whether a hospital admission resulted from failure to properly treat the chronic condition, from a complication of treatment, or from an unrelated acute illness. These algorithms are imperfect, partly due to limitations of the source data, but as payers attempt to evaluate providers and provider organizations on the quality and resource efficiency of the care they provide, it is important to characterize—and properly attribute to physicians—care for distinct episodes of illness. Moving from discrete hospital admis-sions to longitudinal patient records may seem like a subtle transition, but it has far-reaching implications for the design of databases and analytic models.

ENABLING DATA-DRIVEN IMPROVEMENT

Provider organizations and individual providers are often graded by payers or in public accountability initiatives on how consistently they follow accepted guidelines for treating a certain condition and the outcomes their patients achieve. Most pay-for-performance (P4P) plans are also based on such measures. A common process measure is the proportion of a physician's diabetic patients who are tested periodically for glycated hemoglobin (HbA1c) to evaluate their long-term blood glucose control. A corresponding outcome measure is the fraction of patients who are (known to be) in good control. Many factors other than quality of care can influence outcomes, such as the severity or complexity of the patient's disease; comorbid conditions; lifestyle; and compliance with prescribed therapy, level of education, socioeconomic status, family and other support systems, and even values and beliefs that cause some patients to opt for aggressive therapy where others may choose a more conservative course. Seldom do retrospective data include information about all of these, but if outcomes are to be interpreted as reflecting quality of care, we must try to account for all factors other than quality that can affect outcomes.

Risk adjustment refers to statistical methods used to account for patient factors associated with a greater risk of certain outcomes. There are two general approaches to using a large database for risk adjustment. One is to develop a multivariate regression model that reflects the contribution of each (measured) factor to the patient's risk of a particular outcome. After validation of the model, the regression equation is then used to estimate risk for individual patients. The other general approach is to identify, within the data warehouse, a cohort of patients who are similar to the measured population in terms of patient factors and compare outcomes in the measured population to those in the matched cohort. Regardless of the approach, risk must be evaluated separately for each outcome. A patient at high risk for a particular complication may not be at greater risk for a different outcome. Statistical risk adjustment is often used in hospital performance measures, but measures for physicians typically focus instead on process elements that should apply to all patients (e.g., that HbA1c should be measured periodically for all patients with diabetes) or on a subset of the patient population (e.g., applying targets for HbA1c levels and blood pressure control only to patients younger than a certain age). **Patient attribution** is also important for credibility. Measures reflecting a given physician's management of chronic conditions should include only patients for whom the physician is designated as the primary care provider and patients whose pattern of visits indicate that the physician is providing most of the patient's care. No approach to risk adjustment is without disadvantages, but simply having a thorough and open discussion about the selected approach can be an important step toward a culture of data-driven quality and performance improvement.

Risk adjustment is vitally important for measures published as "report cards," used as a basis for payment, or used to direct patients to certain providers through a narrow network or tiered copayments. Without credible risk adjustment in these settings, providers may be reluctant to accept high-risk patients, and this can create a barrier to access for the sickest patients. Risk adjustment is less critical when data are used for quality improvement (QI) within a provider organization, where the goal is to identify opportunities for improvement, not to judge providers. Variation in care processes or patient outcomes—across an organization, across multiple organizations, or over time—suggests opportunity. Although risk adjustment is not essential for QI, it is still useful: the more successful we are in accounting for patient factors that contribute to variation, the more likely the remaining variation points to real opportunity. Integrating patient-reported health status and data on patients' perception of their care experience add important dimensions.

An important change over the past decade is moving from treating each provider's performance data as confidential to understanding the value of internal transparency in engaging physicians in improvement. Not every organization is yet comfortable with it, but P4P programs and public reporting of quality measures have led to greater acceptance, and with meaningful comparative data, many physicians report positive experiences asking colleagues how they approach certain clinical situations in order to achieve better outcomes.

One subtle aspect of analytics for improvement deserves attention. Many initiatives focus just on patient outcomes (e.g., did a physician or care team achieve good glycemic control in their patients with diabetes?). There may be modest variation in average HbA1c if it is being monitored as an outcome, but there is often much greater variation in the process of care that leads to the outcome. And care process elements—diabetes education, nutritional counseling, the pattern of office visits, specialist consultations, and medications used—drive the cost. Overall cost per patient may vary as much as tenfold across physicians or care teams, even within the same provider organization, for patients who are achieving essentially the same outcome in terms of glycemic control.[16] Outcome measures are important, but datasets that capture only the outcome measure, not additional data elements reflecting details of the care process, will be unable to identify or pursue these substantial opportunities for improving cost efficiency.

As noted at the bottom of Figure 12-2, EHRs and registries play an essential role in implementing what is learned from data warehouses and improvement initiatives about which care processes work best for different subgroups within a patient population. EHRs and registries ensure that improved care processes are carried out consistently.

There is great value in data warehouses that span multiple provider organizations and thus are likely to reflect a variety of approaches to care and the corresponding outcomes, as well as differences in the overall cost of achieving those outcomes. De-identified Medicare claims data have been used to demonstrate glaring geographic variation in the distribution and use of medical resources in the United States, in *The Dartmouth Atlas of Healthcare*.[17,18] Other sources of claims data include state Medicaid programs and datasets resulting from various state programs—some mandated, some voluntary—for reporting de-identified, patient-level data. Large health plans and provider organizations, such as the Veterans Health Administration and Kaiser Permanente, make extensive use of system-wide clinical and administrative data for performance improvement and research. Several national organizations of providers have established voluntary data-sharing programs for benchmarking and collaborative shared learning, including the University HealthSystem Consortium, the Premier alliance, the American Medical Group Association, and the High Value Healthcare Collaborative. These groups employ a mix of techniques, from formal **health services research** to rapid-cycle quality improvement. The federally funded Patient-Centered Outcomes Research Institute (PCORI) is creating PCORnet, a national patient-centered clinical research network, which includes provider-oriented clinical data research networks (CDRNs), as well as patient-powered research networks (PPRNs).

HEALTH INFORMATION EXCHANGES

Federal policy has focused not just on EHR adoption but also on taking steps toward an interoperable, standards-based nationwide health information network made up of state or regional **health information exchanges** (HIEs). Governance principles are established by the **Office of the National Coordinator for Health Information Technology** (ONC),[19] and HIEs are currently operated by a variety of local, state, and regional organizations. When a primary care physician refers a patient to a specialist, the referral letter could be sent electronically via an HIE, and the specialist's consult letter could automatically appear in the primary care physician's EHR. Both physicians could also see, if they queried the HIE, that the patient had visited the emergency room of a local hospital in the interim. The primary care physician might have been notified of the ED visit via the HIE, and the ED physician could have determined that there was a pending consultation with a specialist at the time of the visit. Orders for, and results of, lab tests and imaging studies already travel across many HIEs. For patients, ONC is promoting the **Blue Button initiative**, a set of standards designed to allow patients to access their health information held by providers, payers, and government agencies. Initial implementations allow Medicare beneficiaries to access their claims data, and patients of the Veterans Health Administration can use the MyHealtheVet portal.

We have a long way to go before this vision of a semantically interoperable healthcare system can be fully realized, but there has been progress in adopting the standards that it will require. HIPAA established a **national provider identifier** (NPI) for individual and institutional healthcare providers, but it stopped short of establishing a national patient identifier. Most observers believe this concept is not politically feasible in the United States, given our national culture, but the lack of a uniform patient identifier imposes a substantial burden on an HIE to identify data from different providers that refer to the same patient. They are forced to use secondary identifiers and probabilistic matching methods (e.g., assigning greater significance to a match on an uncommon name than to a match on a common name). In addition to technical challenges, HIEs have struggled to develop business models that ensure sustainability. Many are now succeeding, and some are providing a forum that fosters even broader collaboration among provider organizations within the region.[20]

We must be realistic, however, about the benefits we expect from connecting EHRs. Key to managing population health is a focus on care coordination by creating a medical home for each patient. But achieving effective care coordination in our fragmented healthcare system can be a staggering challenge. For just the Medicare patients of a typical primary care physician, there are 229 other physicians, working in 117 practices, with whom care must be coordinated.[21] Clearly, it is unrealistic to expect that simply connecting EHRs, even through a sophisticated HIE, will cause independent physician practices to spontaneously coalesce into medical homes. Multispecialty medical groups have learned that even with a single, shared EHR and a strong group culture, they need to hire, train, and support people whose job it is to provide care coordination and disease management for patients with chronic conditions. They also need predictive analytics, shared protocols, and highly trained clinical personnel to provide case management for complex patients.

PUBLIC HEALTH INFORMATICS

Applied epidemiology is the foundation of public health. From tracking patterns of disease and population needs for health services to prioritizing interventions and evaluating their results, data are essential. It must be remembered, however, that the population view assembled in typical provider or payer data warehouses reflects the *patient* population, that is, those people who have received care. It is not a view of the population as a whole. Thus, public health informatics also relies on survey data, including census data and several surveys conducted by the National Center for Health Statistics, which is part of the Centers for Disease Control and Prevention. Most states also maintain registries for pediatric immunizations; some of them exchange data electronically with providers' EHRs or registries.

Surveillance is an important theme in public health, tracking everything from risk factors, like obesity and smoking, to influenza epidemics and patterns of infection with methicillin-resistant *Staphylococcus aureus* (MRSA). Since September 11, 2001, surveillance for bioterrorism has also become very important. Data sources range from "reportable diseases," which providers are required by various state laws to report, to real-time data shared voluntarily by emergency departments and other frontline care providers. More effective surveillance has been touted as a major benefit of HIEs, providing data that are both broader and richer than those currently available. Patterns of ED visits and even patterns of Google search terms can be used to gauge influenza activity in real time.[22]

An important application of active surveillance is **pharmacovigilance**, aimed at detecting, understanding, and preventing adverse effects of drugs and biologic products. Because clinical trials typically involve a few thousand patients at most, uncommon side effects and adverse reactions may not be known when a drug enters the market. Manu-facturers report to the FDA any adverse events that are reported to them, but patients and providers may fail to recognize the connection to the drug. A potentially powerful method is to use very large databases, assembled from claims and EHRs, to detect patterns of adverse events among patients taking a new drug. The FDA's Sentinel Initiative is the focus of considerable effort to create suitable federated databases and to develop statistical methods for "signal" detection.[23]

"BIG DATA" AND COGNITIVE SYSTEMS

Two promising new technologies deserve mention. First is "big data." We have discussed several ideas to which this buzzword could be applied—aggregating data from multiple source systems to build data warehouses, particularly across multiple provider organiza-tions; data normalization and mapping to common terminology; and using these large datasets to build models that providers can use to risk stratify patient populations and to identify patients for proactive intervention. But these applications involve traditional methods of health services research, where the structure of the model is driven by known or suspected relationships among the variables. Most industries apply the term *big data* to a different set of methods that collect massive datasets from diverse sources *without* careful mapping but carrying along extensive metadata describing the source of each data element and the context in which it was collected. Automated "knowledge discovery" methods identify empirical relationships in the data. The goal is still to distinguish signal from noise, even without a clinical hypothesis. Because the data are collected as by-products of clinical care and billing, noise may be dominant and signals difficult to detect. Big data techniques have been used to identify genetic variants that predispose to certain diseases, but use of these methods in a context as complex as healthcare delivery and population health is relatively new.

Second is a promising way to deal with the explosion of new information and increas-ingly nuanced practice guidelines. With more than 5,000 new articles published in the peer-reviewed medical literature every weekday,[24] routine medical care is beginning to exceed the limits of human cognition. This is especially true in areas like oncology, where therapies are tailored for each patient's **genomic profile** and specific tumor markers. Researchers have long explored application of artificial intelligence techniques in medi-cine, and recent advances in computing have created a commercially practical cognitive system, IBM Watson. The system gained wide attention by beating two of the all-time winningest contestants on the television quiz show *Jeopardy!* in February 2011. Watson assimilates information from unstructured data sources ranging from Wikipedia to papers published in peer-reviewed journals, and it develops a semantic network—not just map-ping content to an existing ontology but recognizing new concepts as they are introduced and identifying relationships among concepts.[25] Watson builds on **natural language**

processing (NLP) to infer concepts from free text and accommodates conflicting and updated information, recognizing gradations in level of confidence and applying evidence-based reasoning techniques to answer questions. In early clinical use, Watson identified a contraindication to a standard chemotherapy regimen, based on an obscure tumor marker and a paper published 18 months earlier that the patient's physicians had been unaware of.[26] The current uses of Watson are limited, but it offers a glimpse into the future of clinical decision support.

PRACTICAL ISSUES OF IT IMPLEMENTATION AND ADOPTION

Industry analysts estimate that health IT currently consumes 25 to 35% of hospital capital budgets,[27] and half of hospitals and integrated delivery systems said in a survey that IT would be their largest capital investment in 2014, ahead of facilities and clinical equipment.[28] Many provider organizations are rushing to implement EHRs while they can still obtain Meaningful Use incentive payments and before the CMS begins to assess penalties for the lack of an EHR. But analysts expect investments in IT will continue to grow. This reflects a growing recognition that all three major categories of systems shown in Figure 12-2 will be essential to deliver improved outcomes at lower overall cost.

PRIVACY AND SECURITY

The HIPAA Privacy and Security Rules, which have been extended by subsequent legislation, have had a profound effect on management of health information, including its use for research. The HIPAA Privacy Rule applies to all individually identifiable health information, regardless of form, and the Security Rule applies to information in electronic form.

IMPORTANCE OF PROCESS REDESIGN AND COGNITIVE SUPPORT

Clinical and operations leadership are the most critical factors for a successful EHR implementation, but redesign of care processes to take advantage of IT is the most important step in realizing efficiencies and improvements in quality and safety. Distributing documentation tasks among care team members and using the system for worklists and messaging within a practice are common areas of emphasis. Clinical decision support and access to context-appropriate reference material are important for patient safety, but these features require careful calibration to ensure that important issues are addressed without creating **alert fatigue**. If clinicians receive a barrage of alerts and reminders about things they already know, such as obvious or trivial drug–drug interactions, they may come to resent inappropriate alerts and reminders, clicking through them without thinking carefully about each one and potentially missing an important alert about something they might not otherwise be aware of. Alerts must also be appropriate for the setting. Nearly all of a nephrologist's patients may have some degree of renal failure, so an alert about an elevated creatinine level, which could be useful to a primary care physician, would not provide new information to a nephrologist. The more data that are captured in structured form, the more precisely alerts and reminders can be tailored to the patient's situation and the physician's practice. This requires a new organizational function for knowledge management to maintain ontologies and clinical content within the organization's systems.

Regardless of the strategic imperative to move to an EHR, observers of such initiatives often say that "culture eats strategy for lunch." It is important to recognize the scope and depth of the transformation that implementing a modern EHR entails, making explicit issues that would otherwise never have surfaced. It is not uncommon for physicians within a practice to take different approaches to treating a certain condition, but the differences may not be recognized when using paper medical records. Creating a standard protocol and decision support rules brings the issue to light. Even more basic is the fact that physicians may be uncomfortable with the visibility that an EHR or a data warehouse gives every clinical decision. Some may feel that they are "practicing in public" or that elaborate documentation is required to justify each decision. This may expose fundamental issues of trust among clinical colleagues. To gain the full benefit of an EHR, provider organizations must develop a sustainable capability for continual improvement and a team-based model of care. For many organizations, this is a big culture change.

Implementation of an EHR should be viewed not as a technology project, but as a strategic change-management initiative, with attention to the sociology and psychology of behavior change. Organizations often have an unrealistic view of such initiatives, thinking the most difficult decision involves selecting the right vendor. While certain vendors and products may be a better match for some organizations than for others, success is much more than simply making the right choice. Major systems typically remain in place for 10 to 20 years, so the ongoing relationship with a vendor becomes a vital element. Implementation is sometimes viewed simply as a matter of good project management—maintaining disciplined focus and avoiding "scope creep." Those are important, but organizations should also approach the initiative with an open mind, anticipating some experimentation and learning.

UNINTENDED CONSEQUENCES

Some organizations have observed unintended adverse consequences of implementing CPOE and EHR systems, including more work or new work for clinicians; unexpected changes in workflow, communication patterns, and the power structure; and generation of new kinds of errors.[29,30] For example, entering medication orders via pulldown lists eliminates illegibility and ambiguity, but it provides the opportunity to mistakenly select an adjacent item from the pulldown list.[31]

More fundamentally, there is a growing recognition that system designs must evolve to reflect the complex nature of clinical work:

There is quite a large mismatch between the implicit theories embedded in these computer systems and the real world of clinical work. Clinical work, especially in hospitals, is fundamentally interpretative, interruptive, multitasking, collaborative, distributed, opportunistic, and reactive. In contrast, CPOE systems and decision support systems are based on a different model of work: one that is objective, rationalized, linear, normative, localized (in the clinician's mind), solitary, and single-minded. Such models tend to reflect the implicit theories of managers and designers, not of frontline [clinical] workers.[32]

Fortunately, the industry is assimilating these lessons into system design and implementation methods. We still have a long way to go, but there is reason for optimism that progress will continue toward effective use of systems and data to improve health and health care for individuals and populations.

CONCLUSION

Provider organizations, researchers, and policy makers are becoming more sophisticated users of a growing body of data about health and health care. Adoption of IT will enable better decision making in caring for individual patients and also in managing population health. Patients are using IT to transform health care from a passive to an active experience. Research based on richer, more real-time data will inform policy decisions in all parts of the healthcare system. This chapter has provided a foundation for wise interpretation of data for any use—an understanding of the source systems and the care processes where the data originate, as well as the mechanisms by which they are aggregated and analyzed.

STUDY AND DISCUSSION QUESTIONS

1. Describe four distinct benefits of an electronic health record (EHR).
2. Explain the relationship between point-of-care systems, surveillance and tracking systems, and retrospective analytic systems.
3. Discuss the challenges of integrating data collected by a patient's mobile apps into a provider organization's EHR.
4. List some of the strengths and weaknesses of clinical and administrative data for health services research.
5. Discuss two ways in which provider organizations can use population-level analyses for performance improvement.
6. Describe the potential of cognitive systems in assisting healthcare providers with identifying and applying new clinical knowledge in caring for their patients.
7. List some critical success factors for EHR implementation and unintended consequences of inserting information technology into healthcare workflows.

SUGGESTED READINGS AND WEBSITES

READINGS

Arlotto P, Irby S, eds. *Rethinking Return on Investment: The Challenge of Accountable Meaningful Use.* Chicago: Healthcare Information and Management Systems Society; 2012.

Bates DW, Saria S, Ohno-Machado L, et al. Big data in health care: using analytics to identify and manage high-risk and high-cost patients. *Health Aff.* 2014;33(7):1123-31.

Han YY, Carcillo JA, Venkataraman ST, et al. Unexpected increased mortality after implementation of a commercially sold computerized physician order entry system. *Pediatrics.* 2005;116(6):1506-12.

Hoyt RE, Yoshihashi A, eds. *Health Informatics: Practical Guide for Healthcare and Information Technology Professionals.* 6th ed. Available in several formats through www.informaticseducation.org.

Kelly JE III, Hamm S. *Smart Machines: IBM's Watson and the Era of Cognitive Computing.* New York: Columbia University Press; 2013.

Krumholz HM. Big data and new knowledge in medicine: the thinking, training, and tools needed for a learning health system. *Health Aff. (Millwood).* 2014;33(7):1163-70.

Larson EB. Building trust in the power of "big data" research to serve the public good. *JAMA.* 2013;309(23):2443-44.

Sittig DF, Singh H. A new socio-technical model for studying health information technology in complex adaptive healthcare systems. *Qual Saf Health Care.* 2010; 19(Suppl 3):i68-i74. http://www.ncbi.nlm.nih.gov/pmc/articles/PMC3120130/. Accessed October 30, 2014.

Topol E. *The Creative Destruction of Medicine: How the Digital Revolution Will Create Better Health Care.* New York: Basic Books; 2012.

Wallace PJ, Shah ND, Dennen T, et al. Optum labs: building a novel node in the learning health care system. *Health Aff.* 2014;33(7):1187-94.

WEBSITES

AcademyHealth (health services research): http://www.academyhealth.org

American Medical Informatics Association: http://www.amia.org

Healthcare Information and Management Systems Society: http://www.himss.org

Informatics Education: http://www.informaticseducation.org

National Institutes of Health Big Data to Knowledge initiative (BD2K): http://bd2k.nih.gov/index.html#sthash.Bxk5aaHS.dpbs. Accessed October 30, 2014.

Office of the National Coordinator for Health Information Technology (ONC): http://www.healthit.gov/newsroom/about-onc. Accessed October 30, 2014.

Oregon Health and Science University Clinical Informatics Wiki: http://www.informatics-review.com/wiki. Accessed October 30, 2014.

REFERENCES

1. i2b2 (Informatics for Integrating Biology and the Bedside). https://www.i2b2.org/. Accessed October 30, 2014.

2. Stewart WF, Shah NR, Selna MJ, et al. Bridging the inferential gap: the electronic health record and clinical evidence. *Health Aff.* 2007;26(2):w181-91.

3. McGlynn EA, Asch SM, Adams J, et al. The quality of health care delivered to adults in the United States. *N Engl J Med.* 2003;348(26):2635-45.

4. Boyd CM, Darer J, Boult C, et al. Clinical practice guidelines and quality of care for older patients with multiple comorbid diseases: implications for pay for performance. *JAMA.* 2005;294(6):716-24.

5. James PA, Oparil S, Carter BL, et al. 2014 Evidence-based guideline for the management of high blood pressure in adults: report from the panel members appointed to the Eighth Joint National Committee (JNC 8). *JAMA.* 2014;311(5):507-20.

6. The World Health Organization is responsible for the ICD system. The National Center for Health Statistics and CMS maintain the Clinical Modification, an adaptation for use in the United States. The Current Procedural Terminology (CPT) system is maintained by the American Medical Association. The Medicare program often needs codes for new procedures or concepts that have not yet been officially adopted in CPT, so the CMS maintains a superset of CPT-4, called HCPCS (often pronounced "hick-picks").

7. Office of the National Coordinator for Health Information Technology (ONC). Health IT dashboard: share of physicians, physician's assistants, and nurse practitioners that received a CMS EHR Incentive Program payment. April 2014. http://dashboard.healthit.gov/quickstats/PDFs/Health-IT-Quick-Stat-Health-Care-Professional-EHR-Incentive-Payment-Scorecard.pdf. Accessed October 30, 2014.

8. Hsiao C-J, Hing E. Use and characteristics of electronic health record systems among office-based physician practices: United States, 2001–2013. NCHS data brief 143. Hyattsville, MD: National Center for Health Statistics. January 2014. http://www.cdc.gov/nchs/data/databriefs/db143.pdf. Accessed October 30, 2014.

9. Care protocols developed by provider organizations tend to be more specific than guidelines published by specialty societies. Guideline developers are usually careful not to go beyond the evidence and thus may recommend only a class of medications, but a provider organization may recommend a specific drug within the class, recognizing additional benefits from consistent use of the same medication. Choosing a specific combination of hypertension meds simplifies patient education materials and allows health coaches and nurse call personnel to provide patients with clear and concise guidance about medications.

10. Conwell LJ, Cohen JW. Characteristics of people with high medical expenses in the U.S. civilian noninstitutionalized population, 2002. Statistical Brief #73. March 2005. Agency for Healthcare Research and Quality, Rockville, MD. http://meps.ahrq.gov/mepsweb/data_files/publications/st73/stat73.pdf. Accessed October 30, 2014.

11. Optum white paper. Predictive analytics: Poised to drive population health. May 2014. http://www.optum.com/thought-leadership/predictive-analytics-drive-population-health.html. Accessed October 30, 2014.

12. See, for example, Microsoft HealthVault (https://www.healthvault.com/us/en) and Dossia Health Manager (http://www.dossia.com/products/health-manager). Accessed October 30, 2014.

13. We use the term *registry* for an operational system for active management of a defined patient population. The term is also used for a passive system used to collect a standardized dataset, over time, on a defined population, such as patients who have received a specific drug, implanted device, or surgical procedure or patients who have been diagnosed with cancer (tumor registry). See Gliklich RE, Dreyer NA, Leavy MB, eds. *Registries for evaluating patient outcomes: A user's guide.* 3rd edition. AHRQ Publication No. 13(14)-EHC111. Agency for Healthcare Research and Quality. April 2014. http://effectivehealthcare.ahrq.gov/index.cfm/search-for-guides-reviews-and-reports/?pageaction=displayproduct&productid=1897. Accessed October 30, 2014.

14. HealthPartners total cost of care (TCOC) toolkit. https://www.healthpartners.com/public/tcoc/. Accessed October 30, 2014.

15. Optum white paper. Getting from big data to good data: Creating a foundation for actionable analytics. March 2014. http://www.optum.com/content/dam/optum/CMOSpark%20Hub%20Resources/White%20Papers/OPT_WhitePaper_ClinicalAnalytics_ONLINE_031414.pdf. Accessed October 30, 2014.

16. Unpublished data on variation in standardized cost across 21 medical groups for patients with type 2 diabetes achieving similar improvements in glycemic control. AMGA's Anceta collaborative. April 2013.

17. The Dartmouth Atlas of Health Care. http://www.dartmouthatlas.org/. Accessed October 30, 2014.

18. Newhouse JP, Garber AM, Graham RP, et al., eds. *Variation in health care spending: target decision making, not geography*. Institute of Medicine. Washington, DC: National Academies Press. 2013. http://www.iom.edu/Reports/2013/Variation-in-Health-Care-Spending-Target-Decision-Making-Not-Geography.aspx. Accessed October 30, 2014.

19. Office of the National Coordinator for Health Information Technology (ONC). Connecting health and care for the nation: a 10-year vision to achieve an interoperable health IT infrastructure. 2014. http://healthit.gov/sites/default/files/ONC10yearInteroperabilityConceptPaper.pdf. Accessed October 30, 2014.

20. See, for example, HealthBridge, in the greater Cincinnati area. http://www.healthbridge.org/. Accessed October 30, 2014.

21. Pham HH, O'Malley AS, Bach PB, et al. Primary care physicians' links to other physicians through Medicare patients: the scope of care coordination. *Ann Intern Med*. 2009;150(4):236-42.

22. Google.org flu trends. http://www.google.org/flutrends/us/#US. Accessed October 30, 2014.

23. Psaty BM, Breckenridge AM. Mini-Sentinel and regulatory science: big data rendered fit and functional. *N Engl J Med*. 2014;370:2165-7.

24. Priem J. Medline literature growth chart. Published online October 18, 2010; data updated for this chapter. http://jasonpriem.org/2010/10/medline-literature-growth-chart/. Accessed October 30, 2014.

25. Kelly JE, Hamm S. *Smart Machines: IBM's Watson and the Era of Cognitive Computing*. New York: Columbia University Press; 2013.

26. Schwartz SA, at IBM briefing, Transforming healthcare with IBM Watson. New York, February 8, 2013.

27. Herman B. EHRs and health IT projects: are they battering hospitals' financial profiles? *Becker's Hospital Review*. January 6, 2014. http://www.beckershospitalreview.com/finance/ehrs-and-health-it-projects-are-they-battering-hospitals-financial-profiles.html. Accessed October 30, 2014.

28. Premier. Economic outlook, Spring 2014: Healthcare trends from the C-suite. May 2014. https://www.premierinc.com/about-premier/publications/economic-outlook/ Accessed November 12, 2014.

29. Campbell EM, Sittig DF, Ash JS, et al. Types of unintended consequences related to computerized provider order entry. *J Am Med Inform Assoc*. 2006;13(5):547-56.

30. Ash JS, Sittig DF, Poon EG, et al. The extent and importance of unintended consequences related to computerized provider order entry. *J Am Med Inform Assoc*. 2007;14(4):415-23.

31. Koppel R, Metlay JP, Cohen A, et al. Role of computerized physician order entry systems in facilitating medication errors. *JAMA*. 2005;293(10):1197-203.

32. Wears RL, Berg M. Computer technology and clinical work: still waiting for Godot. *JAMA*. 2005;293(10):1261-3.

Chapter 13

DECISION SUPPORT

MATTHEW C. STIEFEL

Executive Summary

Measurement provides decision support and drives innovation.

This chapter focuses on the measurement and analysis tools used to support decision making in population health. The tools and methods used depend on the kinds of decisions needing support. The three main purposes of measurement in population health—improvement, accountability, and research—provide the overarching framework for how to develop a strategy. The measurement for improvement section provides an overview of the Model for Improvement[1] and the useful tools associated with it. Predictive modeling is another decision-support mechanism that contributes to effective population health management. The measurement for accountability section describes a framework for assessing value in health care, including metrics for the Triple Aim of population health, per capita cost, and care experience. The chapter concludes with a brief discussion of measurement for research and the distinctions between efficacy and effectiveness research and between comparative and cost effectiveness. Decisions in the areas of improvement, accountability, and research require different types of decision support.

Learning Objectives

1. Distinguish among the three purposes of population health measurement and the various approaches for each purpose.
2. Describe the Model for Improvement and its associated tools.
3. Learn about the key metrics for the Triple Aim.
4. Provide a framework for assessing value in population health.
5. Learn about the major types of population health and health services research.

Key Terms

comparative effectiveness research	predictive modeling
cost effectiveness	quality-adjusted life years
effectiveness	return on investment
efficacy	Triple Aim
efficiency	value
healthy life expectancy	

INTRODUCTION

THREE MAIN PURPOSES FOR MEASUREMENT IN POPULATION HEALTH

Improvement, accountability, and research are the three main purposes of measurement.[2] Approaches to measurement differ according to purpose. In measurement for improvement, the general strategy is to measure just enough to learn. This approach is characterized by limited data and small, sequential samples. Hypotheses are flexible and are apt to change as learning takes place. Trend data are typically analyzed, and the data are used by those doing the improvement.

Measurement for accountability focuses on reporting, oversight, comparison, choice, reassurance, or motivation for change. It is not about hypothesis testing but rather about evaluation of current performance. It is important to make adjustments to reduce bias in comparisons through approaches such as severity indexing and equally important to collect all available, relevant data so that the analysis is significant and credible.

Measurement for research seeks to discover new knowledge that may have broad application, where the standard of evidence is beyond doubt. In the research context, tests are carefully blinded and controlled, and the experimental design seeks to eliminate bias. Hypotheses are fixed, with a single, large test that typically employs traditional statistical techniques.

Because the purpose of measurement should determine the methods, mismatching purposes and methods can have adverse consequences. For example, applying traditional research methods in an improvement setting can slow down the learning process and, more importantly, set the bar for statistical significance too high to detect potentially useful changes. Alternatively, applying improvement methods to research questions can lead to inappropriate generalization of findings. While there are three main purposes of measurement, there are many differences in the methods used for each purpose (Table 13-1).

MEASUREMENT FOR IMPROVEMENT

THE MODEL FOR IMPROVEMENT

Measurement for improvement is built on a rich tradition of quality improvement measurement methods dating back to the early 1900s and was led by the pioneering work of Deming, Shewhart, and Juran. Developed by Associates in Process Improvement, the Model for Improvement incorporates many of the tools and techniques introduced by these pioneers.[1] It is a simple but powerful tool for accelerating improvement.

Table 13-1   The Three Purposes of Measurement

Aspect	Improvement	Accountability	Research
Aim	Improvement of care	Comparison, choice, reassurance, spur for change	New knowledge
Methods:			
Test observability	Test observable	No test, evaluate current performance	Test blinded or controlled
Bias	Accept consistent bias	Measure and adjust to reduce bias	Design to eliminate bias
Sample size	"Just enough" data, small sequential samples	Obtain 100% of available, relevant data	"Just in case" data
Flexibility of hypothesis	Hypothesis flexible, changes as learning takes place	No hypothesis	Fixed hypothesis
Testing strategy	Sequential tests	No tests	One large test
Determining if a change is an improvement	Run charts or Shewhart control charts	No change focus	Hypothesis, statistical tests (t test, F test, chi-square), p values
Confidentiality of the data	Data used only by those involved with improvement	Data available for public consumption and review	Research subject's identities protected

Data from Solberg L, Mosser G, McDonald S. The three faces of performance measurement: improvement, accountability, and research. *Jt Comm J Qual Improv.* 1997;23(3):13–147.

Provost L, Murray S. *The Data Guide: Learning from Data to Improve Health Care.* Austin, TX: Associates in Process Improvement; 2007.

The Model for Improvement consists of two parts. The first part focuses on three basic questions used to frame the improvement journey:

- What are we trying to accomplish?
- How do we know that a change is an improvement?
- What change can we make that will result in an improvement?

The second part consists of continual cycles of plan, do, study, and act (PDSA) to test and implement changes in real-world settings.

A clear goal statement is essential to answer the first question concerning what we are trying to accomplish. A useful technique for developing goal statements is to make them SMART: specific, measurable, attainable, realistic, and timebound.

The tools of statistical process control were developed to answer the question of whether a change is an improvement. In general, the process involves plotting data over time and applying tests to determine whether there has been a change in the underlying results of a process. The first step is to gather data on performance. The data-collection tool needn't be sophisticated but should include basic information about the process and outcomes, and observations about barriers or new ideas to test. The data should then be plotted in a run chart (i.e., a trend graph that includes a median line). Simple rules are used to analyze the data in a run chart to determine special cause variation as opposed to common cause variation, or chance. These rules are illustrated in Figure 13-1.

The control chart is a more sophisticated version of a run chart and is used to detect special-cause variation. This chart adds upper and lower control limits to a run chart and includes rules about the behavior of the data in relation to the control limits to determine whether a process is in control. After the run or control charts are developed, it is important to prominently display them for review by all those involved in the process and to include the charts in the improvement process.

Armed with the tools to determine improvement, the next logical step is to identify process changes that will result in an improvement. The PDSA cycle is a time-tested framework for generating and testing ideas for improvement. The *plan* step involves developing objectives, predictions, and plans to carry out the cycle. The *do* step involves carrying out the plan and documenting data and observations. The *study* step involves analyzing the data, comparing results to predictions, and summarizing what was learned. The *act* step involves determining the changes to be made in the next cycle, after which the cycle repeats. A key feature of the Model for Improvement is the rapid and repeated use of the PDSA cycle. In significant contrast to measurement for research, PDSA cycles might be measured in days or even hours.

The driver diagram developed by the Institute for Healthcare Improvement (IHI) is another useful tool for designing changes that will result in an improvement. This diagram organizes the theory of improvement for a specific project, visually connecting the outcome or aim, key drivers, design changes, and measures. Typical key drivers include performance of a component of the system, an operating rule or value, or some element of system structure. A driver diagram template is shown in Figure 13-2.

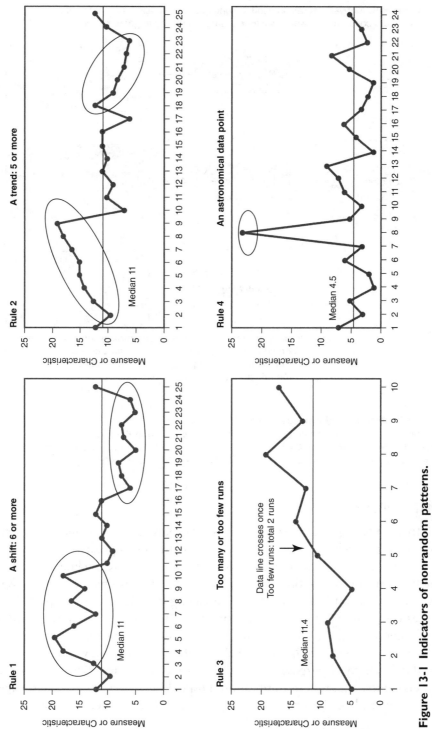

Figure 13-1 Indicators of nonrandom patterns.

Definition: A driver diagram is used to conceptualize an issue and determine its system components, which will then create a pathway to get to the goal.

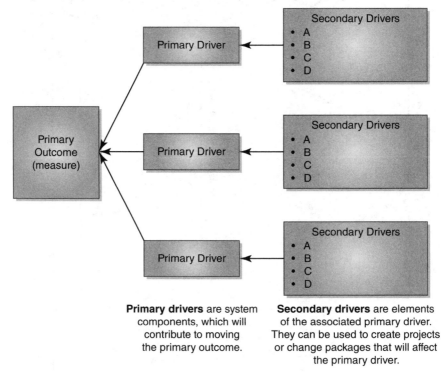

Primary drivers are system components, which will contribute to moving the primary outcome.

Secondary drivers are elements of the associated primary driver. They can be used to create projects or change packages that will affect the primary driver.

Figure 13-2 Driver diagram template.
Reproduced from Institute for Healthcare Improvement, Stiefel M, Nolan K. A Guide to Measuring the Triple Aim: Population Health, Experience of Care, and Per Capita Cost. IHI Innovation Series white paper. Cambridge, Massachusetts: Institute for Healthcare Improvement; 2012. (Available on www.IHI.org)

PREDICTIVE MODELING

Predictive modeling is another powerful set of tools for performance improvement. In general, this approach relies on mathematical algorithms to predict the probability of an outcome. It is used in many industries other than health care, including insurance (e.g., to predict cost) and marketing (e.g., to predict what consumers will buy). Within the context of population health, predictive modeling is typically used to predict such outcomes as cost, resource utilization, or mortality by population segments. The ultimate goal of using a predictive model is to deliver tailored interventions and resources to a specific population segment based on their specific needs. Predictive models in health care are used for a variety of purposes, including identification of individuals at risk for adverse health outcomes, high resource utilization, hospital stays/days/readmissions, expensive or risky procedures, large healthcare-related costs, and disenrollment from a health plan.

The traditional approach to population care management has been to intervene with those individuals who historically have the worst outcomes or the highest utilization. This threshold approach assumes that members with poor outcomes this year are the most likely to have poor outcomes next year. Accuracy of predictions depends on correlation between outcomes now and outcomes in the future. This assumption of correlation has two major shortcomings. First, natural progression of an acute condition or the effect of treatment tends to cause people to get better over time unless they have a progressively deteriorating condition. Second, the statistical phenomenon of regression toward the mean causes outliers in one period to move closer to the mean in the next period due to stochastic or random variation. Because of these two phenomena, most high utilizers in a general population are likely to have *lower* utilization in the next period, even in the absence of any intervention. The predictive modeling approach addresses this problem by looking retrospectively at patterns (see Box 13-1). The model is typically built with data from a prior period and applied to current data to forecast future patterns.

BOX 13-1 KEY PREDICTIVE MODELING QUESTIONS

Modeling questions include the following:

- What are you predicting?
- Why are you predicting it?
- How accurate is your prediction?
- What actions are taken based on the prediction?

The quality of predictive models is assessed through the performance metrics of sensitivity and specificity. Sensitivity (the true positive rate) measures the percentage of high-risk individuals who are correctly identified by the model, and specificity (the true negative rate) measures the percentage of individuals *not* at high risk who are correctly identified by the model. Figure 13-3 illustrates the concepts of sensitivity and specificity. In a population of 100,000 people, 5,000 end up having a given condition, and 95,000 end up not having the condition. In Figure 13-3a, the predictive model correctly predicts all 5,000 individuals who end up with the condition (100% sensitivity) and correctly identifies all 95,000 individuals who do not end up with the condition (100% specificity). Figure 13-3b presents a more realistic example of predictive model performance. In this case, the model correctly predicts 1,000 of the 5,000 people who actually end up with the condition (20% sensitivity) and correctly predicts 91,000 of the 95,000 people who do not end up with the condition (96% specificity); hence, there are 4,000 false positives and 4,000 false negatives.

The performance of a predictive model depends on the threshold selected for identifying those at risk for a condition, as well as population demographics and data quality. Sensitivity and specificity are *competing* objectives. Ensuring that everyone with the condition is included (higher sensitivity) increases the likelihood that people without the

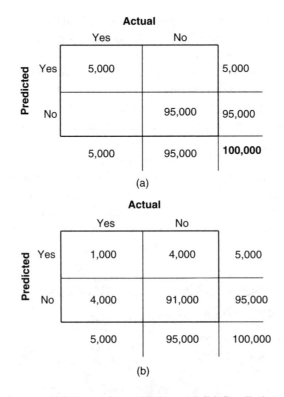

Figure 13-3 (a) Perfect sensitivity and specificity and (b) Realistic sensitivity and specificity.

condition are incorrectly predicted to have the condition (lower specificity). If the model identifies the entire population (specificity = 0%), then no high-risk members will be overlooked (i.e., sensitivity = 100%). If the model identifies no one in the population (sensitivity = 0%), then there will be no false positives (i.e., specificity = 100%). A perfect model would have sensitivity *and* specificity equal to 100%, but in reality, there are no perfect models.

The main challenge with predictive modeling is identifying those individuals who can be helped among those identified as high risk. This challenge is known as impactibility, or targeting people with the highest probability of benefit from an intervention. Figure 13-4 illustrates the impactibility question.

In a predictive model identifying high-cost individuals, the cost trajectory can be influenced only for a subset. Therefore, it is necessary to also predict high-cost individuals whose cost trajectories can be reduced through the use of evidence-based and cost-effective interventions. Nationally recognized guidelines for care assist in establishing these action plans and provide significant decision support to population health efforts.

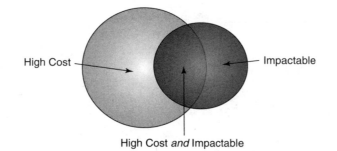

Figure 13-4 Impactability.

MEASUREMENT FOR ACCOUNTABILITY

TRIPLE AIM MEASUREMENT FRAMEWORK

The second step in identifying needs is determining accountability. The IHI's **Triple Aim** provides a framework for measuring accountability,[3] which focuses on three main components—improving population health, per capita cost, and the care experience. This section covers measurement of each of the three aims and discusses how they can be combined to assess overall value.

Population Health Measurement Framework

Many frameworks and models have been developed to illustrate the relationships among the determinants and outcomes of population health. The model shown in Figure 13-5 is based on one originally published by Evans and Stoddart. In their landmark paper (1990),[4] they expanded the relationship between health care and disease by describing broader determinants of health, including genetics, physical and social environment, and behavior. They also broadened the concept of health beyond the absence of disease to include well-being and prosperity.

The model elaborates on the causal pathways and relationships described by Evans and Stoddart and provides a framework for measurement by distinguishing between determinants (upstream and individual factors) and outcomes. Within outcomes, the model distinguishes between intermediate outcomes and health outcomes (states of health).

Following the original Evans and Stoddart model, Kindig and Stoddart later added the important dimension of the *distribution* of health in a population to differentiate it from individual health.[5] McGinnis and colleagues then estimated the relative effects of the various determinants of health described by Evans and Stoddart.[6] These effects are shown in Figure 13-6.

A provocative conclusion of their analysis is health care's relatively small contribution to population health when compared to the contributions of behavioral, environmental,

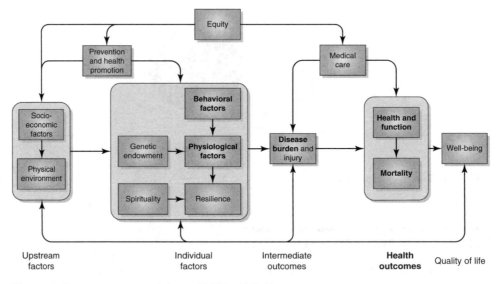

Upstream factors   Individual factors   Intermediate outcomes   **Health outcomes**   Quality of life

Measures in the measurement menu below are highlighted in **bold**

Figure 13-5 Population health.
Reproduced from Stiefel M, Nolan K. A Guide to Measuring the Triple Aim: Population Health, Experience of Care, and Per Capita Cost. IHI Innovation Series white paper. Cambridge, Massachusetts: Institute for Healthcare Improvement; 2012, Available on www.IHI.org.

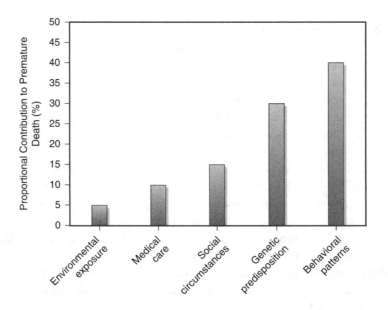

Figure 13-6 Determinants of health.
Data from McGinnis JM, Williams-Russo P, Knickman JR. The case for more active policy attention to health promotion. *Health Aff (Millwood)* 2002;21:78–93.

and genetic determinants. Kindig later operationalized this framework in a measurement system, ranking the counties in Wisconsin on both the determinants and outcomes of population health, as shown in Figure 13-7.[7]

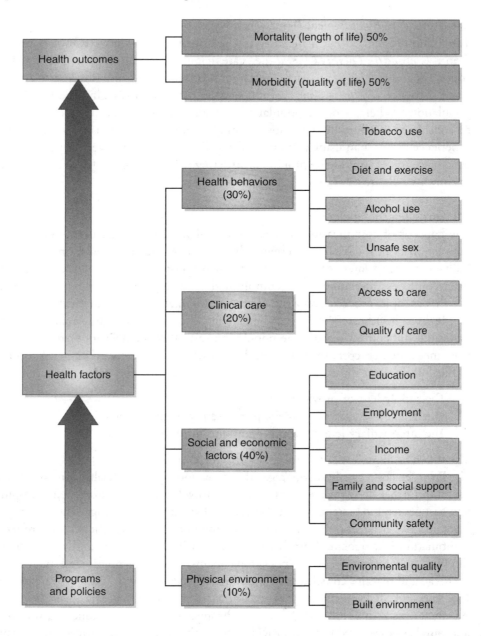

Figure 13-7 Determinants and outcomes of population health in the United States by state.
© 2014 UWPHI, County Health Rankings Model.

The contributions of the healthcare delivery system shown in the model (i.e., prevention, health promotion, and medical care) are discussed later in the chapter as part of the frameworks for the care experience and cost elements of the Triple Aim.

Care Experience Measurement Framework

The six aims for health care articulated by the Institute of Medicine (IOM) in its landmark report, *Crossing the Quality Chasm*[8] (i.e., care that is safe, effective, patient centered, timely, equitable, and efficient), are useful as a framework for measuring the determinants of the care experience and providing decision support for those managing the health status of populations. When used as a population strategic outcome measure, the six aims should be considered as a bundle (i.e., most if not all should be included as the measure of care experience rather than using just one or two). Together with an overall measure of patient experience, these aims are helpful in constructing a driver diagram for the care experience, as shown in Figure 13-2.

Cost Measurement Framework

The concept of cost measurement is more straightforward than is the measurement of population health and care experience, because there are common monetary units with built-in exchange rates that easily can be rolled up or drilled down. That being said, the practice of cost measurement is complicated by a number of factors. Like population health, per capita cost requires a population denominator for measurement; however, most of the U.S. healthcare delivery and financing data are stored and analyzed separately, making it difficult to identify the population served by the delivery system. In addition, it is unclear which costs to include and from whose perspective. Figure 13-8 provides a framework for cost measurement that includes three lenses on cost:

1. The supply lens of providers
2. The demand lens of consumers, purchasers, and the general public
3. The intermediary lens of health plans and insurers

The different lenses assist in understanding the costs being measured.

Provider costs can be disaggregated into various types of health care as shown. It is useful to further disaggregate provider costs into volume and unit cost (e.g., hospital days and cost per day) to better understand sources of variation and change. The sum of provider costs and overhead and margins equals the total costs of care. These costs are paid by a combination of payments from health plans and insurers, public and private payer self-funding, and consumer out-of-pocket payments. These payments and their associated overhead and margins constitute the premium costs paid by public and private payers (e.g., Medicare and Medicaid, employers and union trusts, and individual consumers). Medicare Advantage payments to health plans flow through this pathway. Public and private payers also purchase care directly from providers through self-funding; however, these payments are often administered by insurers through third-party administrator services.

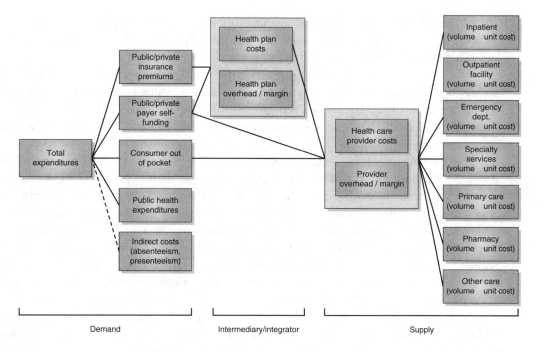

Figure 13-8 Per capita cost.
Reproduced from Stiefel M, Nolan K. A Guide to Measuring the Triple Aim: Population Health, Experience of Care, and Per Capita Cost. IHI Innovation Series white paper. Cambridge, Massachusetts: Institute for Healthcare Improvement; 2012. (Available on www.IHI.org)

From a broad public policy perspective, total costs include public health expenditures as well as direct healthcare costs. Finally, employers increasingly recognize that the indirect costs of poor health (e.g., absenteeism, loss of productivity) may exceed direct healthcare expenditures and must be taken into account when assessing the value of their health promotion and healthcare programs.

The cost of care has been used as a proxy for illness burden. Although this can be directionally correct, great care must be taken when comparing costs between regions because there is significant variation in utilization of services and unit costs from one region to another.[9]

OVERALL VALUE MEASUREMENT FRAMEWORK

Value and return on investment are important decision support metrics to those purchasing health care for a population. A common definition of **value** is "worth, utility, or importance in comparison with something else."[10] This definition highlights an important characteristic of value—that it is relative. Value is more than finding something desirable. It requires a determination of what would be given up in exchange for something. For market goods, value is indicated by the amount of money a person is willing to pay.

The ultimate test of value is choice—people "vote with their feet" if given an opportunity. Another key characteristic of value is that it is subjective. There is no one right answer, and different stakeholders have different perspectives on value.

Taken together, the three parts of the Triple Aim provide a useful framework for measuring *value* in health care, as shown in Figure 13-9. Value can be conceptualized as the optimization of the Triple Aim, recognizing that different stakeholders may weigh the three parts differently. Cost measurement in isolation has little utility; to be useful, it must be combined with measures of the other parts of the Triple Aim.

The combination of cost and care experience enables measurement of **efficiency**, a term that has been both hotly debated and loosely defined in recent years. The AQA alliance, formerly known as the Ambulatory Care Quality Alliance, has developed a useful definition of efficiency in health care that was subsequently endorsed by the National Quality Forum: "Efficiency of care is a measure of the relationship of the cost of care associated with a specific level of performance measured with respect to the other five IOM aims of quality."[11] Similarly, the combination of health outcomes with the care received enables measurement of *effectiveness* of care, or *comparative effectiveness* of alternative treatments. Combining all three parts of the Triple Aim enables measurement of *cost effectiveness*, or overall value.

Trade-offs among the objectives are made differently by different stakeholder groups. Although all three aims are important, purchasers place a priority on cost, consumers focus on health outcomes and the care experience (and cost because they bear an increasing responsibility for costs), and clinicians hone in on the quality of care and service provided. For health plans, the challenge is to develop products that balance these aims to be able to compete successfully in the marketplace.

Another concept related to value, **return on investment** (ROI) for health care is especially important from the purchaser's perspective. ROI describes the size of a return relative to an investment. The ROI measure has some important limitations in that projects with the same ROI can have very different total savings. For any two projects, the

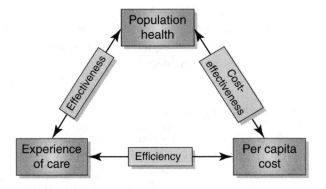

Figure 13-9 Overall value.
Reproduced from Martin LA, Neumann CW, Mountford J, Bisognano M, Nolan TW. Increasing Efficiency and Enhancing Value in Health Care: Ways to Achieve Savings in Operating Costs per Year. IHI Innovation Series white paper. Cambridge, Massachusetts: Institute for Healthcare Improvement; 2009.

one with the lower ROI may actually have the higher total savings. This issue is particularly important to purchasers evaluating disease management programs. For example, a program costing $1 million and returning $3 million in savings has a 3:1 ROI and $2 million in net savings. In contrast, a program costing $10 million and returning $20 million in savings has a 2:1 ROI and $10 million in net savings. Of course, budget constraints are relevant, but the program with the lower ROI in this case produces $8 million more in savings. For this reason, the Population Health Alliance recommends net savings over ROI in the evaluation of disease management programs.[12]

TRIPLE AIM MEASUREMENT GUIDE

A menu of population outcome measures has evolved within the IHI Triple Aim Collaborative, with consideration given to the measurement frameworks outlined in the previous section (Table 13-2).

This menu is based on a combination of the analytic framework presented earlier and the practical experience of participating organizations in the IHI Triple Aim Collaborative. Selection of measures depends in part on data availability, resource constraints, and overall objectives. The ultimate outcome measures for population health (i.e., mortality and health and functional status) can be combined to create a measure of **healthy life expectancy**, representing both length and quality of life. This has become a standard for assessing health outcomes for countries around the world.[13,14] Measures of disease burden and behavioral and physiological factors are included because they are direct causes of health outcomes and are generally more available than true outcome measures.

Table 13-2 Potential Triple Aim Outcome Measures

Dimension of the IHI Triple Aim	Outcome Measures
Population health	Health outcomes: • Mortality: Years of potential life lost, life expectancy, standardized mortality ratio • Health and functional status: Single-question assessment (e.g., from CDC HRQOL-4) or multidomain assessment (e.g., VR-12, PROMIS Global-10) • Healthy life expectancy (HLE): Combines life expectancy and health status into a single measure, reflecting remaining years of life in good health Disease burden: • Incidence (yearly rate of onset, average age of onset) and prevalence of major chronic conditions

Reproduced from Stiefel M, Nolan K. A Guide to Measuring the Triple Aim: Population Health, Experience of Care, and Per Capita Cost. IHI Innovation Series white paper. Cambridge, Massachusetts: Institute for Healthcare Improvement; 2012. (Available on www.IHI.org)

There are two important perspectives on the experience of care: (1) the perspective of the individual who interacts with the healthcare system (i.e., patient experience surveys) and (2) the perspective of the healthcare system focused on designing a high-quality experience for its patients as defined by the IOM's six aims.

Patient surveys are a good source to determine the individual perspective. The measurement menu includes two commonly used assessments: the Consumer Assessment of Healthcare Providers and Systems (CAHPS) family of surveys and the "How's Your Health?" survey.[15,16] Some health systems utilize an overall measure of "likelihood to recommend" as an indirect measure of care quality.

Total cost per member of the population per month is the desirable measure for cost. Sources for per capita cost measurement include the relative resource use measures from the National Committee for Quality Assurance Healthcare Effectiveness Data and Information Set and the Dartmouth Atlas.[17,18]

A healthcare system that doesn't serve a defined population is not able to use population-based measures. In that case, organizations often use a high-cost services measure (e.g., inpatient utilization and costs). Because these services account for a substantial share of healthcare expenditures, such a measure is a good surrogate measure for cost. In addition, episode-based costing is more commonly used today. The unit of analysis—the episode of care—is defined as "a series of temporally contiguous health care services related to the treatment of a given spell of illness or provided in response to a specific request by the patient or other relevant entity."[19]

MEASUREMENT FOR RESEARCH

A full review of research methods for health services and population health research is beyond the scope of this chapter. See Suggested Readings and Websites for texts on health services research methods.

One important high-level topic for decision support is the distinction between efficacy and effectiveness research. Both are focused on whether a particular intervention works. The term **efficacy** refers to whether an intervention can work under ideal conditions. The pragmatic question of whether an intervention works in routine clinical care is addressed by the term **effectiveness**.

Clinical trials are examples of efficacy research. They are designed to isolate the effect of a particular intervention by controlling, to the extent possible, for other factors of potential influence. In real life, these factors *do* intervene and influence the effectiveness of the intervention (e.g., patients enrolled in clinical trials usually have no health problems other than the ones under investigation, and compliance is carefully controlled). In contrast, patients treated in routine clinical practices often have multiple conditions and may fail to follow medical advice. The questions addressed by efficacy research and effectiveness research are both meaningful and complementary, but it is important to be clear about which question is being addressed in a particular research study.

Comparative effectiveness and **cost-effectiveness** are two related and important types of health services research. The IOM defines **comparative effectiveness research** (CER) as:

> the generation and synthesis of evidence that compares the benefits and harms of alternative methods to prevent, diagnose, treat, and monitor a clinical condition or to improve the delivery of care. The purpose of CER is to assist consumers, clinicians, purchasers, and policy makers to make informed decisions that will improve health care at both the individual and population levels.[20]

Cost-effectiveness research views economic considerations in relation to effectiveness. It is a construct closely related to efficiency, measuring the cost of a program or intervention associated with a given level of effectiveness. In health services research, **quality-adjusted life years**, or QALYs, is the measure of individual health most commonly used in cost-effectiveness analysis. The QALY is the individual health building block of the population health measure of healthy life expectancy. It is defined as a year of life lived in less-than-perfect health compared to a year of life in perfect health (e.g., a year lived with blindness may be equated to half a year in perfect health). Healthcare regulatory agencies in many countries (e.g., the National Institute for Health and Clinical Excellence in the United Kingdom) use cost-effectiveness analysis explicitly in their evaluations of new drugs and technologies. In the context of the Triple Aim value framework, cost-effectiveness can also be seen as a combination of two elements of the Triple Aim: cost and health.

CONCLUSION

The decision support tools and methods used in population health are dictated by the kinds of decisions needing support. Decisions in the areas of improvement, accountability, and research require different types of decision support, and the distinctions have been highlighted in this chapter for clarity. However, the boundaries are not as distinct in practice, and it is important to consider how they fit together in an integrated analytic and evaluation system. For example, the Triple Aim framework, while used here to illustrate accountability measurement, is also useful for improvement.

Local improvement efforts frequently reach a point at which a large investment or change is required for widespread implementation. At that point, more tightly controlled research methods may be required to enhance confidence in the investment decision. As clinical information systems and electronic medical records become more widespread, there is increasing opportunity to thoughtfully design data systems that can be used for all three purposes of process improvement, external reporting, and research. As knowledge expands in health informatics and healthcare delivery, clinical decision support increasingly will be built into the electronic process with embedded clinical guidelines and alerts. With such an integrated decision-support infrastructure, it is possible to envision improvement projects generating ideas for research, research findings more quickly implemented in practice, and reporting requirements fulfilled through automated extractions from electronic data systems. Data could seamlessly roll up to the board of directors and external reporting agencies for accountability, down to frontline teams for improvement, and over to research teams to generate new knowledge and insights.

STUDY AND DISCUSSION QUESTIONS

1. What are the three main purposes of population health measurement?
2. What are the three basic questions in the Model for Improvement?
3. What are the primary outcome measures of population health?
4. What are the key determinants of population health?
5. How can value and efficiency be measured in population health?
6. How do key stakeholders' perspectives differ?

SUGGESTED READINGS AND WEBSITES

READINGS

Aday LA, Begley CE, Lairson DR, et al. *Evaluating the Healthcare System: Effectiveness, Efficiency, and Equity.* 3rd ed. Chicago, IL: Health Administration Press; 2004.

Berwick DM, Nolan TW, Whittington J. The Triple Aim: care, health, and cost. *Health Aff.* 2008;27(3):759-69.

Evans RG, Barer ML, Marmor TR, eds. *Why Are Some People Healthy and Others Not? The Determinants of Health of Populations.* Hawthorne, NY: Aldine De Gruyter; 1994.

Evans RG, Stoddart GL. Producing health, consuming health care. *Soc Sci Med.* 1990;31(12):1347-63.

Langley GJ, Moen RD, Nolan KM, et al. *The Improvement Guide: A Practical Approach to Enhancing Organizational Performance.* San Francisco, CA: Jossey-Bass; 2009.

McGinnis JM, Williams-Russo P, Knickman JR. The case for more active policy attention to health promotion. *Health Aff.* 2002;21(2):78-93.

Mullner RM, ed. *Encyclopedia of Health Services Research.* Thousand Oaks, CA: SAGE Publications; 2009.

Murray CJL, Evans DB, eds. *Health Systems Performance Assessment: Debates, Methods and Empiricism.* Geneva, Switzerland: World Health Organization; 2003.

Osheroff J, Pifer E, Teich J, et al., eds. *Improving Outcomes with Clinical Decision Support: An Implementer's Guide.* Chicago: Healthcare Information and Management Systems Society; 2011.

Solberg LI, Mosser G, McDonald S. The three faces of performance measurement: improvement, accountability, and research. *Jt Comm Qual Improv.* 1997;23(3): 135-47.

Stiefel M, Nolan K. *A Guide to Measuring the Triple Aim: Population Health, Experience of Care, and Per Capita Cost.* IHI Innovation Series white paper. Cambridge, MA: Institute for Healthcare Improvement; 2012. http://www.ihi.org/resources/Pages/ IHIWhitePapers/AGuidetoMeasuringTripleAim.aspx. Accessed October 31, 2014.

WEBSITES

Dartmouth Atlas of Health Care: http://www.dartmouthatlas.org/

Healthy People 2020: http://www.healthypeople.gov/

Réseau Espérance de Vie en Santé (REVES): http://reves.site.ined.fr/en/home/ about_reves/

University of Wisconsin Population Health Institute: http://uwphi.pophealth.wisc.edu/

REFERENCES

1. Langley GJ, Moen RD, Nolan KM, et al. *The Improvement Guide: A Practical Approach to Enhancing Organizational Performance.* San Francisco, CA: Jossey-Bass; 2009.

2. Solberg LI, Mosser G, McDonald S. The three faces of performance measurement: improvement, accountability, and research. *Jt Comm Qual Improv.* 1997;23(3):135-47.

3. Berwick DM, Nolan TW, Whittington J. The Triple Aim: care, health, and cost. *Health Aff.* 2008;27(3):759-69.

4. Evans RG, Stoddart GL. Producing health, consuming health care. *Soc Sci Med.* 1990;31(12): 1347-63.

5. Kindig D, Stoddart G. What is population health? *Am J Public Health.* 2003;93(3):380-3.

6. McGinnis JM, Williams-Russo P, Knickman JR. The case for more active policy attention to health promotion. *Health Aff.* 2002;21(2):78-93.

7. Taylor KW, Athens JK, Booske BC, et al. *2008 Wisconsin County Health Rankings.* Madison, WI: University of Wisconsin Population Health Institute; 2008. https://uwphi.pophealth.wisc.edu/ programs/match/wchr/2008/rankings.pdf. Accessed October 31, 2014.

8. Institute of Medicine. *Crossing the Quality Chasm: A New Health System for the 21st Century.* Washington, DC: National Academies Press; 2001.

9. Marder B, Carls GS, Ehrlich E. et al. *Geographic Variation in Spending and Utilization Among the Commercially Insured.* Thomson Reuters white paper, July 27, 2011. http://archive.rgj.com/assets/pdf/ J7178046812.PDF. Accessed October 31, 2014.

10. Merriam-Webster Word Central. Value. http:// www.wordcentral.com/cgi-bin/student?value. Accessed October 31, 2014.

11. AQA Alliance. AQA Principles of "Efficiency" Measures. http://www.aqaalliance.org/files/Principlesof EfficiencyMeasurement.pdf. Revised June 2009. Accessed October 31, 2014.

12. DMAA: The Care Continuum Alliance. *DMAA Outcomes Guidelines Report.* Washington, DC: DMAA: The Care Continuum Alliance; 2008; 4:80.

13. World Health Organization. *World Health Statistics 2009.* Geneva, Switzerland: World Health Organization; 2009. http://www.who.int/whosis/ whostat/EN_WHS09_Full.pdf. Accessed October 31, 2014.

14. European Commission. Healthy life years. http://ec.europa.eu/health/indicators/healthy_life_years/index_en.htm. Accessed January 1, 2015.

15. Agency for Healthcare Research and Quality. *CAHPS Pocket Reference Guide for Adult Facility Surveys.* https://cahps.ahrq.gov/consumer-reporting/measures/CAHPS_FAC_PG_041310.pdf. Accessed October 31, 2014.

16. FNX Corporation and Trustees of Dartmouth College. How's Your Health website. http://www.howsyourhealth.org/. Accessed October 31, 2014.

17. New HEDIS® measures allow purchasers, consumers to compare health plans' resource use in addition to quality [news release]. Washington, DC: National Committee for Quality Assurance; February 22, 2006.

18. The Dartmouth Institute for Health Policy and Clinical Practice. The Dartmouth Atlas of Health Care. http://www.dartmouthatlas.org/. Accessed October 31, 2014.

19. Hornbrook MC, Hurtado AV, Johnson RE. Health care episodes: definition, measurement and use. *Med Care Rev.* 1985;42(2):163-218.

20. Institute of Medicine. *Initial National Priorities for Comparative Effectiveness Research.* Washington, DC: National Academies Press; 2009.

chapter 14

POPULATION HEALTH IN ACTION: SUCCESSFUL MODELS

RONI CHRISTOPHER AND GINA HEMENWAY[*]

[*] This chapter is based on contributions made by Paul Wallace, MD, from the first edition.

Executive Summary

Success = Better care, lower cost, better patient experience.

As rising healthcare costs—and the national focus on managing them—continue to provide fodder for political and public debate, a common denominator among the varied potential solutions can be found within the science of population health. Recently, there has been a greater focus on standardizing the approach of healthcare quality interventions and meeting the need for new strategies that utilize electronic clinical decision support tools with evidence-based guidelines to better manage chronic conditions and promote wellness. Likewise, there is growing recognition that social determinants, community supports, and education are predictors of health outcomes. Understanding health care as a combination of many factors—not just the presentation of a disease, condition, or acute healthcare need—is at the core of population health science. Responsibility for creating opportunities and testing strategies that will fulfill the goals of the Triple Aim[1]—better care for lower costs and better patient experiences—rests with providers, patients, healthcare systems, payers, and employers. This collaborative core will build the right environment for improved patient care, decreased healthcare spending, and satisfied consumers of healthcare services.

Durable models of population health must provide broad access to care across the whole population while reliably improving critical health outcomes over time. Successful models will be those that are actionable by healthcare professionals and valuable to the funders of healthcare services. Success varies based on financial and human resources and the degree of an organization or practice's commitment to supporting the work and effectiveness of tools used. While policy makers' and payers' decision criteria to allocate resources may both be evidence based, differences in decision-making rules and perspectives on the need for change may lead these entities to draw different conclusions. Regardless, policy support for population health management is necessary to drive the healthcare system toward sustainable changes. Similar to the chronic care field, policy approaches may leverage more than one model to meet the needs of both the purchaser and provider environments.

Learning Objectives

1. Identify key characteristics of a successful population health model.
2. Understand the key components of population health in practice.
3. Characterize the differences between chronic care and preventive care management.
4. Define the role of clinical decision support systems in creating a sustainable population health strategy.

Key Terms

access

accountable care organizations

bundled payments

Chronic Care Model

clinical decision support

fee-for-service

patient engagement

patient-centered medical home

practice redesign

risk stratification

INTRODUCTION

With the implementation of healthcare reform incentives for primary care and clinically integrated systems to produce efficient healthcare delivery models, the focus on population health has never been more prominent. The challenge ahead is to create a well organized healthcare system that utilizes evidence-based care, **clinical decision support** tools, and community supports to deliver the right care (clinical perspective) at the right time (patient perspective) for the right cost (payer perspective). For this reason, it is impossible to think of population health as a strategy solely in terms of the healthcare delivery system; rather, we must think about how the payer, the patient, and the delivery system work together toward a comprehensive viewpoint that is necessary for success. Without reconciling quality indicators with cost and claims data, we cannot fully appreciate what is needed to move a population toward better health.

In this chapter, we introduce the concept of practice redesign as a key mechanism for delivery system change and explore its central strategies that support population-based care. We apply these strategies to chronic and preventive care practices and provide examples of real-world success. Finally, we highlight recent payment innovations to show how these initiatives affect population-based care strategies.

PRACTICE REDESIGN PRINCIPLES

In recent years, substantial efforts have been made to better equip and position healthcare providers to directly meet the needs of patients and the populations they serve through internal redesign of clinical practices. Practice redesign focuses on a continuum of population care interventions. Prominent examples include the **Chronic Care Model**, proposed in 1998 by Wagner and colleagues,[2] and the **patient-centered medical home** (PCMH) model, endorsed by several national accrediting bodies such as the National Committee for Quality Assurance (NCQA), the Joint Commission (JC), and the Utilization Review Accreditation Commission (URAC), as a framework for patient-centered care. Additionally, there have been notable efforts within integrated healthcare delivery systems and clinical "safety net" and community-based providers since the mid-1990s. Although each model is unique in certain aspects, all of them promote core competencies that are critical to population health management.

ACCESS

Access to the right care at the right time is the most foundational concept for **practice redesign**. From a healthcare delivery system's perspective, access includes having sufficient providers and offering sufficient services to the market it serves. From a patient's perspective, access is something much more personal as indicated by typical patient satisfaction measures:

- Was I able to get a convenient appointment?
- Did I feel taken care of while at the appointment?
- Do I have confidence that I matter to the providers and health delivery system?

There are three main types of access that drive patient care: (1) acute access (i.e., I have an urgent or immediate healthcare need), (2) maintenance access (i.e., I have a chronic or preventive care need that requires provider input), and (3) personal access (i.e., I want to seek advice from providers or systems for something that is important to me about my own health). In the case of personal access, a payer, an employer, or a public service announcement may lead a patient to reach out for services.

CLINICAL DECISION SUPPORT

The national effort to encourage adoption of electronic health records (EHRs) through meaningful use[3,4] has greatly enhanced providers' ability to use electronic health data to support clinical decisions. Although the healthcare system continues to pursue data as a means to identify opportunity, the reality is that EHRs are not always robust enough to yield the actionable data required to improve care and control costs. Population health strategies rely on identifying patients who are due or overdue for and would benefit from an intervention, a process that is made significantly more efficient by the use of electronic data but requires aggregation and query capabilities of a registry not found in most EHRs. For an individual patient, data are only one piece of the overall picture. Risk stratification techniques and patient engagement strategies play equally important roles in a healthcare delivery system's ability to manage populations.

RISK STRATIFICATION

Risk stratification is a technique used to identify patients with a greater need for care over the course of their healthcare journey. For example, a patient with a hemoglobin A1c (HbA1c) of 14 has a far greater risk of complications secondary to diabetes than does a patient with an HbA1c of 7.9. In either scenario, such patients would benefit from clinical interventions and likely from community supports such as diabetic education or support groups. Risk stratification techniques that identify patients with a priority need allow the system to balance resources against patient needs while simultaneously assuring no one group or population is neglected.

Identifying the two types of patients who might benefit from an intervention for diabetes management is essential to the concept of risk management. Risk management occurs when a healthcare delivery system works with the payer system to share clinical and cost data to assess value (value = quality/cost). A clear understanding of how payers enter into risk management contracting is useful for healthcare delivery systems as they allocate resources and set priorities. At the core of risk management is the concept of value-based payment models, which are discussed later in this chapter.

PATIENT ENGAGEMENT

Patient engagement is the art and science of understanding the readiness of a patient to make a commitment to his or her own health. The body of work most closely aligned with patient engagement strategies is motivational interviewing (MI).[5] MI, a foundational approach to assessing a patient's ability and willingness to manage his or her health when not receiving active care from the healthcare delivery system, is considered essential to reducing healthcare costs over the long term. As a science, patient engagement is often measured through the use of surveys. In fact, patient satisfaction surveys are now mandated by several payers, including Medicare and Medicaid, because of substantial evidence suggesting that satisfied patients are often more compliant with care plans and are active participants in their own healthcare journey. As an art, patient engagement entails understanding how to gain insight into a patient's personal agenda as it relates to any clinical agenda that may exist on the part of the provider. Within the purview of population health, the art of patient engagement may be the most difficult concept to grasp because it exists outside of traditional clinical data sets. Improvement in this area goes beyond the interpretation of lab values or the execution of evidence-based practice guidelines—it is built on relationship management.

BUILDING AND TRACKING RELATIONSHIPS

A healthcare delivery system or payer network must be able to build and track relationships to be able to provide cohesive, complementary, and collaborative care for all patients. Although tracking a patient across a system is beneficial to everyone, it can be difficult to execute because of complex privacy requirements and technical challenges and established provider and patient perspectives. Traditional medical school training is designed to create content experts rather than collaborators and systems thinkers. Patients generally assume that any one physician or provider group is aware of the patient's health journey. In reality, without a formal commitment from a healthcare delivery system or provider network, communications among providers often do not occur outside of a traditional unilateral referral process. In the ideal setting, patient EHRs would be viewable by all healthcare providers who serviced the patient as well as to the patient. As providers exchange information about a patient's healthcare needs, they would also highlight the areas of greatest concern and complexity. Likewise, the patient would offer his or her own perspective and document areas of personal interest (e.g., setting self-management goals, updating status on progress, requesting additional information from the provider). The most robust clinical decision support systems would provide population health management techniques to help organize patient needs for all providers. As a provider made referrals to other clinical experts, the referring provider would be able to track and react to issues (e.g., access to services, outstanding or overdue tests) in a timely manner.

MEASURING AND IMPROVING OVER TIME

A healthcare delivery system must be able to improve its performance on evidence-based outcome and process measures, with a high degree of belief that improvement in these measures will yield a positive clinical outcome. Guided by data graphed over time, healthcare delivery systems implement measures at various system levels to ensure that goals are met. In this system-thinking approach, it is important to recognize what types of outcomes or processes should be measured at each level of the organization.

System-level thinking about measurement is critical for proper allocation of resources and enables an actionable approach. It divides the system into three different measurement categories: macro, meso, and micro. A macrolevel goal sits at the highest level of the organization; this type of goal can be found on an executive scorecard (e.g., 30-day hospital readmissions). Although the goal is likely to have the broadest effect, it may not be sufficiently actionable to mobilize providers toward real change. A mesolevel (midlevel) goal is intended to bridge the gap between the macro- and microlevels. These goals generally reside within middle management and allow administrators to look across practices or individual providers to globally assess progress and highlight strong and poor performers (e.g., Which provider within the system has the best overall diabetes control?). A microlevel goal is generally provider, unit, or practice specific and can be immediately implemented at the front line. Microlevel goals support achievement of both the meso- and macrolevel objectives (e.g., follow up within 48 hours of a hospitalization and priori- tize discharged patients for an in-practice visit).

Example

A health system's macrolevel goal is to reduce 30-day readmissions by 20%. Review of data for hospital readmissions highlights chronic heart failure (CHF) readmissions as a driver of overall readmissions in both volume and frequency. The mesolevel measures become general quality indicators for management of CHF that allow administrators to see which provider is managing the condition best and how that translates to readmission rates. Information systems are then mined, and evidence-based practices are examined to determine what type of CHF patients are likely to be readmitted and for what reason. The system uses clinical decision support tools to identify the population of patients that fits the established criteria. Interventions are put in place to manage performance against the established criteria. The defined interventions create the microlevel measures and produce an actionable way for providers to approach the more global issue of hospital readmission rates.

CHRONIC CARE MANAGEMENT

WHY FOCUS ON CHRONIC DISEASE?

Meeting the full needs of patients with chronic health conditions remains a major goal for formulating effective health policy and restructuring healthcare services and their delivery. Patients with chronic medical conditions consume the majority of U.S. health- care resources, and yet quality, service, and cost outcomes lag behind what is required to meet clinical and administrative goals for U.S. population health.

THE CHRONIC CARE MODEL

Wagner's Chronic Care Model (CCM) predicts that improved health outcomes will ensue as the product of increasingly effective interactions between patients and their primary care clinicians. Key design features include the development of an interdisciplinary prac- tice team led by the primary care clinician and improved patient engagement and educa- tion about patient health care and options. Policy and operational support for this core clinician–patient interaction is achieved by refining the design of overall care delivery and physician payment; improving primary and specialty care interaction; and building health information technology capabilities to record and track care, communicate well with patients (with an emphasis on patient self-care), and expand linkages to community health resources.[2,6,7]

The model assumes a distinct relationship between community supports, primary care supports, and the patient's own ability to self-manage care between medical visits.[2] The conceptual framework is based on the premise that chronic care management cannot occur in a single sector of the healthcare delivery system and that, quite often, it relies on complementary services to effect a change in a patient's outcome. In a more traditional chronic care model, the medication regimen and physician-driven orders take priority. In Wagner's and other contemporary models, the concept of patient-centered care with involvement from community or social supports takes precedence in driving change.[8]

PRACTICE REDESIGN PRINCIPLES IN CHRONIC CARE MANAGEMENT

The aim of practice redesign in chronic care management is to minimize disease and maximize health among patients with conditions such as diabetes, asthma, and heart disease. Redefining practice approaches and the processes that drive performance is essential to achieving desired outcomes. A commitment to reviewing the current healthcare delivery model, both operationally and clinically, is critical to the realization of tangible improvements (i.e., standardizing chronic care management through evidence-based guidelines, using clinical decision support tools, engaging patients in self-management, and operating within a financially successful model). When these strategies are reviewed and refined, the population health strategy for any organization becomes more obvious and attainable.

Spotlight
Kaiser Permanente (KP), a multiregional, fully integrated healthcare system, which serves more than 8 million members (including approximately 1 million patients with coverage through Medicare Advantage), offers an example of the effectiveness of practice redesign in achieving integrated care and improved quality of care delivery. KP consists of the Kaiser Family Foundation health insurance plan (based on prepaid, globally capitated care services) in mutually exclusive partnership with the self-governing and independent Permanente Medical Groups (PMGs). The PMGs are multispecialty practices employing salaried physicians. KP has operated internally developed programs for improving chronic condition care since the early 1990s. The design of programs aligns closely with the elements of the Chronic Care Management model.[9] Formal evaluation of programs in the Northern California region of KP, which focus on the care of patients with diabetes, heart disease, and asthma, demonstrated substantial quality improvement and reductions in apparent cost trends for the population of managed patients but was unable to show net cost savings for the programs evaluated.[10] Models that do not employ a closed-system

approach must depend on strong affiliated and network contracts to create the governance and standardization to meet the goals of population health.

PREVENTIVE CARE MANAGEMENT

WHY FOCUS ON PREVENTIVE CARE?

The traditional approach to health care has undoubtedly created a system that focuses more on "sick care" than on "health care" and that fails to effectively encourage healthy living and early detection of preventable health conditions. Preventive services can reduce the prevalence of a targeted disease or condition and help people live longer, healthier lives. Moreover, many preventive services, when targeted appropriately, come at a relatively low cost and help stretch the value of our increasingly scarce healthcare dollars.[11]

THE PATIENT-CENTERED MEDICAL HOME MODEL

As defined by the NCQA, one of the most widely recognized accrediting bodies in the country, the PCMH model is a way of organizing primary care that emphasizes care coordination and communication to transform primary care into what patients want it to be. The model enlists the core principles of population health and primary care redesign as they relate to chronic care. It extends beyond chronic disease management, emphasizing elements such as same-day scheduling, after-hours access, comprehensive health maintenance, and patient outreach for preventive care that enhance the quality and the care experience for chronic care patients and well patients alike.[8]

PRACTICE REDESIGN PRINCIPLES IN PREVENTIVE CARE

Where the Chronic Care Model focuses on a population health strategy aimed at maintaining or improving health for a chronic condition, preventive care management arms patients with the best opportunity to stay well. Preventive care management entails the ability to scan a population and identify when an intervention is warranted. Interventions are defined by regulatory clinical bodies that set parameters and guidelines of care. Most often, preventive care triggers are identified because of age, personal or family history of a certain condition, and unintended exposure to or risk of a potentially harmful situation. To manage prevention successfully, a healthcare delivery system and its partners must be able to perform effective outreach and encourage patients to participate in prevention services. Both the preventive model and the Chronic Care Model require engaged patients, access to data that helps identify patient populations who would benefit from interventions, and the ability of the healthcare system to manage patient health journeys. The use of evidence-based guidelines and clinical decision support tools further accelerates and standardizes interventions to catalyze success.

COMMUNITY-BASED CARE

While the previous examples predominantly apply to practice redesign within the primary care setting, there has also been tremendous success applying the same principles within the community setting. The practice of "hot-spotting," or targeting the small minority of high-cost cases that account for the majority of healthcare spending, has gained significant traction in recent years. These medically and socially complex patients require a frequency and depth of interaction beyond the traditional healthcare system. Such patients can be identified by frequent emergency department or inpatient use, noteworthy claims costs, or other qualifying criteria established in each model. Once identified, a community-based care team, care coordinator, or community health worker is often deployed to establish a relationship with the patient and provide support for an array of physical, emotional, and social needs. Programs may exist as part of the primary care or health delivery system or as an independent resource that works collaboratively with healthcare providers, hospitals, and physician practices to improve care and coordination while simultaneously decreasing costs.

SPOTLIGHT

The most touted example of the hot-spotters model, the Camden Coalition of Healthcare Providers, has experienced unprecedented success by deploying a community-based approach to address the needs of high-cost patients in Camden, New Jersey. Camden is a small city with three hospitals in 9 square miles and ranks as one of the poorest cities in the United States. Using readily available claims data, the Camden Coalition of Healthcare Providers determined that 99% of costs were being incurred by only 20% of patients. The coalition designed and implemented an innovative case management intervention to address the specific needs of the small group of patients who were consuming a disproportionate quantity of medical care. The coalition located the superusers, obtained their consent to join the program, and extended the necessary services to them in their home settings to reduce or eliminate their need to use Camden's emergency departments for nonemergent medical care. Each team consisted of a nurse practitioner; a social worker, who served as case manager; and a community health worker. A program evaluation revealed that the charges incurred per month for the 36 identified patients fell by slightly more than 56% and the number of monthly visits to hospitals and emergency departments for this group declined by roughly 40% per month.[12–14]

GAUGING SUCCESS

To gain momentum and create reliable systems, a successful population care model must achieve a passing grade on two key tests:

- Access: Is the model feasible and meaningful to its stakeholders (i.e., patients, providers, systems)?

- Outcomes: Does the model improve the critical health outcomes of quality, service, and cost for individual patients and the population served?

A sustainable approach for the whole population must meet the professional require-ments of clinicians and deliver adequate value to satisfy the one who pays the bill. Payers include employers, patients as consumers of services, federal and state governments as providers of benefits, and private insurance organizations. Although no single practice model can currently deliver results that meet the expectations of all payer and care delivery settings, there is a growing body of work that supports primary care as a cornerstone of redesign efforts. The distinct focus on patient-centered care, bold strategies for chronic condition management, preventive care management, and discipline in measuring improvement of interventions form a strong foundation for population health models in the future. There is also growing interest among employers and insurance companies in determining whether this redesigned approach to care can in fact reduce the costs of the current system. For this reason, meaningful use[3] recognition by third-party reviewers that endorse population health strategies[4] and payer incentives for measures specifically related to the Triple Aim[1] have been introduced in most national markets.

PAYMENT MODELS AND POPULATION HEALTH

The introduction of new payment models that facilitate improved quality at lower costs, while offering standards for achievement, requires a robust population health strategy to be successful. Moving from a volume-based or **fee-for-service** model to a value-driven payment model requires considerably more collaboration and interdisciplinary care. This section highlights two very popular payment models.

AMBULATORY EPISODIC–BASED PAYMENT

An episode is the collection of care provided to treat a particular condition for a given length of time. The payment model reimburses for episodic treatment. Therefore, a pay-ment threshold is set for a bundle of services associated with a specific procedure or disease state. The payment threshold includes all aspects of the care from acute to ambulatory to postacute services, meaning the delivery system needs to have an interdisciplinary approach to providing and billing for services. The model encourages strong care coordination across the entire continuum of services and a delivery system. As a patient utilizes services for those conditions or diseases, the delivery system is either paid a precontracted, finite sum for the care or continues to bill in accordance with the traditional fee-for-service model and retroactively receives savings or penalty payments based on total cost of care and achievement of minimum quality measures. Delivery systems that choose this model can set contract rates with a specified time period (e.g., 30, 60, or 90 days) for preapproved conditions or diseases.

This payment mechanism is being considered by many for acute episodes (e.g., acute myocardial infarction), acute procedures (e.g., hip and knee replacements), perinatal care, management of complex chronic conditions (e.g., cancer), and populations with intensive care needs (e.g., behavioral and developmental disabilities). Management of multidisciplinary care against the payment threshold is critical in this model and requires a primary accountable provider or designated individual to shepherd the entire care process. This individual will vary based on the episode (e.g., orthopedist for hip and knee replacements) and will be the primary risk bearer and recipient of payment incentives. For some conditions, there will be significant crossover for successful management of the chronic nature of the condition and its potential for acute exacerbation (e.g., asthma). In every circumstance, there should be a deliberate and appropriate hand-off between the primary care provider and the specialist or acute care service line. Currently, there are limited **bundled payments**, although both Medicare and Medicaid have endorsed this value-based payment model as an option for cost containment and as an indicator of quality of care.[15] The model is being tested in the Medicaid environment, with Arkansas leading the state initiatives nationally.[16]

ACCOUNTABLE CARE ORGANIZATIONS

Accountable care organizations (ACOs) and the Medicare Shared Savings Program put the management of a Medicare patient's condition or disease in the hands of the primary care provider. This model requires that all aspects of a person's chronic and preventive care be managed and guided through a longitudinal relationship with a primary care provider who helps the patient navigate the system and access other services as needed. Savings in this model are realized when a combination of quality metrics, patient experience metrics, utilization metrics, and proper acuity coding meet certain thresholds. Unlike the bundled payment model, the ACO does not have a finite time limit and the provider is expected to manage both preventive and chronic conditions. If successful with this model, the delivery system can reap significant savings and share those savings with Medicare.[15] Although this model is currently being tested within the Medicare population, there is an opportunity to expand to other payers if successful.

Population health strategies that prepare the clinician and his or her team to provide the necessary care are key to managing within a contracted dollar amount under a bundled payment model. For the ACO model, access to primary care, using population health strategies that identify patients who are in need of services for prevention or chronic disease management, and ensuring that the patient has a positive experience during a visit are critical to success.[15] Elements that must be standardized and useable in either model include the following:

- Ability for the delivery system to have current and historical electronic data for its patient population

- A commitment to quality improvement and the ability to put evidence-based practice into play
- Longitudinal relationships with patients to mitigate unexpected catastrophic incidents
- Pleasant patient experiences

CONCLUSION

Population health strategies and techniques are essential to meeting the goals of the Triple Aim: better care for lower costs and better patient experiences. With the onset of healthcare reform and national interest in creating clinically integrated networks or delivery systems, population health techniques must be mastered and used at all points in the patient health journey. A focus on strategies that increase access to lower-cost providers, manage and identify high-risk patients, coordinate care, and engage patients in self-management is a core tenet of population health. Social factors and community supports are indicators for identifying population health needs, and there should be equal focus on preventive care and chronic conditions management for patients. Clinical decision support tools are increasingly helpful in efficiently managing populations over time. Although primary care is at the forefront in implementing population health strategies, the effort must extend to specialist and acute care settings.

As payers continue to support new payment models that will shift the focus from volume-based to value-based care, delivery systems must give thought to redefining their scope of care and services for success. Creating collaborative and narrow networks of providers will allow systems to identify a payment model that will yield the best results. Regardless of the model selected, meeting quality objectives and goals (which include utilization and experience measures) is required and expected. Employing a strategy for system thinking to identify the right goals for the right portions of the delivery system will ensure that quality services are provided.

STUDY AND DISCUSSION QUESTIONS

1. What are the key tenets of any population health model?
2. What would macro-, meso-, and microlevel goals be for the following measure: reduce emergency department visits?
3. Describe the differences between the bundled payment and ACO payment models.
4. Despite the differences in the bundled payment and ACO models, what does each of these models have in common as necessary for success?
5. What are the three most common operational models used to create a value-based delivery system?

SUGGESTED READINGS AND WEBSITES

READINGS

Chronic Condition Care

Coleman K, Mattke S, Perrault PJ, et al. Untangling practice redesign from disease management: how do we best care for the chronically ill? *Annu Rev Public Health.* 2009;30:385-408.

Schoen C, Osborn R, How SK, et al. In chronic condition: experiences of patients with complex health care needs, in eight countries, 2008. *Health Aff.* 2009;28(1):w1-w16.

Practice Redesign and the Chronic Care Model

Bodenheimer T, Wagner EH, Grumbach K. Improving primary care for patients with chronic illness. *JAMA.* 2002;288(14):1775-9.

Bodenheimer T, Wagner EH, Grumbach K. Improving primary care for patients with chronic illness: the chronic care model, Part 2. *JAMA.* 2002;288(15):1909-14.

Institute for Healthcare Improvement. *The Breakthrough Series: IHI's Collaborative Model for Achieving Breakthrough Improvement.* Boston, MA: Institute for Healthcare Improvement; 2003. http://www.ihi.org/resources/Pages/IHIWhitePapers/TheBreakthrough SeriesIHIsCollaborativeModelforAchievingBreakthroughImprovement.aspx. Accessed November 1, 2014.

Population Care in Publicly Funded Programs

Bott DM, Kapp MC, Johnson LB, et al. Disease management for chronically ill beneficiaries in traditional Medicare. *Health Aff.* 2009;28(1):86-98.

Kaiser Family Foundation, the Kaiser Commission on Medicaid and the Uninsured. Top 5 Things to Know about Medicaid. February 2011 [chartpack]. Texas Association of Community Health Centers (TACHC). https://www.tachc.org/content/Top_5_ Things.pdf. Accessed November 1, 2014.

Rosenbaum S, Markus A, Sheer J, et al. *Negotiating the New Health System at Ten: Medicaid Managed Care and the Use of Disease Management Purchasing.* Hamilton, NJ: Center for Health Care Strategies Inc.; May 2008. http://www.chcs.org/media/Negotiating_ the_New_Health_System_at_Ten.pdf. Accessed November 1, 2014.

WEBSITES

Brookings Institution: http://www.brookings.edu/
Center for Health Care Strategies, Inc.: http://www.chcs.org/
Centers for Medicare and Medicaid Services: http://www.cms.hhs.gov/
Community Care of North Carolina: http://www.communitycarenc.com/

HealthIT.gov: http://www.healthit.gov/
Improving Chronic Illness Care: http://www.improvingchroniccare.org/
Institute for Healthcare Improvement: http://www.ihi.org/
Kaiser Permanente Care Management Institute: http://www.kpcmi.org/
National Business Group on Health: http://www.businessgrouphealth.org/
National Committee for Quality Assurance: http://www.ncqa.org/
Partnership to Fight Chronic Disease: http://www.fightchronicdisease.org/
Patient-Centered Primary Care Collaborative: http://www.pcpcc.org/

REFERENCES

1. Barwick DM, Nolan TW, Whittington J. The Triple Aim: care, health, and cost. *Health Aff.* 2008;27(3):759-69.

2. Wagner EH, Austin BT, Von Korff M. Organizing care for patients with chronic illness. *Milbank Q.* 1996;74(4):511-44.

3. Blumenthal D, Tavenner M. The "meaningful use" regulation for electronic health records. *N Engl J Med.* 2010;363:501-4.

4. Blumenthal D. Launching HITECH. *N Engl J Med.* 2010;362:382-5.

5. Miller W, Rollnick S. *Motivational Interviewing: Helping People Change* (3rd ed.). New York, NY: Guilford Press; 2013.

6. Bodenheimer T, Wagner EH, Grumbach K. Improving primary care for patients with chronic illness. *JAMA.* 2002:288(14):1775-9.

7. Bodenheimer T, Wagner EH, Grumbach K. Improving primary care for patients with chronic illness: the chronic care model, Part 2. *JAMA.* 2002;288(15):1909-14.

8. National Center for Quality Assurance. Patient-Centered Medical Home. http://www.ncqa.org/medicalhome.aspx. Published 2011. Accessed September 4, 2013.

9. Wallace PJ. Physician involvement in disease management as part of the CCM. *Health Care Financ Rev.* 2005;27(1):19-31.

10. Fireman B, Bartlett J, Selby J. Can disease management reduce health care costs by improving quality? *Health Aff (Millwood).* 2004;23(6):63-75.

11. Cohen J, Neumann, P. The cost savings and cost-effectiveness of clinical preventive care. Robert Wood Johnson Foundation. The Synthesis Project. September 2009. http://www.rwjf.org/content/dam/farm/reports/issue_briefs/2009/rwjf46045/subassets/rwjf46045_1. Accessed November 1, 2014.

12. Green S, Singh V, O'Brynne W. Hope for New Jersey's city hospitals: the Camden Initiative. *Perspect Health Inf Manag.* 2010;7(Spring):1d.

13. Gwande A. The hot spotters: can we lower medical costs by giving the neediest patients better care? *The New Yorker.* January 24, 2011. http://www.newyorker.com/reporting/2011/01/24/110124fa_fact_gawande. Accessed November 1, 2014.

14. Brenner J. Reforming Camden's health care system—one patient at a time. *Prescriptions for Excellence in Health Care.* 2009;(5) Summer:14-5.

15. Sanghavi D, George M. Payment and delivery reform case study: congestive heart failure. http://www.brookings.edu/research/opinions/2014/04/15-payment-delivery-reform-sanghavi. Published April 2014. Accessed November 1, 2014.

16. Emanuel E, Tanden N, Altman S, et al. A systematic approach to containing health care spending. *N Engl J Med.* 2012;367:949-54.

15

THE LEGAL IMPLICATIONS OF HEALTH REFORM

HENRY C. FADER

Executive Summary

Legal counsel—working to meet the patient's, healthcare provider's, and institution's goals.

This chapter discusses the role that legal risk plays as new directions in patient care are developed to better foster the health of patient populations. In particular, the **U.S. Supreme Court**'s decision with respect to the legalities of the **Patient Protection and Affordable Care Act** (ACA) and the rapid advances in medical and data technology increasingly affect the risk manager. An inherent requirement to understanding risk is to incorporate an appreciation for the laws that govern healthcare policy and healthcare delivery. This necessitates the development of a relationship between legal counsel and risk management.

To understand how laws, regulations, and court opinions affect population health initiatives, one must consider constitutional boundaries and their effects on an organization's and society's collective goals. Understanding how laws govern healthcare policy and delivery is instrumental in developing a framework for population health, especially structures such as **accountable care organizations** (ACOs). Through a review of a few specific risks as they relate to protected populations, medical errors, safety concerns, licensure, professional liability, health care, privacy, nonprofit tax laws, and employer wellness plans (including the effect of genetic information), this chapter provides an overview of relevant legal considerations for addressing population health.

Learning Objectives

1. Understand how legal and risk management affect population health.
2. Learn the importance of legal counsel working with risk managers to create a collaborative environment.
3. Appreciate how the U.S. Supreme Court decision on the ACA affects the separation of powers essential to promulgating and enforcing laws and regulations at the state and federal levels.
4. Reflect on specific areas of the law that appear to affect population health strategies.
5. Understand how lawyers assist providers with reduction of risk from potential claims arising from clinical errors and how an apology program might be of use in risk reduction.
6. Learn how employer wellness initiatives may affect population health strategies.

Key Terms

accountable care organization
American Recovery and Reinvestment
 Act of 2009
apology law
breach notification rules
Emergency Medical Treatment and
 Active Labor Act
Employee Retirement Income Security
 Act of 1974
Genetic Information Nondiscrimination
 Act of 2007
health information exchange
Health Information Technology for
 Economic and Clinical Health Act

Health Insurance Portability and
 Accountability Act
meaningful use
medical legal partnerships
Medicare Advantage
negligence
Nurse Licensure Compact
Patient Protection and Affordable Care Act
readmission rules
risk management
tax-exempt status
tort system
U.S. Supreme Court

INTRODUCTION

With change there is generally increased legal risk. This chapter demonstrates the effect of legal risk for initiating new directions for the health of patient populations. It focuses on the provider's role in caring for patients and resultant risks involved, how risks can be mitigated, and the necessary partnerships that must be formed among lawyers, healthcare institutions, and individual providers. Legal risk can be quantified in litigation and result in financial loss, but it also can be professionally damaging to providers when it results in disciplinary proceedings, lost or suspended licenses, or damaged reputations. There are inherent legal risks in providing quality healthcare services, especially under new models of care, and risk must be considered when new approaches to patient care are introduced.

An understanding of laws that govern healthcare policy and healthcare delivery is instrumental in developing a framework for focusing on the implementation of population health strategies. Lawyers provide guidance on the application of law and, when required, challenge the status quo through advocacy for their direct clients and beneficially in better outcomes for patients. Risk managers also play an important role in loss prevention at the individual provider and institutional provider levels. Through identification and prevention of potentially high-risk situations and timely mitigation, risk managers can prevent unnecessary loss from unfavorable situations as they arise.

The partnership among healthcare providers, lawyers, and risk managers is useful not only when an occurance requires guidance from legal counsel but also when it prevents untoward events through training and **risk management**. A legal risk manager assesses the relative risks of a particular activity under the applicable laws, regulations, and court decisions within the jurisdiction of the patient or provider, as the case may be.[1] Although consultation from legal counsel is not required, it is preferred to ensure appropriate and complete mitigation of risk. Because our U.S. legal system is based on legal argument of precedent and interpretation of complex laws, risk managers are wise to engage legal counsel to prepare for the expected challenge to the providers' actions. In a planning context, legal counsel can provide insight into how the proposed implementation of new concepts or ideas meets or exceeds current legal guidelines and protections expressed in court decisions and written laws and regulations.

Healthcare services are so highly regulated in the United States that introducing population-focused approaches adds legal exposures. When change in the manner of care affects a particular population, there will be other stakeholders who may attempt to modify or stop the chosen initiative through legal action, regulatory change, or legislation. A healthcare delivery change (e.g., the formation of patient-centered medical homes and ACOs) calls for proactive anticipation and response to the potential reactions of all of the affected stakeholders that will contribute to reduction of risk. Not all stakeholders will be obvious, but collaboration will be essential.

This chapter will touch on many important areas of the law that affect education in population health, but space does not permit a review of all possible legal areas. The law literally changes every day as courts make rulings, new directives are issued, administrative tribunals issue decisions and interpretations, and legislators seek compromise solutions to community-wide problems. After a brief review of the role law plays on behalf of patients, providers, and healthcare institutions, some of the key legal risk areas in population health will be discussed. Finally, developing approaches to legal risk management and avoidance or mitigation will be illustrated.

ROLE OF LAW

One of the important teachings of the field of population health is to move away from an individual patient focus to an emphasis on the needs of a particular community, such as those with a particular disease or characteristic.[2] When introducing initiatives that affect population health, policy makers must consider how a proposed action will affect the overall health of the targeted population. Because our legal system focuses on provider identification and risk assessment of those providers, one must understand how the laws of the United States operate and the challenges they present to devise strategies to adequately address them.

Under the U.S. Constitution and most state constitutions, government is organized into three branches: legislative, executive, and judiciary, all of which have influence over any changes to the focus, structure, and delivery of care as we know it today.[3] The legislative branch passes laws after deliberating on the views of various stakeholders to proposed legislation. The executive branch regulates and licenses professionals and facilities and issues regulations as required by state and federal laws. Enforcement of all laws and regulations also falls to the executive branch of government. The judicial branch is represented by the state and federal court system. Under the U.S. Constitution, the jurisdiction of certain legal proceedings is mandated to the federal courts, and others are left to state courts, an important distinction because state and federal courts have different political constituencies. In health care, important constitutional issues are typically part of any mechanism of change, so a thorough understanding of U.S. and state constitutional law is essential. All three branches play an important role in creating and enforcing regulations that protect healthcare providers and patients in the provision of healthcare services.[3]

An excellent example of how the three branches of government work under the U.S. Constitution was the U.S. Supreme Court's decision in *National Federation of Independent Business v. Sebelius*, which was decided on June 28, 2012.[4] In a thorough review of Congress's legislative actions and the executive branch's regulatory initiatives, the U.S. Supreme Court upheld the ACA[5] but allowed the states to decide individually as to whether they wanted to participate in the health insurance exchanges and Medicaid expansion. The holding by the U.S. Supreme Court on the ACA was a major support for many of the concepts for the expansion of population health.

Laws, regulations, and court decisions at the institution level affect how care is delivered by that institution, whereas laws, regulations, and court decisions at the provider level affect how providers practice. At the patient level, laws, regulations, and court decisions serve to protect the rights of the patient in all matters related to receiving healthcare services. All such restrictions and directives have an effect on the provider's practice and the patient's ability to receive safe care that is timely, efficient, and equitable. Although laws and regulations are necessary for protection and risk mitigation, it is ultimately individual clinicians' behaviors that have an effect on outcomes.

Many policy makers believe that appropriate incentives can change the behaviors of patients, providers, and institutions and will guarantee improved clinical results. Healthcare risk managers can play an important role in developing and implementing safe and effective patient care practices, preserving financial resources, and maintaining safe working environments.[6] The American Society for Healthcare Risk Management (ASHRM) provides support in this area. Although they typically play a role in policy making and regulation at the institutional level, risk managers are often engaged in training and education efforts to mitigate risk within an institution or particular provider group and can serve as patient advocates.[6] In a perfect world, all professionals would be properly trained, similarly aligned, and agree upon the same goals. Because this is not the case, strategies must be devised to administer incentives with the interests of the institution, providers, and especially the patients in mind.[7]

The population health agenda includes providing comprehensive care and treatment for chronically ill patients, which changes the manner in which patients are treated by their physicians and supporting clinicians over the years. This trend prompted the **Medicare Advantage** program, which provides bundled payment incentives for insurance companies to sell managed care products to Medicare beneficiaries.[8] The primary aim of Medicare Advantage is to provide plans with an incentive for providers to better coordinate care; it remains unclear whether a bundled payment provides sufficient compensation to actually affect outcomes with respect to the coordination of care goals. Some researchers believe that penalties may be more effective. One example of the limitations of incentives is the past failure of many physicians to adopt electronic medical records in medical office practices. Legislation was enacted in 2009, and the Office of the National Coordinator was established to carry out the directives contained in the **American Recovery and Reinvestment Act** (ARRA)[9] and the **Health Information Technology for Economic and Clinical Health** (HITECH) **Act**.[10] ARRA and HITECH provide incentives for physicians to implement electronic health records and then financial penalties if they fail to adopt them. Although many physicians finally did adopt electronic health records through the **meaningful use**[11] program, that effort may falter as compliance becomes more expensive and difficult. Given competing concerns about the adequacy of the physician workforce, policy makers must consider whether a penalty will influence physicians to make the investment required or drive them to leave medical practice. Regardless of the decision to impose an incentive or penalty, one must not lose sight of what is best for the population as a whole. Although incentives may not be the answer, penalties run the risk of leaving institutions without sufficient resources for improvement activities.

Another approach to consider is a combination of incentives and penalties aimed at achieving the desired changes and deterring inefficient or lower quality practice. To have a true picture of the effect of an incentive or a penalty, it should be applied as a community-based standard across the broad population. As U.S. health reform efforts focus on what levels of care and provider behaviors are appropriate for different population groups, incentives and penalties could play an important role. As a critically important component of policy analysis, leaders must determine the associated legal risks arising from each and make appropriate choices.

PATIENT ADVOCACY

Regardless of what motivates behavior change, there is an inherent need for advocacy at the patient, provider, and health institution levels. Risk managers serve to mitigate risk at each of these levels, and lawyers advocate for the best interests of their respective clients.

All three branches of government are sensitive to the need to protect the most vulnerable populations. Not only does government display compassion for those less fortunate, it also provides affirmative protections for those who cannot otherwise protect themselves. Populations with mental or physical disabilities, those with AIDS or who are HIV positive, and individuals with drug and alcohol addictions have been protected from disclosure under an umbrella of state and federal laws and court opinions for decades.[12] These areas of protection most recently have been extended to the patient information contained in medical and pharmaceutical records and the prohibition against mining such data at the individual patient and physician levels.[13] Appropriate attention to training and compliance with laws is necessary to protect institutions and providers from legal risk in determining the type and level of treatments applicable to particular patient populations, especially those with chronic diseases.

Although an analysis of each protection afforded for special populations under laws, statutes, regulations, and court cases is not within the purview of this chapter, most federal and state laws and agencies that oversee protected special populations have sought to expand these laws widely to encompass the most vulnerable populations. Although protection is not guaranteed to all special populations, regulation affords protection to many more individuals than would have received it otherwise. Constitutional law and congressional action have played a significant role in advocacy for and expansion of healthcare and legal protections afforded these special populations.

In recent years, there has been a growth in the institution of **medical legal partnerships**.[14] These are organizations of physicians and lawyers working collaboratively to identify and ameliorate environmental and social risks that will contribute adversely to a patient's health. Some examples include damp, moldy living quarters that exacerbate a child's asthma or a recalcitrant landlord who refuses to remove lead paint from the walls of a house. Once the medical legal partnership identifies the issue and its effect on patient health, the legal side of the partnership commences appropriate actions, usually on a pro bono or volunteer basis.

In addition to risk mitigation at the government level, risk managers within institutions serve as patient advocates. Risk managers track and trend errors and other occurrences and work closely with legal counsel for guidance on the law with the ultimate goal of ensuring safe patient care.

PROVIDER ADVOCACY

Handling delicate situations associated with provider behaviors requires careful thought and, in most cases, legal consultation. When a medical error occurs or is discovered, procedures are usually in place to mitigate risk either through error reporting systems that document the occurrence or through policies that direct the healthcare provider to the institution's risk management officer for anonymous error reporting. Complicating matters in such instances are the extensive compliance programs in existence to combat fraud and designated compliance officers who take on a risk preventive role for a health-care organization.

Risk managers within institutions also serve as provider advocates. Internal to the organization, risk managers have an understanding of the provider and institution and are sensitive to their needs. When high-risk situations present themselves, the risk manager is available for consultation, and when error occurs, timely mitigation is provided. Risk managers work closely with legal counsel for guidance on the law with the ultimate goal of minimizing loss from unintentional or poor outcomes.

Heightened awareness of medical errors has caused institutional providers to change their behavior to embrace compliance and codes of ethics. Fear of financial loss (even with adequate insurance coverage), as well as threats to licensure and certification, has led such providers to be more cognizant of their behavior and how they handle poor outcomes. Education on reporting poor outcomes and compliance with safety initiatives have progressed significantly. Although being forthright about a medical error may not always result in avoidance of financial loss, it demonstrates the provider's obligation to patients and dedication to the role of advocate, a fine line for the risk manager. Because patients are increasingly expected to be active participants in their health care, open, honest conversations with individual providers must be the cornerstone of the physician–patient relationship, and a two-way dialogue will hopefully emerge. This is becoming more evident with the growth of joint decision making in choosing medical procedures and treatments.

Professional Licensure

Many observers believe that a national certification and licensing system for all professionals is a vital element to establishing a system of health care that focuses on the health of the general population and distinct population subsets. Today, most professionals must be licensed under the state laws where they practice, and although reciprocity is common, it is more focused on basic requirements than actual skills and certification of competency. Numerous national societies and associations provide national certification across state lines but have no standing under state licensing laws. The nursing profession has made the most progress in national licensure by developing a federal compact approach (like a driver's license) that would permit nurses to practice across state lines. Today, at least 24 states are part of the **Nurse Licensure Compact** for registered nurses.[15,16] However, progress and change in the area of professional licensing and accreditation are stymied by the insistence of constitutional state police power advocates that only state law govern professionals within their borders.

As we work toward reforming health care to focus on collaboration and population-based approaches, we must consider the current processes and procedures that prepare and certify healthcare providers for practice. For example, licensure is an archaic system that has been used for centuries to evaluate a provider's knowledge and competency based on standards. Traditional licensing procedures do not support a culture of safety in healthcare systems. Currently, professionals are investigated and disciplined by peers, which raises serious questions and concerns (e.g., implications regarding collegiality and referral patterns, potential barriers to clinical staff members questioning their superiors on issues of quality and safety).[13] The emerging population health agenda includes reviewing the procedure for licensing.

As expectations for health professionals change, so should the procedures and legal sanctions that enforce their licensure and certification. Population health requires standardization of treatment. For example, as national quality standards evolve, there should be a parallel movement that encompasses national licensing status. The most successful improvements in quality of care for patients come about as a result of peer review by applying national standards in areas such as anaesthesia[17] and radiology.[18] From a legal perspective, such a dramatic shift will require the cooperation of many stakeholders, including the licensed professionals and their representative organizational bodies, to remediate years of administrative and court decisions under state and federal laws.

Professional Liability and Negligence

A change in the focus of America's health system usually calls for reform of the country's **tort system**, which defines what constitutes injury and the circumstances under which the responsible party should be held accountable.[19] This discussion typically places providers and healthcare institutions on one side and patients' rights advocates on the other. The current tort system encourages practicing "defensive medicine," which significantly drives healthcare costs. Providers argue that without placing financial limits on the current tort system, expenses incurred for unnecessary testing and procedures will continue to increase the cost of care.[20] The ACA's focus on population health and coordinated care of patients will require a new look at traditional tort law concepts.

The tort system also provides an opportunity to correct the "wrongs" that result from professional **negligence**. For negligence to be determined, injury must have occurred, typically physical, and the provider must have breached the duty to perform a procedure or make a diagnosis and direct treatment correctly. Negligence is typically governed by the standards developed in a particular jurisdiction, which causes duties, standards, and definitions of injury to vary from one jurisdiction to another.[21]

When an unexpected adverse event or condition occurs in a hospital or other healthcare facility, the medical staff and risk management departments often investigate the facts and circumstances, as well as the professional competency of the individual(s) involved. In the past, the professional peer review process has been relied upon to improve quality of care in institutions and to assist physicians and other professionals in improving their skills. To allow this process to serve both professionals and the community, special statutes are in place to protect internal peer-review proceedings from discovery in litigation.[22,23]

Today, serious misadventures must be reported to state licensing boards, accrediting orga-nizations, and patient safety authorities. In some states (e.g., Minnesota), misadventures are also publicly reported.[24] This shift in the direction of greater transparency and account-ability continues to highlight the evolution of the relationship between individuals and their healthcare providers, which is necessary for population health improvement.

The issue of standard of care is also evolving. Many courts require that expert testi-mony on the standard of care be related not only to the standard of practice in the state but also to the community in which the injury occurred.[25] As a result, determinations of whether the standard of care was met are inconsistent because they depend on the juris-diction where the incident occurred. Expert witnesses must be considered qualified (under special evidentiary rules that vary by jurisdiction) to comment upon local practice in the community wherein the alleged malpractice occurred, notwithstanding the possibility that a higher level of care and treatment may be provided by medical professionals in another geographic location in an adjoining state or county.

What should be the standard of care for professional negligence? Options for consid-eration include development of a set of standards by (1) national boards or clinical experts, (2) subgroups that reflect local practice differences associated with the patient's location in a rural community or in a region of the county with a lower experience level for a particular approach, or (3) some other evolving standard.

Many healthcare professionals and institutions argue that because of defensive medi-cine practices and the costs of defending lawsuits, the current tort system adds a huge financial burden and negatively affects the relationship of professional and patient when procedures or treatments do not go as planned. There is a movement afoot to reform the tort system and develop an alternative. One alternative, adopted in some states and under discussion in many legal jurisdictions, is the **apology law**.[26–29] Under today's tort system, an admission of error is an enormous gamble for the individual professional or institution. Because it is an admission against interest and purely voluntary, it can be used as evidence in a court of law. The apology movement requires that the individual professional and institution provide the specifics of what happened to the patient and the patient's family immediately after discovering the problem. Such action is typically carried out with the involvement of the institution's risk manager. The apology includes a description of the steps being taken to avoid a recurrence. The clinician or institution might agree not to charge the patient and his or her family for the costs of the procedure or medical treat-ment in exchange for the patient's and family's agreement not to sue for damages. The notion is one of respect for the patient and the family, and the goal is to reduce the incalculable costs of litigation that affects healthcare delivery.

To many, it seems essential that to reduce the costs of defensive medicine and the real and threatened liability payouts for judgments against doctors and institutions, tort reform must be a part of any change in care delivery. Without an alternative, professionals may continue to migrate to jurisdictions where tort laws have less effect, to the detriment of communities where tort reform is not a tenable option.

Healthcare Confidentiality and Privacy Law

All providers are required to protect patient information through confidentiality and privacy laws. Healthcare privacy laws will have an effect on new programs directed at preventive and chronic care treatment in a population health framework. An examination of the ethical and licensure standards that professionals are bound to follow is germane to the discussion of patient confidentiality and privacy. These ethical and legal standards are generally applicable to professionals such as physicians, nurses, and other skilled clinicians. Prior to 1996, the right to privacy primarily referred to legal decisions and laws designed to control the media and its invasion of private lives; it did not specifically outline the special status of health information in our society, and case decisions concerning primarily confidential information were from state courts.

In 1996, the **Health Insurance Portability and Accountability Act** (HIPAA) was enacted by Congress to protect health information held by providers and employers.[30] Regulations implementing HIPAA were issued in 2000.[31] HIPAA's purpose was to protect all electronic health records, but it was soon interpreted to cover all records in any format, including printed records. Under HIPAA provisions, state law protections preempt federal law where HIPAA requirements are less stringent.[32] Although institutions and medical providers generally have become compliant with the privacy protections of HIPAA, concerns remain over breakdowns in the security and protection for health records, especially electronic information.

HIPAA uses the term *protected health information* (PHI) when referring to patient data and information that must be protected by law.[33] One important use of de-identified PHI (i.e., stripped of those elements that would permit a viewer to determine the identity of the individual) is that researchers are permitted to utilize available data to follow trends and conduct comparative effectiveness studies in population health.[34] In February 2009, the HITECH provisions of ARRA included a number of changes to HIPAA and its regulations that tightened the security requirements for data stored by providers.[9] HITECH changed who is covered, what is covered, and how interactions with state law operate. It also set forth new rules for compliance and enforcement of HIPAA generally. The HIPAA regulations under HITECH will continue to expand the focus on the protection of PHI.

The HITECH Act introduced a new focus on promoting physicians' widespread use of electronic health records. To meet the cash incentives for new provisions known as meaningful use, physicians are required to purchase certified vendor-developed systems that have sufficient privacy and security protections built into them and that include interoperability and patient communication standards. All providers and others known as business associates will be subject to **breach notification rules** and will have to meet more stringent standards for security as well.[35]

As electronic data become more commonplace in health care, compliance with healthcare privacy laws will continue as a high-risk area. Actions are being brought in both the state and federal courts (including class actions) when there are breaches or failures to properly secure PHI.[36] Although there is still no federal private right of action for violations of HIPAA, the U.S. Department of Justice, Office of Civil Rights, and the Federal Trade Commission are taking on new responsibilities for breach notification and other alleged violations of HIPAA and privacy and security laws.[37] Personal responsibility of physicians, physician practices, and institutions to properly protect this information will continue to develop.

An essential outgrowth of the risk of protecting PHI for patients in a population health setting is the formation of **health information exchanges** (HIEs).[38] Currently, HIEs operate locally or regionally, but national HIEs have been advocated. HIEs permit providers to share PHI across boundaries—within facilities and among providers—wherever the patient seeks care. Perhaps the most important advantage of a population health setting is that it permits coordination of care and assists in avoiding duplicative tests and procedures. With expanded use of PHI comes an expanded risk of a privacy or security breach; some states now require providers to obtain specific opt-in permissions prior to sharing information on an HIE. For risk management, the issues are assessing the risk of a security or privacy breach and making certain that state laws for opting in or opting out are properly followed based on legal advice.

ADVOCATING FOR PATIENT CARE IN THE AGE OF THE ACA

Two important areas of the law that require consideration as the healthcare system's focus is redirected to population health are (1) not-for-profit provider tax status and (2) employer-based health insurance.

TAX STATUS

The development of acute care hospitals as mission-based, not-for-profit or charitable organizations is a unique characteristic of the U.S. hospital system. These hospitals serve large numbers of uninsured patients and create clinics and outreach programs, often without payment, out of a strong sense of service. Because some have criticized the not-for-profit sector as being profit motivated,[39] the sector has been subjected to increasing scrutiny since 2006 (in terms of governance, executive compensation, and the level of community benefit provided) as a condition of maintaining tax-exempt status.[39]

The key to the existence of any not-for-profit organization is a determination of **tax-exempt status** by the Internal Revenue Service (IRS) under myriad complex requirements.[40] The more complicated the healthcare corporate structure being examined, the more complex the requirements for continuing obligations to maintain that tax exemption. Tax-exempt status granted by the IRS exempts the organization from payment of taxes on earnings derived from its operations and investments.[40] Tax-exempt organizations have a significant advantage in that they are permitted to finance capital and operating expenses through tax-exempt indebtedness sold to the public and large financial institutions at lower rates. IRS tax exemption also translates into state and local tax exemptions, providing relief from state income and sales taxes as well as local real estate and business taxes.

Studies comparing the level of care and treatment provided by not-for-profit organizations to that provided by for-profit organizations have not produced conclusive evidence that one is superior to the other. For-profit organizations consistently bemoan the fact that they lack the tax and financing opportunities provided to not-for-profit organizations, especially when the organizations are in direct competition.[41] Depending on the level of payment associated with particular groups of patients, not-for-profit status could continue to work to the financial benefit of not-for-profit providers under the ACA because of "community benefit" levels of care being delivered in return for retained tax-exempt status.[42] Although the ACA added certain requirements to be met by not-for-profit hospitals, these institutions will most likely continue to serve the general health of their current populations.[42]

EMPLOYER-BASED HEALTH INSURANCE

Another important area of the tax law relates to employer-provided employee benefits. Aside from the Medicare and Medicaid programs and other federal and state payment programs, the majority of individuals receive coverage through private plans provided by employers. These plans are regulated by the federal **Employee Retirement Income Security Act of 1974** (ERISA).[43] State laws also govern private employer plans in the areas of insurance regulation, state mandates, and required coverage that must be offered to employees by employers in their benefit plans. These are extremely technical and highly regulated areas of federal and state law jurisdiction. Employers have traditionally provided options from which employees can choose along the spectrum from health maintenance organizations, to preferred provider organizations, to health savings accounts, the latter with high deductibles and copays. Employers have always been fearful of being too involved in their employees' care. For this reason, many large employers have sought to establish employer-funded, ERISA-qualified plans,[43] which shield employer sponsors against malpractice actions that can lead to damage awards for pain, suffering, lost earnings, and costs of future medical care as a result of withholding care or treatment. Another benefit of ERISA self-insured plans is that they typically are able to bypass state-mandated benefits, one of the cost drivers of higher healthcare costs for employees.[44]

Most ERISA plans, as well as other plans that meet state law requirements, are structured in such a way that payments are made directly to providers for only the care rendered to the beneficiaries. This keeps medical costs lower for self-funded plans because they do not share in costs for other community members whom they do not employ or fund under the plan. Private insurers and third-party administrators are permitted to take into account the medical conditions of the participants in the employer's plan when making their underwriting decisions. This practice has changed the way that plans are written, from a community-wide basis to a medical underwriting model. Abuses associated with the medical underwriting model (e.g., dropping participants from coverage after policy issuance and after the fact denying coverage for undisclosed preexisting conditions) have led many to call for federal laws to protect against such practices.

The growth of employer-sponsored health plans is also rooted in taxation. The primary benefit of employer sponsorship is the ability granted to employees to exclude the cost of health coverage from their incomes when determining their federal and state income taxes.[43] As costs have continued to rise in this area, and as a result of the recession that dates back to December 2007, these tax laws have exacerbated the need for change.

Although it was primarily targeted to providing insurance coverage for those individuals without coverage, the ACA has begun to change the landscape for health insurance coverage.[5] Mandates that working individuals of certain income levels have health coverage led to the ACA's initiative of setting up health insurance exchanges to provide subsidized coverage. Many states expanded their Medicaid programs to accommodate the millions of uninsured. Risk management will be required to broaden its focus to ensure that the complex coverage rules of the ACA are maintained and that those seeking emergency room coverage under the **Emergency Medical Treatment and Active Labor Act** (EMTALA) are stabilized in accordance with the law. Under the ACA, Medicare has begun to penalize or reward hospitals based on their meeting certain **readmission rules**. These are all new risk areas for population health clinical providers. The ACA also eliminated preexisting conditions as a reason for denying coverage and provided for free preventive care under most health plans.[5]

Many employers who are dedicated to improving employee health and limiting the increases in employee healthcare costs have overcome some of their fears about being involved in their employees' healthcare management. An emerging area of reform is an employer-based approach to prevention and greater personal responsibility for wellness through the use of incentive plans.[44-47] Putting aside concerns about malpractice liability, employers are experimenting with incentives for their employees to take better care of their health. Employer-sponsored fitness memberships, monitoring of health indicators (e.g., blood pressure, blood sugar, weight), and programs that address smoking cessation and other lifestyle issues are not uncommon today.

It remains unclear how the court system and regulators will view these changes. Will they support employers' efforts, or will they feel that such involvement in employee health is an invasion of privacy? For example, employees could bring charges under claims that employers discriminated against those who did not meet health-related goals or that as disciplinary measures, employers used private information about their employees' genetic makeup, inability to stop smoking, or inability to lose weight. Although employees may consent to this intrusion into their lives, it is unclear whether the participation is indicative of a perceived need for assistance or a perceived threat of intimidation or reprimand for nonparticipation.

Recent legislation affords even more protection for employees who participate in wellness programs. The **Genetic Information Nondiscrimination Act of 2008** (GINA)[48] protects employees from employers who might utilize personal genetic testing information for hiring and firing decisions. As patients increasingly demand genetic testing for current or future disease predictions and counseling, these become new risks for providers. Risk managers and attorneys who advise hospitals and other providers who counsel patients after genetic testing need to establish standards and policies for the release of this most sensitive information.

Tax law, especially tax-exempt status and employee benefits for health insurance coverage, is in need of reexamination. The success of the population health agenda rests on having support rather than impediments for better health and wellness.

CONCLUSION

The United States has a great opportunity to affect the health of its population. This chapter has been devoted to how the law intersects for patients, providers, and institutions, as well as the management of risk. Any reform to the fragmented and complex healthcare system must give careful consideration to the legal concepts that provide guidance and oversight. As many change advocates have learned over the years, the U.S. healthcare system is tremendously complex; its growth and transitions over the years have been sensitive to balancing myriad legal concepts. As a result, any attempt to refocus delivery of health care on populations must be guided by a thorough understanding of the prevailing laws and regulations. Looking ahead, population health has yet to be considered by the myriad inconsistent laws and regulations on the state and federal levels. For example, ACOs violate traditional notions of antitrust, fraud and abuse, and patient referral laws. Telemedicine is a growing technology, but crossing state boundaries can be problematic in a population health setting due to restrictive state-by-state licensing. Scope of practice and the use of independent health centers at pharmacies are challenges in redesigning a legal and regulatory system to support population health initiatives.

STUDY AND DISCUSSION QUESTIONS

1. Describe how legal counsel should work with a risk manager at an institution to achieve a collaborative environment for both professionals.
2. Provide a schematic diagram of the separation of powers under the U.S. Constitution and describe how each branch affects healthcare providers.
3. Select one area of the law and describe how population health innovations will be implicated.
4. From an employee's viewpoint, describe how wellness initiatives would affect his or her employer's health plan. What legal pitfalls do you perceive?

SUGGESTED READINGS AND WEBSITES

READINGS

Antieau CJ, Rich WJ. *Modern Constitutional Law*. Vols. 1–3. 2nd ed. New York, NY: Thomson West Publishers; 2009.

Dunkle DS. *VEBAs and Other Self-Insured Arrangements (Portfolio 395)*. Arlington, VA: BNA Tax & Accounting; 2009.

Gue DG, Fox SJ. *Guide to Medical Privacy & HIPAA*. Washington, DC: Thompson Publishing Group, Inc.; 2009.

Humo T. *Employer's Guide to Self-Insuring Health Benefits*. Washington, DC: Thompson Publishing Group, Inc.; 2009.

Journal of Law, Medicine & Ethics. Boston, MA: American Society of Law, Medicine & Ethics.

Sanbar SS, American College of Legal Medicine, eds. *Legal Medicine*. 7th ed. Philadelphia: Mosby; 2007.

Scheutzow SO. State medical peer review: high cost but no benefit—is it time for a change? *Am J Law Med*. 2009;25(7):7-60.

Teitelbaum JB, Wilensky SE. *Essentials of Health Policy and Law*. 2nd ed. Burlington, MA: Jones & Bartlett; 2013.

WEBSITES

American Health Lawyers Association: http://www.ahla.org

American Society for Healthcare Risk Management: http://www.ashrm.org/

Center for Studying Health System Change: http://www.hschange.com

The Joint Commission: http://www.jointcommission.org

REFERENCES

1. Teitelbaum JB, Wilensky SE. *Essentials of Health Policy and Law*. Sudbury, MA: Jones & Bartlett; 2007:153.
2. Kindig D, Stoddart G. What is population health? *Am J Public Health*. 2003;93(3):380-3.
3. Teitelbaum JB, Wilensky SE. *Essentials of Health Policy and Law*. Sudbury, MA: Jones & Bartlett; 2007:14-15.
4. *National Federation of Independent Business v. Sebilius*, U.S. Supreme Court, 11-393, (2012).
5. Patient Protection and Affordable Care Act of 2010, P.L. 111-148.
6. American Society of Healthcare Risk Management. http://www.ashrm.org. Accessed November 1, 2014.
7. American Society for Healthcare Risk Management. Data for safety: turning lessons learned into actionable knowledge. http://www.ashrm.org/ashrm/education/development/monographs/Mono_ActionKnowledge.pdf. Accessed November 1, 2014.
8. Centers for Medicare and Medicaid Services. Medicare Advantage Plans. http://www.medicare.gov/sign-up-change-plans/. Accessed April 30, 2014.

9. American Recovery and Reinvestment Act of 2009. Pub. L. No. 111-115, H.R. 1, 123 Stat. 115.

10. Health Information Technology for Economic and Clinical Health Act § 13, Pub. L. No. 111-115, H.R. 1 (2009), codified at 42 USC § 300jj et. seq.

11. 45 CFR Part 170, RIN 0991-AB58, Health Information Technology (2010).

12. Teitelbaum JB, Wilensky SE. *Essentials of Health Policy and Law*. Sudbury, MA: Jones & Bartlett; 2007:148-50.

13. *IMS Health, Inc. and Verispan, LLC v Kelly A. Ayotte*, 550 F3d 42 (1st Cir 2008), *cert. denied*, 77 USLW 3708 (2009).

14. Retkin R, Brandfield J, Hoppin M. Medical legal partnerships: a key strategy for mitigating the negative health impacts of the recession. *The Health Lawyer*, 2009;22(1). http://medical-legalpartnership.org/wp-content/uploads/2014/03/MEDICAL-LEGAL-PARTNERSHIPS-A-KEY-STRATEGY-FOR-MITIGATING-THE-NEGATIVE-HEALTH-IMPACTS-OF-THE-RECESSION.pdf. Accessed November 1, 2014.

15. National Council of State Boards of Nursing. Nurse Licensure Compact. https://www.ncsbn.org/34.htm. Accessed November 1, 2014.

16. National Council of State Boards of Nursing. Model Legislation for States to Enact the Nurse Licensure Compact (NLC). https://www.ncsbn.org/95.htm. Accessed November 1, 2014.

17. American Society of Anesthesiologists. Standards, Guidelines, and Statements. https://www.asahq.org/. Accessed November 1, 2014.

18. American College of Radiology. Practice Guidelines and Technical Standards and RADPEER. http://www.acr.org. Accessed November 1, 2014.

19. Miller RD. *Problems in Health Care Law*. 9th ed. Sudbury, MA: Jones & Bartlett; 2006:251-70.

20. Miller RD. *Problems in Health Care Law*. 9th ed. Sudbury, MA: Jones & Bartlett; 2006:587-622.

21. American Medical Association. Health System Reform Bulletin—Sept. 10, 2009.

22. U.S. Chamber of Commerce. Medical Liability Reform. http://www.uschamber.com/issue-brief/medical-liability-reform. Accessed November 1, 2014.

23. Bremer WD. Scope and extent of protection from disclosure of medical peer review proceedings relating to claim in medical malpractice action. *American Law Reports* 5th. 2009;69(559).

24. Minnesota Adverse Event Reporting Law. Minn. Stat. 144.7063 et. seq.

25. Pearson JO, Jr. Modern status of "locality rule" in malpractice action against physician who is not a specialist. *American Law Reports* 3rd. 2009; 99(1133).

26. Segal J, Sacopulos MJ. Apology laws: a variety of approaches to discussing adverse medical outcomes with patients and others. *AHLA Connections*. 2009;13(11):26-9.

27. Apology laws in Maine: 24 Me. Rev Stat Ann § 2907.

28. Apology laws in Colorado: Colo Rev Stat Ann § 13-25-135(1).

29. Apology laws in Vermont: Vt Stat Ann title 12 § 1912(a).

30. Pub. L. No. 104-191 (1996).

31. *Fed Regist*. 2000;65(82):461. *Fed Regist*. 2002; 67(53):181.

32. Miller RD. *Problems in Health Care Law*. 9th ed. Sudbury, MA: Jones & Bartlett; 2006: 440-52.

33. Definition of protected health information. http://www.hipaasurvivalguide.com/hipaa-regulations/160-103.php. Accessed November 1, 2014.

34. Miller RD. *Problems in Health Care Law*. 9th ed. Sudbury, MA: Jones & Bartlett; 2006:452-5.

35. Omnibus HIPAA Rulemaking. http://www.hhs.gov/ocr/privacy/hipaa/administrative/omnibus. Accessed November 1, 2014.

36. Conn J. Breach law uncovers shortfalls: experts say problems exist keeping data secure. *Mod Healthc*. 2009;39(d49):10, 12.

37. New penalties and procedures under HIPAA were issued by the Department of HHS. See note 35.

38. Health Information Exchange (HIE). What is HIE? http://www.healthit.gov/providers-professionals/health-information-exchange/what-hie. Accessed November 1, 2014.

39. Furrow BR, Greaney TL, Johnson SH, et al. *Furrow, Greaney, Johnson, Jost and Schwartz' Health Law: Cases, Materials, and Problems*. Abridged 6th ed. New York, NY: Thomson West; 2008:498-504.

40. 26 USCA. § 501(c)(3).

41. 29 USCA Title I, § 1132 (preemption of state law) and § 1144 (exclusive federal court jurisdiction) relating to exemptions applicable to employee benefit plans.

42. Internal Revenue Code of 1986, as amended, Section 501(r).

43. Fronstin P, Salisbury D. Health insurance and taxes: can changing the tax treatment of health insurance fix our health care system? *EBRI Issue Brief.* 2007;(309):1-25.

44. The Leapfrog Group. http://www.leapfroggroup .org/. Accessed November 1, 2014.

45. Partnership for Prevention. http://www.prevent .org. Accessed November 1, 2014.

46. U.S. Chamber of Commerce. Workplace Wellness. http://www.uschamber.com/health-reform/ workplace-wellness. Accessed November 1, 2014.

47. U.S. Department of Labor. Employee Benefits Security Administration. The Affordable Care Act and Wellness Programs. http://www.dol.gov/ esba/newsroom/fswellnessprogram.html. Accessed November 1, 2014.

48. GINA, Pub. L. No. 0-233 and Final Rule, 75 FR 68912 (November 9, 2010).

chapter 16

MAKING THE CASE FOR POPULATION HEALTH MANAGEMENT: THE BUSINESS VALUE OF A HEALTHY WORKFORCE

FIKRY ISAAC AND DEBORAH GORHAN

Executive Summary

Good health is good business.

Although nearly everyone recognizes the intrinsic value of improving population health, the *business* case for improving employee health is acknowledged less often. This chapter explores why good health is good business. Specifically, the authors define the cost and causes of poor health, the effect of the hidden costs of poor health to business, and the potential profit of improving workforce health. Proven approaches that organizations can use to embark on the difficult—but critical—mission of improving employee health care are also explored.

Learning Objectives

1. Understand the economic effect of preventable health conditions.
2. Recognize that scientific and economic data support the business case for improving workforce health.
3. Identify how workforce health has an effect on an organization.
4. Understand the roles of the health plan, purchaser, consultant, and specialty vendors in workforce health improvement.
5. Identify proven strategies to promote good health and increase employee engagement.

Key Terms

absenteeism	presenteeism
accountable care organization	prevention
health and wellness program	value-based insurance design
health risk assessment	wellness
noncommunicable disease	

INTRODUCTION

Healthcare expenditures are often described using terms such as "crisis" and "impending disaster"—and it's easy to see why:

- Recent U.S. National Health Expenditure (NHE) data show a continued rise in the cost of health care. NHE grew 3.7% to $2.8 trillion in 2012, which is $8,915 per person.[1] That's up from $8,086 in 2009.[2] NHE accounted for a whopping 17.2% of the gross domestic product (GDP) in 2012.[3]
- Private health insurance spending grew 3.8% in 2011 or 33% of total NHE, and out-of-pocket spending grew 2.8% to $307.7 billion in 2011.[4]

In past decades, healthcare costs were largely due to communicable diseases. Many of today's healthcare costs can be attributed to lifestyle factors (e.g., inactivity, poor nutrition choices, tobacco and alcohol usage) and **noncommunicable disease**s (NCDs), including cardiovascular disease, cancers, chronic respiratory diseases, and diabetes. Consider the following statistics:

- Often a precursor to metabolic illness (e.g., heart disease, diabetes), obesity has been estimated to cost between $147 billion[5] and $190 billion a year in pharmacy and medical costs alone.[6]
- People with diagnosed diabetes, on average, have medical expenditures approximately 2.3 times higher than what their expenditures would be in the absence of diabetes.[7]
- According to the World Health Organization (WHO), NCDs were responsible for two-thirds of all deaths globally in 2011, which is up from 60% in 2000.[8]

- In high-income countries, 87% of all deaths are caused by NCDs. In upper-middle income countries, 81% of deaths are caused by NCDs.[9]
- Worldwide, approximately 44% of all NCD deaths occurred before the age of 70.[10]

Of greatest concern, most premature deaths are linked to *preventable* risk factors (see Figure 16-1).[11] The World Health Organization (WHO) estimates that 80% of heart disease and stroke, 80% of type 2 diabetes, 90% of chronic obstructive pulmonary disease, and 40% of cancer could be prevented if people would do just three things: eat healthy diets, increase physical activity, and stop smoking.[12] Experts believe that "worldwide, healthy life expectancy can be increased by 5–10 years if governments and individuals make combined efforts against the major health risks," such as poor eating habits, lack of exercise, tobacco use, and alcohol misuse.[13]

When she addressed the Global Forum in 2010, Dr. Margaret Chan, director general of the WHO, said of the rise of chronic NCDs that "it is no exaggeration to describe the situation as an impending disaster . . . for health, for society, and most of all for national economies."[14] The Clinton Global Initiative, the World Economic Forum, and the UN General Assembly have similarly categorized the increase in NCDs as a "global epidemic" with serious consequences.

Mental illness has an economic effect as well. The 2010 Global Burden of Disease Study showed that mental disorders account for 7.4% of the world's burden of health conditions in terms of disability-adjusted life years.[15] The global economic costs of mental disorders were estimated at $2.5 trillion in 2010; that number is projected to reach $6.0 trillion by 2030.[16]

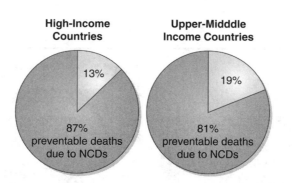

Figure 16-1 In terms of proportion of deaths that are due to NCDs (non-communicable diseases), high-income countries have the highest proportion with 87% of all deaths caused by NCDs, followed by upper-middle income countries with 81%. Deaths due to NCDs are largely preventable.
Reproduced from The top 10 causes of death. World Health Organization. http://www.who.int/mediacentre/factsheets/fs310/en/index2.html. Updated May 2014. Accessed June 13, 2014.

WORKFORCE ISSUES: THE EFFECT OF NCDS ON EMPLOYERS

The burden of providing healthcare services for chronic conditions such as depression, obesity, heart disease, and diabetes is undermining the profitability of employers and endangering the fiscal future of the United States and other nations. As a result, some organizations have sought to improve profitability by passing on more costs to employees (e.g., increased copays or coinsurance). However, this strategy may have hidden costs. When chronically ill individuals (e.g., those with lipid disorders or diabetes) experience higher copayments or higher cost sharing, their use of inpatient and emergency medical services increases.[17] Also, when the focus is on reducing health *costs* rather than reducing health *risks*, an employer's costs for **absenteeism**, **presenteeism**, and disability tend to increase (see Figure 16-2).

Health-related productivity losses, such as substandard performance on the job (presenteeism) and employee absences caused by illness, injury, and other factors (absenteeism), are a significant hidden cost burden for employers:

- For every dollar of medical and pharmacy costs, employers are burdened with two to three dollars in health-related productivity losses (presenteeism and absenteeism).[18]
- For every absent employee (absenteeism), three more employees are present but not maximally productive because of illness (presenteeism).[19]

Absenteeism and presenteeism are even more worrisome when coupled with current trends of downsizing and increased stress on employees who are being asked to do more with less. In other words, we live and work in an era that requires full engagement and greater productivity from employees.

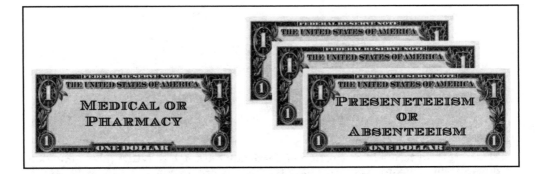

Figure 16-2 For every dollar of medical or pharmacy costs, employers are burdened with two to three dollars in health-related presenteeism and absenteeism costs.
Data From Loeppke R, Taitel M, Haufle V, et al. Health and productivity as a business strategy: a multiemployer study. *Journal of Occupational and Environmental Medicine.* 2009; 51(4): 411–428.

WHY A FOCUS ON HEALTH AND PERFORMANCE IS CRITICAL TO BUSINESS PERFORMANCE

HEALTH AND WELLNESS PROGRAMS: AN INVESTMENT THAT DECREASES HEALTHCARE SPENDING

With more than 2.9 billion people in the labor force,[20] public and private sector employers have an enormous opportunity to reduce health risks by reinforcing positive health behaviors. It is up to individuals, of course, to take responsibility for their own health—to put down their cigarettes, increase their activity levels, schedule preventive care screenings, and maintain a healthy diet and weight—but because we spend so much of our lives at work, the work environment can help shape a desire to adopt healthy habits. In fact, several studies in recent years have proven that **wellness** programs are a good investment toward managing healthcare costs through positive behavior changes.

A 2007 study of 355 large employers showed that organizations with strong wellness programs achieved remarkably lower total healthcare costs than other employers, with shorter sick leaves, reductions in short- and long-term disability, and improved general health coverage.[21] In 2010, Baicker and colleagues conducted a meta-analysis of the return on investment from work-site wellness programs. They reported cost savings at a rate of $3.27 for every one dollar spent. In other words, their savings exceeded program expenses.[22]

Looking beyond cost savings, Phillips[23] argues that the increasing sums paid by large, self-insured corporations for health care may have an effect on the U.S. economy, because, to offset this burden, they will be forced to charge higher prices for services and manufactured goods and reduce the number of jobs. Phillips notes that corporations have an increasing interest in controlling rising healthcare costs and containing corporate financial responsibility through establishing preventive healthcare programs.

In their 2011 evaluation of the effect of Johnson & Johnson's **health and wellness program** on employees' health risks and medical care costs, Henke and colleagues found that the company's annual average increase in medical and drug costs was 1% compared with an average increase of 4.8% in 16 comparative companies similar in industry and size (Figure 16-3). The program also yielded a savings of $565 per employee annually. With an average annual program cost ranging from $144 to $300 per person, the return on investment for the program ranged from $1.18 to $3.92 saved for every dollar spent.[24]

Another study, published in the *Journal of Occupational and Environmental Medicine*, found that Johnson & Johnson employees who maintain a healthy weight have average annual medical costs of $285 per year compared with average annual medical costs of $1,267 for those who gain weight and are at risk for obesity (Figure 16-4). These numbers make it easy to see why Johnson & Johnson makes numerous weight-management resources available to employees as part of its health and wellness program.[25]

Edington has demonstrated that companies experience increased health risks and health costs when they do not manage health status.[26] Within nonmanaged populations,

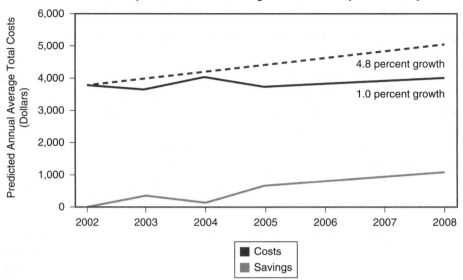

Figure 16-3 Health & Wellness programs can bend the healthcare cost curve. Average savings 2002–2008 = $565/employee per year. Estimated ROI: $1.88 to $3.92 to $1.00.
Reproduced from Copyrighted and published by Project HOPE/Health Affairs as Henke R, Goetzel R, McHugh J, Isaac F. Recent experience in health promotion at Johnson & Johnson: lower health spending, strong return on investment. *Health Affairs.* (Project Hope) 2011; 30(3):490–9. The published article is archived and available online at www.healthaffairs.org.

the low-risk cohort diminished by approximately 5%, whereas the moderate- and high-risk segments increased by approximately 8% and 11%, respectively, over a 3-year period. Edington also demonstrated that this trend can be improved through work-site risk-reduction programs.[27]

WELLNESS PROGRAMS: A KEY TO IMPROVED PROFITABILITY

Although lowered medical costs are a desirable result of wellness programs, it has been questioned whether health and wellness programs can affect businesses' bottom lines in other positive ways.[28] An interesting study was developed to test the hypothesis that when companies create an environment for their employees that (1) reinforces healthier lifestyle choices and (2) provides more effective access to appropriate health care, the companies are not only more productive, but increased productivity drives business performance in a way that can be reflected in the price of their stock.

To test the hypothesis, companies with proven health, safety, and environmental programs (i.e., companies that had previously received the Corporate Health Achievement

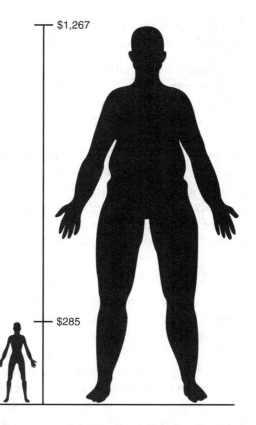

$1,267

$285

Figure 16-4 Johnson & Johnson employees who maintain a healthy weight have average annual medical costs of $285 per year compared with those who gain weight and are at risk for obesity who have average annual medical costs of $1,267.
Data from Goetzel R, Ozminkowski R, Bruno J, Rutter K, Fikry I, Wang S. The long-term impact of Johnson & Johnson's Health and Wellness Program on employee health risks. *Journal of Occupational and Environmental Medicine*. 2002. http://content.healthaffairs.org/content/30/3/490.full. Accessed June 13, 2014.

Award [CHAA] from the American College of Occupational and Environmental Medicine [ACOEM]) were tracked. CHAAs are presented to organizations in manufacturing and service sectors, including city health departments, federal agencies, and healthcare systems, in recognition of their providing effective health and lifestyle programs to their employees and verifiably lowering workplace illnesses and injuries. Using four hypothetical portfolios and a methodology tested by a well known financial institution's wealth management division using recognized financial tools, the market performance of the ACOEM's CHAA winners consistently outperformed the stock market S&P 500 average:

- One hypothetical portfolio outperformed the S&P 500 with a total return of 78.72% during a period when there was no growth in the S&P 500 ($17,871.52 vs. $9,923.14).

- Another portfolio outperformed the market $24,058.29 vs. $15,389.20.
- A third portfolio outperformed the S&P 500 $19,404.12 vs. $9,923.14.

The performance of publicly traded CHAA-winning companies strongly supports the hypothesis that (1) investing in the health and safety of a workforce is good business and (2) focusing on the health and safety of a workforce yields greater value for investors.[29]

In another study, Towers Watson demonstrated that employers with highly effective health and productivity programs generate 20% more revenue per employee, realize a 16.1% higher market value, and deliver 57% higher shareholder return.[30]

Clearly, when employers view their employees as human capital—and regard health and wellness programs as an *investment* rather than as a *cost*—the economic assets and financial value of the enterprise are enhanced along with the health of the workforce. To summarize, the health of the workforce is inextricably linked to the productivity of the workforce and therefore is linked to the bottom line for corporate America.

WELLNESS PROGRAMS: A KEY TO IMPROVED PERFORMANCE

Personal health has an effect on organizations, schools, communities, and social institutions. The opportunity to influence and *truly* change population health risks requires a concerted effort by consumers, producers, governments, schools, health plans, academics, the media, and workplaces. In the workplace, a concentrated, multifaceted effort is most efficacious. For instance, opportunities for healthy nutrition (e.g., cafeteria offerings, meeting room food, vending machine food) can make the difference between engagement and disengagement or lethargy. Lack of engagement is widespread. A Gallup survey of employee engagement estimated that "of the approximately 100 million people in America who hold full-time jobs, 30 million (30%) are engaged and inspired at work; roughly 20 million (20%) employees are actively disengaged; and the other 50 million (50%) Americans are not engaged."[31] Breaks can also have an effect on workplace engagement and health. An organization that promotes "stretch breaks" or breaks that are coupled with healthy, energy-promoting snacks may have very different outcomes than an organization that, in effect, condones smoking by making it easy for employees to take tobacco breaks.

NCD PREVENTION STRATEGIES

Because the most prevalent NCDs are largely preventable, the consensus of many organizations is that disease **prevention** strategies offer the most cost-effective approach for reversing this deadly global epidemic. Changing people's habits, values, and behaviors can be extremely difficult, but proven success strategies exist, especially among businesses that focus on improved health and wellness as a means to reduced employee healthcare costs.

Successful population health management strategies require an examination of the population's lifestyle risk factors and social constructs that impede or improve an individual's ability to form long-term healthy habits. The goal of health and wellness strategies is to encourage the development of personal accountability for adopting the behaviors that could significantly reduce morbidity and mortality associated with lifestyle-related risk factors and disease. At a minimum, these strategies require:

- Access to healthy food
- Opportunities for safe recreation and physical activity
- Incentives or disincentives that reduce consumption of tobacco and alcohol
- Support of mental well-being by reducing the stigma associated with identification and access to care

It's also important for organizations to define what they mean by "a healthy employee." One recognized definition[32] includes the following characteristics:

- *Healthy*: Employees demonstrate optimal health status as defined by positive health behaviors; minimal modifiable risk factors; and minimal illnesses, diseases, and injuries.
- *Productive*: Employees function to produce the maximum contribution to achievement of personal goals and organizational mission.
- *Ready*: Employees possess an ability to respond to changing demands, given the increasing pace and unpredictable nature of work.
- *Resilient*: Employees adjust to setbacks, increased demands, or unusual challenges by bouncing back to optimal well-being and performance without incurring severe functional decrement.

KEY STAKEHOLDERS IN POPULATION HEALTH MANAGEMENT

The Global Alliance for Health and Performance has suggested[33] that to optimize health, the following principles should be applied:

- Optimize individual, team, and organizational resilience
- Drive successful worker health protection and promotion efforts
- Provide the tools to create systems change in work-site health approaches
- Build scalable and sustainable practices for business and industry

Within a business, collaboration across multiple disciplines is required to create and sustain a successful population health management approach. Engaging a multidisciplined network across the enterprise ensures an approach that can be implemented and *sustained* over time. The disciplines include leadership from health, benefits, human resources, facilities, procurement, finance, and the business operations because they all have a potential stake in the success of a healthier workplace with better employee engagement.

GETTING STARTED

The initiator of an employee population health management approach must identify specific stakeholders and prepare key messages that are relevant to the interests of each potential constituent. For example, finance will be motivated by data describing the value on investment or return on investment experienced by other similar employers. Others in the business will be motivated by understanding the connection between health, employee engagement, and productivity. Facilities and other areas of the business need to understand the effect of any capital improvements that are under consideration, such as:

- Food service improvements affecting the cafeteria, catering, or vending
- Furniture options, such as sit and stand desks
- On-site fitness facilities
- Walking paths
- Safe and attractive stairways to encourage walking

THE PURCHASER'S ROLE

Although the most effective health and wellness programs are characterized by shared, aligned goals between all parties (i.e., employees, employers, providers, and health plans), purchasers play an especially critical role because they are responsible for selecting benefits and services and for ensuring that their purchase decisions provide value, which can be defined as a combination of cost-effectiveness, comprehensiveness, sustainability, and the ability to engage with the target audience.

Purchasers must understand that to be most effective, their purchases should focus on disease prevention as well as on returning employees to work after illness or injury. Prevention encompasses:

- Keeping healthy people healthy
- Supporting health and wellness programs to reduce the likelihood that at-risk populations will become unhealthy
- Using screening and biometric testing for early detection and early treatment
- Facilitating early intervention and evidence-based treatment in an effort to reduce morbidity, mortality, and disability

Whoever the internal stakeholder purchaser is, a formal request for information or request for proposal process enables an organization to objectively compare vendor offerings and expertise in a way that minimizes subjective bias. Midsize or smaller businesses may benefit from relationships with healthcare consultants and health plans to support their own internal data analysis, strategic plan for employee population health improvement, and identification of the most appropriate outside partners to achieve desired outcomes.

THE HEALTH PLAN'S ROLE

Health plans and other commercial insurers have the expertise, structure, staff, and technologies required to help businesses and other organizations develop and implement health and wellness programs. Their responsibilities include improving the health of members while ensuring that copays, coinsurance, and overall plan designs are effective. Health plans typically ensure that a certain standard of care is delivered by its participating providers. Progressive health plans have also developed effective pay-for-performance and other incentive programs that reward positive clinical outcomes and health improvements rather than compensating on the basis of the volume of services provided.

Health plans can provide a wide range of expertise and support, including:

- Recommending a mix of medical coverage and prevention strategies to meet the goals of the employers
- Analyzing medical claims to help an employer understand the health challenges of its employees and their dependents
- Administering a **health risk assessment**, which can help an organization understand its overall workforce health and target particular employees for professional support or interventions

Health plans can influence how and when patients access the healthcare system and can encourage certain access points over others. They can also work with employers to develop a **value-based insurance design**, which incorporates incentives to encourage use of high-value services, adherence to treatment regimens, and support of healthy behaviors.[34]

THE ACCOUNTABLE CARE ORGANIZATION'S ROLE

Health plans and employers have even greater potential to improve population health management by collaborating with or including **accountable care organization**s (ACOs) in their provider networks. In an ACO, physician groups are accountable for their *total* patient populations, not just those who access the system for acute and chronic care. Unlike typical physician practices that are focused on scheduled patients, ACO physicians must become aware of the health risks of their entire patient network through gathering data and statistics and requiring all patients to complete a health risk assessment. In place of the current practice model (i.e., a sick-care system), the ACO model focuses on the long-term positive effect on prevention of NCDs by means of proactive early identification (e.g., biometric screening) and proactive outreach. Early indications are that this model may positively affect workplace interventions.

THE HEALTHCARE CONSULTANT'S ROLE

Consultants' capabilities vary greatly. Some offer intensive data capture and analytics abilities, some are true health plan design innovators, and others have experience and systems that employers generally lack. Regardless, healthcare consultants can provide or complement an employer's expertise in the area of benefit plan design. For instance, health and human resource consulting companies can assist with identifying solutions, locating appropriate providers, and providing technological solutions for:

- Benefit design and administration
- Employee assistance programs
- Talent management
- Rewards
- Financial management
- Wellness and fitness services
- Occupational health

METHODOLOGY INSIGHTS FOR SUCCESSFUL POPULATION HEALTH STRATEGIES

BUILDING A CULTURE OF HEALTH

Despite the well documented difficulties it presents, changing unhealthy behaviors of individuals is the core of effective population health strategies. One proven approach for chipping away at unhealthy behaviors and replacing them with healthier ones is to immerse employees in a "culture of health."

A culture of health is perceived by a population through intangibles, through the delivery of programs and communications, and through reporting on how success toward goals is being achieved. According to the 2013/2014 Staying@Work Survey conducted by Towers Watson, U.S. employers "now point to establishing a culture of health as their top priority and as an essential factor for success."[35] In organizations with the most vibrant cultures of health, a deep and many-faceted devotion to healthfulness is evident almost from the moment a person walks in the door. For instance, healthy food is served at meetings and available in the cafeteria. Employees are encouraged to use fitness facilities and walking paths, even during work hours. Stairways and parking lots are safe and well lit in a way that encourages walking. The organization provides ergonomic or health-promoting furniture, such as standing desks or treadmill desks. There are incentives for desirable behavior, such as getting gender- and age-appropriate screenings or achieving a healthy weight. The organization is always seeking new ways to support healthful choices and new ways to reach the people who are at risk. Simply stated, a culture-of-health organization consistently conveys that it deeply believes in the value of healthful behaviors and is willing to invest in those healthy behaviors.

The Johnson & Johnson culture of health is built on five organizational characteristics, referred to as the Five Pillars for Establishing a Culture of Health (Figure 16-5).

1. Leadership and Commitment

In a successful culture of health, the behaviors, values, and norms of the organization and its members are aligned. There is no "say one thing, but do another" on the part of the

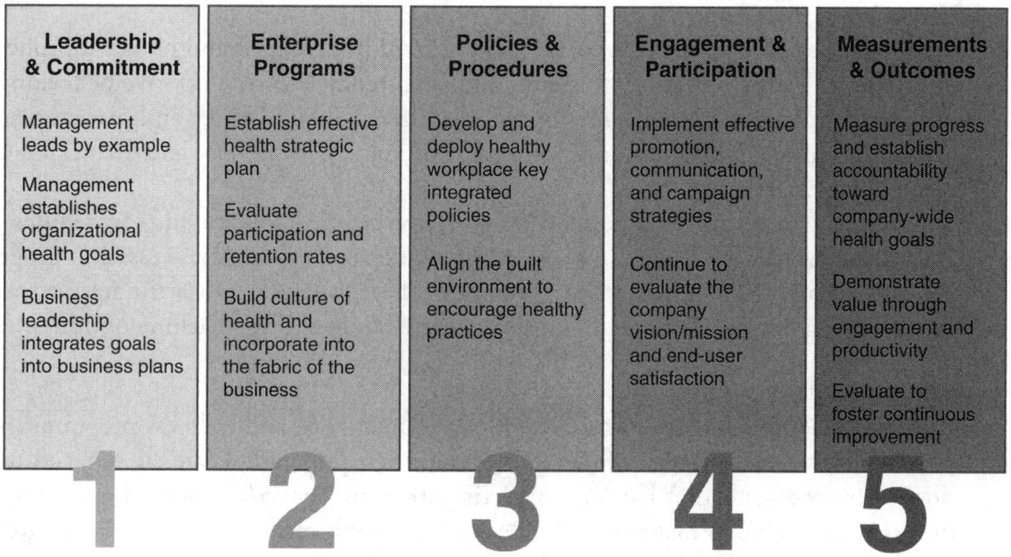

Leadership & Commitment	Enterprise Programs	Policies & Procedures	Engagement & Participation	Measurements & Outcomes
Management leads by example	Establish effective health strategic plan	Develop and deploy healthy workplace key integrated policies	Implement effective promotion, communication, and campaign strategies	Measure progress and establish accountability toward company-wide health goals
Management establishes organizational health goals	Evaluate participation and retention rates	Align the built environment to encourage healthy practices	Continue to evaluate the company vision/mission and end-user satisfaction	Demonstrate value through engagement and productivity
Business leadership integrates goals into business plans	Build culture of health and incorporate into the fabric of the business			Evaluate to foster continuous improvement

1 2 3 4 5

Figure 16-5 The five pillars for establishing a culture of health.

top leadership and middle management. It is imperative that the organization's strategic plan for improving health is embedded in the on-boarding and training of the leadership and other individuals within the organization. Furthermore, improved health of the employee population is a key goal of the organization—one that is integrated into the organization's business plan.

2. Enterprise Programs

The culture of an organization is conveyed in numerous subtle and nonsubtle ways—through health plan design, wellness communications and campaigns, the built environment, and the commitment of employees at all levels. Programs that are developed and introduced into the enterprise must include the following elements:

- A design that solves specific problems or changes specific behaviors
- A distinct set of goals
- Well articulated engagement and participation strategies
- Defined outcomes and measures

According to the 2013/2014 Staying@Work Report, "lack of a clear strategy that is connected to the employee value proposition makes it difficult for employees to understand the purpose of the program and their role in it, which in turn can result in low engagement and participation levels."[36]

3. Policies and Procedures

Population health management goals are best served by *consistent* and *persistent* prohealth, prosafety work experiences. Consistency and persistency reinforce positive behaviors and help outliers conform to the values of the organization. Consistency and persistency also deepen the culture of health over time—contributing to performance and financial returns of the organization.

Successful organizations develop and deploy healthy policies and procedures that conform with their stated goals. They don't provide access to tobacco cessation programs and also permit tobacco use on the premises. They don't emphasize the importance of healthy eating but fail to provide healthy cafeteria and vending machine options.

4. Engagement and Participation

Beyond developing and deploying health communications and wellness programs, organizations must have strategies for ensuring that their populations are encouraged to use those resources—and that barriers to participation are *correctly* identified and removed. Towers Watson reports that although 78% of U.S. employers identify stress as the greatest workforce risk issue for their population,[36] employers and employees have vastly different ideas about what causes their job-related stress. Without understanding the actual causes, it's hard for an organization to drive engagement and participation.

5. Measurements and Outcomes

There's an old saying: "If you can't measure it, you can't manage it." Although an altruistic desire to improve employee health is admirable, organizations must demonstrate that their actions can deliver a return on investment. Employers must approach health and wellness programs with an understanding of what will quantitatively and qualitatively be measured, how they will be measured (i.e., metrics, testimonials) and validated, and what next step(s) will be taken based on what those measurements reveal.

PUSH THE ENVELOPE WITH INNOVATIONS

Employers that provide innovative, integrated health improvement programs are looked upon as employers of choice in their communities; such companies are better able to attract and retain employees. Their employee job satisfaction goes up, and their turnover rates go down.[37] But what is innovation? And how does one decide which innovations to try?

The employee health risk assessment data is a good place to start. Biometric screening may be combined with a health risk assessment, typically a questionnaire completed by employees to capture their self-reported health status and health risks. Biometric screening is defined by the Centers for Disease Control and Prevention as "the measurement of physical characteristics such as height, weight, body mass index, blood pressure, blood cholesterol, blood glucose, and aerobic fitness tests that can be taken at the worksite and used as part of a workplace health assessment to benchmark and evaluate changes in employee health status over time."[38]

Employee health data typically indicate problems with weight, nutrition, inactivity, stress, smoking, and alcohol use. Employee or health plan data may also indicate that employees are not making time for preventive screenings or are not using case managers (if available) to manage chronic illnesses or NCDs. When a pervasive health problem is identified, it is an opportunity for a company to engage in innovative thinking.

Financial incentives are one proven method of increasing an individual's willingness to get healthcare screenings and use a case manager. Commonplace now, paying employees and their dependents to do something that will result in lower healthcare costs was once considered innovative.

New technologies also provide companies with an opportunity to innovate by testing the effect of reimbursing employees for health-related or food and exercise diary apps. Alternately, companies can license existing apps for employee use (faster and more cost-effective than developing apps from scratch). Noteworthy Smartphone and tablet health apps include:

- Apps that can track caloric intake and burn rate and exercise
- Apps that can not only educate but encourage and support users as they seek to improve their nutritional health or change a behavior (such as getting more sleep or drinking alcohol safely)
- Apps that can scan a food bar code and report back on how that food item helps with meeting or sabotaging food goals
- Apps that can support stress management, meditation, journaling, or other methods of coping with the pace of life

Years ago, companies took the then-innovative step of offering pedometers to employees to make them more aware of the number of steps they were taking (10,000 steps a day has been identified as one measure of acceptable daily activity level). Today, the successors to pedometers include electronic wristbands that track far more than the number of footsteps taken.

At the popular Consumer Electronics Show (CES) in Las Vegas in January 2014, wearable health monitoring devices proved to be a popular category. Heart rate earphones, activity goal-setting electronic wristbands, and activity monitoring headbands got as much press as the latest mega-flat-screen TVs. Many of these new devices are wireless enabled or Bluetooth enabled, capitalizing not just on the fact that there are more than 3.2 billion unique mobile users worldwide but also on the "mHealth" phenomenon—part of which is the desire of individuals to capture and monitor their own health and fitness data. According to the *Journal of the American Medical Association*, mHealth takes advantage of the "remarkable capability this [mobile technologies] brings for the bidirectional instantaneous transfer of information."[39]

Technology changes rapidly, but each new technology or health-related trend provides an opportunity for health-conscious organizations to provide innovative ways to engage their employees.

THE IMPORTANCE OF PUBLIC AND PRIVATE PARTNERSHIPS

Companies cannot lead the prohealth charge alone. When businesses, government bodies, schools, and other important institutions use their unique positions to share data and support healthy behaviors, big positive changes can occur.

Consider the story of how tobacco use has declined in the United States. In the late 1950s, the Surgeon General declared a causal relationship between smoking and lung cancer. In 1964, the public health threat of tobacco usage was exposed. More than fifty years later, tobacco still contributes to poor health, but tobacco usage is decreasing.[40] This decrease is the result of many public and private efforts, including press-reported scientific studies, grassroots efforts from citizens, school programs, company tobacco-free workplace policies, and government funding for tobacco-cessation programs. The Surgeon General established mandatory tobacco product label warnings. States and cities have passed legislation that limits where tobacco products can be consumed, limits where and how tobacco products can be marketed, and places taxes on tobacco to discourage tobacco use. Pharmaceutical companies have taken steps to make tobacco-cessation products available to those who cannot afford them.

Tobacco reduction is just one example of how a combined public and private effort can succeed in addressing an important common cause. Helping people understand the dangers of obesity, prediabetes, and diabetes is another excellent example of a public challenge that is worthy of public and private efforts. Public and private organizations could work together, for example, to increase food label literacy, improve safe alcohol consumption awareness, create awareness of the need for safe places for recreation and physical activity, and highlight underserved populations or inequities in the healthcare system.

How can public and private organizations better work together? The Institute of Medicine (IOM) convened a committee of experts in response to a request by the Centers for Disease Control and Prevention (CDC) and the Health Resources and Services Administration (HRSA) to examine the integration of primary care and public health. They came up with a set of principles for public and private integration:

- A shared goal of population health improvement
- Community engagement in defining and addressing population health needs
- Aligned leadership that:
  - Bridges disciplines, programs, and jurisdictions to reduce fragmentation and foster continuity
  - Clarifies roles and ensures accountability
  - Develops and supports appropriate incentives
  - Has the capacity to manage change
- Sustainability, the key to which is the establishment of a shared infrastructure and building for enduring value and effect
- The sharing and collaborative use of data and analysis

The IOM acknowledges that integration of primary care and public health is complex; however, collaboration could enhance the capacity of both sectors to carry out their missions and link with other stakeholders to energize a collaborative, intersector movement toward improved population health.[41]

Though there are challenges whenever governments, private companies, private citizens, and organizations work together, the *mutual need* for progress is clear. According to the Milken Institute, with modest improvements in treating chronic disease, the United States could avoid 40 million cases of chronic disease, decrease costs by $218 billion, reduce the economic effect of disease by $1.1 trillion, and increase GDP by $908 billion.[42]

CONCLUSION

Since the early 1950s, America's health system has been designed to care for the sick. Now is the time to move toward a true health and wellness system. Good health is not only of great value to individuals and populations but also to industry and society. Healthy employees experience higher productivity and lower overall healthcare costs—thus contributing to bottom-line business performance.

In short, wellness works and prevention pays (Box 16-1). Therefore, it is important for stakeholders to look beyond health care as a *cost* that needs to be controlled and instead see health plans and health and wellness programs as an *investment* that can be leveraged. The statement "employees are your greatest asset" must move beyond a simple platitude to become a fundamental guiding principle designed to ensure the health and well-being of employees and the economic viability of employers.

BOX 16-1 COMPANIES WITH HIGHLY EFFECTIVE HEALTH AND PRODUCTIVITY PROGRAMS

- Are nearly 80% more likely to report their financial performance as significantly higher than their peers (20% vs. 11%)
- Are 40% more likely to report financial performance above their peers over the past year than low-effectiveness companies (63% vs. 45%)
- Have unplanned absences that were lower (3.3 vs. 4.0 days per year)
- Have lower annual healthcare costs, giving a company with 20,000 employees a $32 million cost advantage over low-performing organizations
- Have obesity rates (BMI > 30) that are 25% lower than low-effectiveness companies (33% vs. 43%), and the rate of diabetes and high-glucose risks are roughly half (12% vs. 23%)

Data from 2013/2014 Staying@Work Report, Towers Watson/National Business Group on Health.

STUDY AND DISCUSSION QUESTIONS

1. What is the relationship between health and productivity?
2. What are the barriers to achieving a healthier population?
3. What can health plans and employers do to overcome these barriers?
4. What role do absenteeism and presenteeism have on the employer's health-related costs?
5. How can public and private organizations work together better to achieve goals of mutual interest?
6. What innovations can be adopted to improve an individual's accountability for improving his or her health?

SUGGESTED READINGS AND WEBSITES

READINGS

Baicker K, Cutler D, Song Z. Workplace wellness programs can generate savings. *Harvard Business Review*. http://dash.harvard.edu/handle/1/5345879. Accessed November 1, 2014.

Carls GS, Goetzel RZ, Henke RM, et al. The impact of weight gain or loss on healthcare costs for employees at the Johnson & Johnson Family of Companies. *J Occup Environ Med*. 2011;53(1):8-16.

Fabius R, Thayer RD, Konicki DL, et al. The link between workforce health and safety and the health of the bottom line: tracking market performance of companies that nurture a "culture of health." *J Occup Environ Med*. 2013;55(9)339-1000.

Henke R, Goetzel RZ, McHugh J, et al. Employers' role in cancer prevention and treatment-developing success metrics for use by the CEO Roundtable on Cancer. *Popul Health Manag*. 2013;16(5) 296-305.

Isaac F. A role for private industry: comments on the Johnson & Johnson's wellness program. *Am J Prev Med*. 2013;44(1S1):S30-S33.

Kowlessar NM, Goetzel R, Carls GS, et al. The relationship between 11 health risks and medical and productivity costs for a large employer. *J Occup Environ Med*. 2011;53(5)468-77.

Mattke S, Liu H, Caloyeras J, et al. Workplace Wellness Programs Study. RAND Health. Sponsored by the U.S. Department of Labor and the U.S. Department of Health and Human Services. http://www.dol.gov/ebsa/pdf/workplacewellnessstudyfinal.pdf. Accessed November 2, 2014.

Staying@Work™ Survey Report 2013/2014, United States. http://www.towerswatson.com/en-US/Insights/IC-Types/Survey-Research-Results/2013/12/stayingatwork-survey-report-2013-2014-us. Accessed November 2, 2014.

WEBSITES

American College of Occupational and Environmental Medicine: http://www.acoem.org
Centers for Disease Control and Prevention: http://www.cdc.gov/
The Health Enhancement Research Organization: http://www.the-hero.org/
Institute for Health and Productivity Management: http://www.ihpm.org
Institute of Medicine: http://www.iom.edu/
Integrated Benefits Institute: http://www.ibiweb.org
National Business Group on Health: http://www.businessgrouphealth.org
World Health Organization: http://www.who.int/en/

REFERENCES

1. Centers for Medicare and Medicaid Services. National Health Expenditures 2012 Highlights. http://www.cms.gov/Research-Statistics-Data-and-Systems/Statistics-Trends-and-Reports/NationalHealthExpendData/Downloads/highlights.pdf. Page modified May 5, 2014. Accessed November 2, 2014.

2. Centers for Medicare and Medicaid Services. Press Release: CMS Office of the Actuary Issues Annual Report on National Health Spending. http://www.cms.gov/Newsroom/MediaReleaseDatabase/Press-releases/2011-Press-releases-items/2011-01-06.html. Published January 6, 2011. Accessed November 2, 2014.

3. Centers for Medicare and Medicaid Services. National Health Expenditures 2012 Highlights. http://www.cms.gov/Research-Statistics-Data-and-Systems/Statistics-Trends-and-Reports/NationalHealthExpendData/Downloads/highlights.pdf. Page modified May 5, 2014. Accessed November 2, 2014.

4. Centers for Medicare and Medicaid Services. NHE Fact Sheet. http://www.cms.gov/Research-Statistics-Data-and-Systems/Statistics-Trends-and-Reports/NationalHealthExpendData/NHE-Fact-Sheet.html. Page modified May 6, 2014. Accessed November 2, 2014.

5. Finkelstein EA, Trogdon JG, Cohen JW, et al. Annual medical spending attributable to obesity: payer- and service-specific estimates. *Health Aff*. 2009;28(5):w822-31.

6. Cawley J, Meyerhoefer C. The medical care costs of obesity: an instrumental variables approach. *J Health Econ*. 2012;31(1):219-30. doi: 0.1016/j.jhealeco.2011.10.003. Epub 2011 Oct 20. http://www.ncbi.nlm.nih.gov/pubmed/22094013.

7. American Diabetes Association. Economic Costs of Diabetes in the U.S. in 2012. http://care.diabetesjournals.org/content/early/2013/03/05/dc12-2625.abstract. Published March 6, 2013. Accessed November 2, 2014.

8. World Health Organization. The top 10 causes of death. http://www.who.int/mediacentre/factsheets/fs310/en/index2.html. Updated May 2014. Accessed November 2, 2014.

9. World Health Organization. The top 10 causes of death. http://www.who.int/mediacentre/factsheets/fs310/en/index2.html. Updated May 2014. Accessed November 2, 2014.

10. World Health Organization. Premature NCD deaths. http://www.who.int/nmh/publications/ncd_report_chapter1.pdf. Accessed December 1, 2014.

11. World Health Organization. Global status report on noncommunicable diseases 2010. http://www.who.int/nmh/publications/ncd_report_full_en.pdf. Reprinted 2011. Accessed November 2, 2014.

12. World Health Organization. Global status report on noncommunicable diseases 2010. http://www.who.int/nmh/publications/ncd_report_full_en.pdf. Reprinted 2011. Accessed November 2, 2014.

13. Stuckler D. Population causes & consequences of leading chronic diseases: a comparative analysis of prevailing explanations. *Milbank Q.* 2008;86: 273-326.

14. Dr. Margaret Chan, Director-General of the World Health Organization. WHO Global Forum in 2010: Addressing the Challenge of Non-communicable Diseases, Moscow, Russian Federation, 27 April 2011.

15. Whiteford HA, Degenhardt L, Rehm J, et al. Global burden of disease attributable to mental and substance use disorders: findings from the Global Burden of Disease Study 2010. *Lancet.* 2013;382:1575-86.

16. Bloom DE, Cafiero ET, Jané-Llopis E, et al. The global economic burden of non-communicable diseases. Geneva: World Economic Forum, September 2011.

17. Goldman DP, Joyce GF, Zheng Y. Prescription drug cost sharing: associations with medication and medical utilization and spending and health. *JAMA.* 2007;298(1):61-9. http://jama.jamanetwork.com/article.aspx?articleid=207805. Published July 2007. Accessed November 2, 2014.

18. Loeppke R, Taitel M, Haufle V, et al. Health and productivity as a business strategy: a multiemployer study. *J Occup Environ Med.* 2009;51(4):411-28.

19. Serxner SA, Gold DB, Bultman KK. The impact of behavioral health risks on worker absenteeism. *J Occup Environ Med.* 2001;43(4):347-54.

20. McKinsey Global Institute. The world at work: jobs, pay, and skills for 3.5 billion people. http://www.mckinsey.com/insights/employment_and_growth/the_world_at_work. Published June 2012. Accessed November 2, 2014.

21. Watson Wyatt Worldwide. *Building an Effective Health & Productivity Framework: 2007/2008 Staying@Work Report.* New York, NY: Watson Wyatt Worldwide; 2007:1–23.

22. Baicker K, Cutler D, Song Z. Workplace wellness programs can generate savings. *Health Aff.* (Millwood) 2010;29(2):304-11.

23. Phillips J. Using an ounce of prevention: does it reduce healthcare expenditures and reap pounds of profits? A study of the financial impact of wellness and health risk screening programs. *J Health Care Finance.* 2009;36(2):1-12.

24. Henke R, Goetzel R, McHugh J, et al. Recent experience in health promotion at Johnson & Johnson: lower health spending, strong return on investment. *Health Aff.* (Project Hope) 2011; 30(3):490-9.

25. Goetzel R, Ozminkowski R, Bruno J, et al. The long-term impact of Johnson & Johnson's Health & Wellness Program on employee health risks. *J Occup Environ Med.* 2002;44(5):417-24.

26. Edington DW. Emerging research: a view from one research center. *Am J Health Promot.* 2001; 15:341-9.

27. Edington DW. *Zero Trends: Health as a Serious Economic Strategy.* Ann Arbor, MI: University of Michigan Health Management Research Center; 2009.

28. Fabius R, Thayer RD, Konicki DL, et al. The link between workforce health and safety and the health of the bottom line: tracking market performance of companies that nurture a "culture of health." *J Occup Environ Med.* 2013;55(9): 993-1000.

29. Fabius R, Thayer RD, Konicki DL, et al. The link between workforce health and safety and the health of the bottom line: tracking market performance of companies that nurture a "culture of health." *J Occup Environ Med.* 2013;55(9):993-1000.

30. Watson Wyatt/NBGH. The Health and Productivity Advantage: 2009/2010 Staying@Work Report. New York, NY: Watson Wyatt Worldwide; 2009. http://www.towerswatson.com/en/Insights/IC-Types/Survey-Research-Results/2009/12/20092010-North-American-StayingWork-Report-The-Health-and-Productivity-Advantage. Accessed November 2, 2014.

31. Gallup. State of the American Workplace: Employee Engagement Insights for U.S. Business Leaders. http://www.gallup.com/strategicconsulting/163007/state-american-workplace.aspx. Published 2013. Accessed November 2, 2014.

32. Loeppke R. Good health is good business. *J Occup Environ Med.* 2006;48(5):533-7.

33. Global Alliance for Health and Performance. A New Global Perspective on Health, Performance and Sustainability. http://www.globalalliancehp.com/pdfs/J&J_GLOBALALL_whitepaper_pages_Final.pdf. Accessed November 2, 2014.

34. The National Committee for Quality Assurance. Value-Based Insurance Design fact sheet. http://www.ncqa.org/portals/0/Public%20Policy/ValuedBasedInsuranceDesign_8.15.12.pdf. Accessed November 3, 2014.

35. Towers Watson 2013/2014 Staying@Work Report, U.S. Executive Summary. http://www.towerswatson.com/en-US/Insights/IC-Types/Survey-Research-Results/2013/09/2013-2014-stayingatwork-us-executive-summary-report. Accessed June 13, 2014.

36. Towers Watson. 2013/2014 Staying@Work Report, U.S. Executive Summary. http://www.towerswatson.com/en-US/Insights/IC-Types/Survey-Research-Results/2013/09/2013-2014-stayingatwork-us-executive-summary-report. Accessed November 3, 2014.

37. Loeppke R, Nicholson S, Taitel M, et al. The impact of an integrated population health enhancement and disease management program on employee health risk, health conditions, and productivity. *Popul Health Manag.* 2008;11(6):287-96.

38. Centers for Disease Control and Prevention. Workplace Health Promotion: Glossary Terms. http://www.cdc.gov/workplacehealthpromotion/glossary/index.html. Accessed November 3, 2014.

39. Steinhubl SR, Muse ED, Topol EJ. Can mobile health technologies transform healthcare? *JAMA.* 2013;310(22):2395-6.

40. Centers for Disease Control and Prevention. Smoking and Tobacco Use: Tobacco-Related Mortality. http://www.cdc.gov/tobacco/data_statistics/fact_sheets/health_effects/tobacco_related_mortality. Accessed November 3, 2014.

41. Institute of Medicine. Primary Care and Public Health: Exploring Integration to Improve Population Health. http://www.iom.edu/~/media/Files/Activity%20Files/PublicHealth/PrimCarePublicHealth/PCPH-Report-Release-Presentation-03-28-12.pdf. Accessed November 3, 2014.

42. DeVol R, Bedroussian A. *An Unhealthy America: The Economic Burden of Chronic Disease. Charting a New Course to Save Lives and Increase Productivity and Economic Growth.* Santa Monica, CA: The Milken Institute; 2007. http://www.mphaweb.org/documents/Milken-EconomicBurdenofChronicDisease.pdf. Accessed November 3, 2014.

Chapter 17

MARKETING AND COMMUNICATION

ERIC N. BERKOWITZ

Executive Summary

Marketing has the potential for engaging individuals to affect behavioral change and lead to positive health outcomes.

Marketing is a core function utilized by for-profit, commercial organizations in developing competitive strategies for increasing market share and, ultimately, serving customers. In the public health and population health environments, marketing has evolved to encompass the concept of social marketing; however, in many instances the translation of this functional area from the commercial to the not-for-profit environment has been limited in its scope.

At its core, marketing is a structured approach to developing plans and strategies. It involves consumers, patients, and clients in the research from which strategies are developed. Effective strategies result in an exchange between the individual and the organization, be it paying dollars to the organization for a product or altering behavior to improve health status. In both cases the exchange is voluntary. This chapter describes the difference between a market-based and a non-market-based approach to planning and the nature of research in developing these plans.

Inherent in developing a marketing strategy are the concepts of a target market and market segmentation. These core concepts focus on identifying individuals who are most likely to benefit from a behavior change or the purchase of an organization's product. The closer a strategy aligns with a homogeneous group of consumers, the greater the likelihood of affecting a positive response. Marketers develop segmentation strategies based on this premise. In most instances, social marketing has taken a highly constrained perspective (i.e., that marketing is merely communication). Thus, the majority of social marketing approaches have focused on communicating more effectively.

In fact, marketing is based on a "marketing mix" comprising four Ps: product, place, price, and promotion. These four Ps refer to the product or service the organization provides, the price at which the product or service is offered to the market, the accessibility of the place in which it is offered (e.g., location, business hours), and the manner in which the availability of the product or service is promoted within the market. A marketing strategy or plan is based on these elements.

This chapter discusses the four Ps of marketing strategy, the bases for segmentation, and how segmentation is applied in social marketing.

Learning Objectives

1. Appreciate the meaning of marketing and the concept of social marketing.
2. Understand market segmentation and target marketing as it applies to developing plans.
3. Learn the appropriate input of market research in the development of marketing strategy and the evolution of data mining.
4. Recognize each of the four Ps of marketing as they apply to social marketing strategies.
5. Describe the effect of the Web 2.0 environment on the promotional element of the marketing mix.

Key Terms

channel of distribution
data mining
homophily
knowledge discovery
marketing mix
opportunity cost
Pareto's rule

product element
psychographic segmentation
segmentation
social marketing
target market
targeting

INTRODUCTION

Population health has increasingly turned to the discipline of marketing as a potential strategy for engaging individuals to affect behavioral change and lead to positive health outcomes. Marketing is a core discipline in for-profit organizations, and it has become increasingly relevant in not-for-profit organizations since the mid-1970s. The application of marketing in **social marketing** contexts has demonstrated that, effectively implemented, there is significant opportunity for utilizing marketing strategies to positively affect health across unique population groups.

WHAT IS MARKETING?

Contrary to a commonly held belief in the field of public health, marketing is not just communication.[1] The American Marketing Association defines marketing as the activity, set of institutions, and processes for creating, communicating, delivering, and exchanging offerings that have value for customers, clients, partners, and society at large.[2] There are four prerequisites for marketing to occur:

1. There must be two or more parties with unsatisfied needs. For instance, one party might be a consumer seeking to fulfill certain needs and the other might be a company or organization seeking to exchange a service or product for economic gain or other positive result such as improved health status in an individual.
2. There must be the desire or ability of one party to meet the needs of another.
3. Both parties must have something to exchange. A physician, for example, has the clinical skills that meet an individual patient's need to have a torn meniscus repaired, or a health provider has the knowledge and ability to provide instructions that meet an individual's need to manage a chronic condition or improve nutritional status. A consumer must have health insurance or financial resources to exchange for the receipt of these medical services.
4. There must be a means to communicate. To facilitate an exchange between two parties, each party must learn of the other's existence. This aspect of health care has undergone unprecedented development in recent years, becoming more individual specific with the increasing use of social media and technology.

THE EVOLUTION OF MARKETING TO SOCIAL GOOD

Originally utilized in the for-profit setting, marketing's relevance and conceptual possibilities were first expanded from the for-profit to the not-for-profit setting in the late 1960s by Philip Kotler and Sidney Levy. They observed that the concept of exchange was central to these organizations' activities, and it was on this basis that marketing occurred.[3]

Viewing the concept of exchange as the core of marketing, leaders in other areas were moved to consider how marketing might be useful. Fine arts centers and museums, hospitals, and school districts began to see the relevance of marketing strategies and tactics in their settings. For instance:

- A consumer exchanges time and money for the pleasure of seeing a display of fine art.
- A patient pays for medical services provided by a freestanding diagnostic clinic.
- A school district provides education in exchange for public support through tax levies.[4]

In a social marketing context, however, exchange is more complex. Exchange may involve third parties, and the transfer may be values, attitudes, or beliefs.[5] Implicit in this concept of exchange is the recognition that marketing—including social marketing—involves a voluntary action on behalf of the individual customer or consumer (i.e., it is not a regulatory action imposed on a person to change his or her behavior).[6]

Alan Andreasen posited the most relevant definition of social marketing as follows: "Social marketing is the application of commercial marketing technologies to the analysis, planning, execution and evaluation of programs designed to influence the voluntary behavior of target audiences in order to improve their personal welfare and that of society."[7] It is important to note that Andreasen specifically highlighted influencing behavior as the "bottom line" objective of social marketing. He underscored this objective to distinguish it from the commercial goal of marketing (i.e., the production of sales).[8] By this definition, social marketing focuses on behavior and is applicable to population health (i.e., the goal of social marketing is to persuade individuals to change their behavior in measurable ways).[9]

A key similarity between commercial marketing and social marketing is that both have a distinct focus on the consumer. However, commercial marketing focuses on developing strategies to benefit the organization by generating sales that increase profits or return on stockholder equity, whereas social marketing focuses on improving the welfare of individuals.[10]

Andereasen outlined six criteria that distinguish the best social marketing programs as shown in Table 17-1. Several key aspects of this framework are critical in the development of an effective strategy for population health programs:

- Consumer research: Developing effective marketing programs requires an understanding of the consumer.
- Concepts of **segmentation** and **targeting**: Segmentation is at the core of effective marketing strategies. It involves developing tactics and programs that are tailored closely to the individual consumer.
- Marketing mix: A common misconception is that marketing is only communication. Maibach and colleagues noted that much of what is referred to as "social marketing" in the public health domain is constrained to "promotion" or "communication."[11] In fact, an effective marketing plan uses the full range of **marketing mix** elements, commonly referred to as the four Ps—product, price, place, and promotion.
- Competition: Although exchange was discussed earlier in the chapter as a prerequisite, competition is as important a consideration in population health social marketing as it is in designing effective marketing strategies in the for-profit setting.

This approach to social marketing does not utilize the full range of tactics used by commercial organizations in developing marketing plans. The four Ps of commercial marketing include:

- The *product* or bundle of goods or benefits a person receives for the desired behavior
- The *price* of the bundle of goods or monetary, tangible, or intangible costs a person incurs to receive the goods.

Table 17-1 Andreasen's Criteria for Social Marketing

Criterion	Explanation
Behavior change	Intervention seeks to change behavior and has specific, measurable behavioral objectives.
Consumer research	Intervention is based on an understanding of consumer experiences, values, and needs. Formative research is conducted to identify these.
Segmentation and targeting	Different segmentation variables are considered when selecting the intervention target group.
Marketing mix	Intervention strategy is tailored for the selected segment.
Exchange	Intervention considers what will motivate people to engage voluntarily with the intervention and offers them something beneficial in return. The offered benefit may be intangible (e.g., personal satisfaction) or tangible (e.g., rewards for participating in the program and making behavioral changes).
Competition	Forces competing with the behavior change are analyzed. Intervention considers the appeal of competing behaviors (including current behavior) and uses strategies that seek to remove or minimize this competition.

Reproduced from http://www.towerswatson.com/en-US/Insights/IC-Types/Survey-Research-Results/2013/09/2013-2014-stayingatwork-us-executive-summary-report.

- The *place*—the time and location—for the exchange to occur. This can be a benefit or a cost, depending on its convenience.
- The *promotion* messages that announce the proposed exchange (the product, price, place, and desired behavior).[12]

KEY DIFFERENCES BETWEEN SOCIAL MARKETING AND COMMERCIAL MARKETING

In discussing social marketing for the management of population health, it is essential to understand the key differences that make marketing principles more difficult to apply in social marketing than in for-profit settings. The products (or services) tend to be more complex:

- Demand is more varied and often negative.
- Target groups can be more difficult to reach.
- Consumer involvement is more challenging.
- The competition is more subtle and varied.[13]
- Counterdetailing commercial marketing may be required.

In social marketing for population health, the products and services tend to be more complex because they often involve a behavioral change. The abstraction involved (e.g., improved diet, reduced consumption) presents more difficulty, and the desired outcomes are often harder to observe in a near term. The buyer of a tangible product or service can experience the benefit of improved communication through a better cell phone or the immediate pleasure of driving a new car. In an industrial setting (a business-to-business sale), the commercial buyer can tangibly measure the enhanced productivity of the production line with an investment or purchase of new equipment or software for the firm.

The challenge in social marketing is that, frequently, strategies must be developed to target negative behaviors—and the individuals may not view this behavior as negative.[14] When individuals engage in activities that are counter to positive health outcomes, the challenge is to "*de*market" these behaviors, or redirect the consumers' behaviors to more positive effects.

The concept of demarketing was first proposed in 1971 by Kotler and Levy in an industrial context. When there are product shortages or when certain segments are unprofitable for a particular company,[15] a company may strategize to reduce demand for its product or service. Thus, Kotler and Levy defined "demarketing" as "that aspect of marketing that deals with discouraging customers in general or a certain class of customers in particular on either a temporary or permanent basis."[16] For example, a demarketing strategy to combat the significant issue of obesity is the packaging of food products to create an artificial stopping point (e.g., by separating a larger package into subpackages, in essence demarketing the consumption of the entire item). Another example is using internal sleeves in a package of cookies so that a person must consciously decide whether to continue consuming cookies beyond a certain point.[17]

Another issue in population health and social marketing is that individuals in the target groups may be more difficult to reach. Some challenges are a function of socioeconomic status. Health status has been correlated to socioeconomic levels, which may hold distinct attitudes that work against beneficial population health behaviors.

The level of involvement must be considered in the marketing of any item. Although there are many definitions of involvement, it can be considered to be the amount of cognitive effort that will be expended in a given situation.[18] In traditional marketing, a consumer's decision process often varies as a function of the level of involvement—the personal, social, or economic significance of the purchase to the individual. In general, a high-involvement product has one of three characteristics: it is expensive, it can have serious personal consequences, or it can reflect on one's social image. In these situations, a consumer engages in a very deliberate decision process and searches for information. A person may also seek word-of-mouth communication from multiple social sources. In low-involvement purchases (e.g., toothpaste, soap), a consumer uses routine problem solving and few external information sources.

As can be extrapolated from the foregoing, involvement for population health management requires that aspects of social marketing be considered as strategies are developed. Certain behaviors or attitudes may be associated with serious personal consequences or reflect on one's social image (e.g., smoking or the attempt to reduce smoking in teens). On the other hand, it may be difficult to get individuals involved in processing the information communicated for low-involvement issues.

The final difference between commercial marketing scenarios and social marketing is that of competition. Few would question that in the traditional commercial setting, competitors must be taken into consideration as one develops an effective marketing plan or strategy (e.g., Apple faces direct competition from Android operating systems and Microsoft, Mercedes Benz faces direct competition from Lexus). But what competition does a diabetes management program or health educator face? How does a program to curb binge drinking or promote sunscreen protection among college students face competition? Does the same issue or concern come into play when social marketing strategies are being considered or developed?

THE COMPETITION

It is obvious that in the commercial marketing environment, competition must be considered in the development of an effective marketing plan. For example, Toyota develops its marketing plans in consideration of its overt competition from Honda, Ford, and Hyundai. For social marketers in the population health management space, competition is more complex. Competition exists in the fact that individuals enjoy what they are doing or suffer from inertia or believe that few options would effect a positive outcome. Rothschild's definition of competition is particularly pertinent for social marketers: "any environmental or perceptual force that impedes an organization's ability to achieve its goals."

At some level, the competition is fairly overt. When addressing the challenge of obesity in children, the competition is video games, the Web, or what has been described as other comorbid behavior. Alternative behavioral choices in many contexts are, in fact, competition for social marketers. Individuals perform these competing behaviors because they provide some perceived benefit (e.g., enjoyment or diversion from homework by playing a video game) or reduce costs better than the desired behavior.[19] Large, well financed competitors are introducing "reduced risk" tobacco products and sending countermessages that compete with smoking cessation programs (e.g., programs designed to discourage smoking in the adolescent population).[20]

Although competition may take a more abstract form for a social marketer, the reality is that it is an important factor in affecting behavior change.

THE MARKET-DRIVEN APPROACH TO POPULATION HEALTH STRATEGY DEVELOPMENT

The misconception of social marketing as communication may have originated with the National Cancer Institute's document "Making Health Communication Programs Work," first published in 1989 by the Office of Cancer Communications (now the Office of Communications of the National Cancer Institute [NCI]). The purpose of this guide was to affirm the value of communication strategies for promoting health and preventing disease. In 2002, the NCI proposed the Social Marketing Wheel (SMW), a six-step model, shown in Figure 17-1. An examination of each stage of this model as depicted reveals limitations that may have restricted the scope of social marketing strategies for population health by confining them to a single aspect of the marketing mix. All marketing is better described as "a logical planning process involving consumer oriented research, marketing analysis, market segmentation, objective setting and the identification of strategies and tactics."[21]

In Figure 17-2, showing the traditional flow of a market-driven approach to developing strategies, it is important to recognize the difference between strategies and communications.

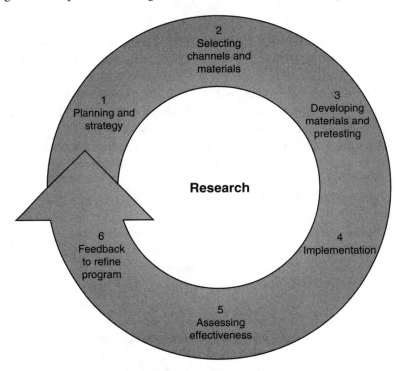

Figure 17-1 The social marketing wheel.
Data from National Cancer Institute (NCI). *Making Health Communication Programs Work: A Planner's Guide*. Bethesda, MA: NCI, 2002.

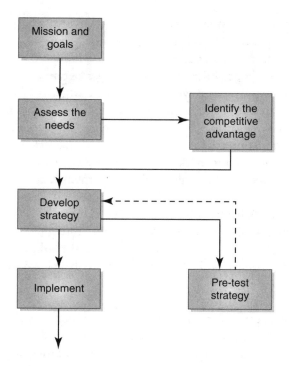

Figure 17-2 A market-driven approach to planning.

In reviewing the mission and goals, a planning committee (step 1) might address new market penetration in a commercial context or behavior modification to improve health outcomes in a population health context. In either scenario, the second step is to assess the needs of the market. It is useful to examine the difference between this market-driven approach and the SMW approach proposed to the NCI.[22] Viewed in the context of the latter, the range of social marketing strategies is limited to promotion (only one of the four Ps) tactics for population health benefits.

Even in the promotion phase, the traditional market-driven approach differs from the SMW in that it attempts to understand the competitive differential advantage. How else can an organization or committee develop a better product, program, or idea, bring it to the market, and persuade an individual or customer to engage in the desired exchange? It is important to recognize that the market will provide the necessary insight through research rather than through the planning committee or the social marketer. It is from this research that the strategies are developed.

At this point, the differences in Figures 17-1 and 17-2 become significant. In the SMW as originally configured, strategies are developed as a first step while commercial marketers work toward understanding the goals and conduct research with the target market to identify key issues, problems, and challenges. In this way, commercial marketers are better able to develop strategies that increase the probability of an exchange whether it be a purchase, an attitude change, or a modified behavior.

Another significant difference between the two models is the step that must be taken prior to a full-scale rollout of the social marketing program for population health management (i.e., the program pretest with the intended target market). This is done in traditional commercial settings, and it should be done in a social marketing context. This step often leads to refinements in a program or changes in the mode of access before implementation (reformulation).

The last two stages of the market-driven approach are the rollout (or implementation) and evaluation. In the commercial environment, the metrics for evaluation are relatively straightforward (e.g., market share, sales revenue gained). In social marketing, evaluation measures are more challenging but nonetheless essential for any program. For instance, metrics are often complicated by the length of time required to measure the effect of a social marketing effort. A systematic review of social marketing effectiveness conducted by Stead, Gordon, Angus, and McDermott reported that across the 54 social marketing interventions reviewed, the period of evaluation ranged from a month to several years, with the majority being a 1- to 2-year follow up.[23]

An interesting approach to developing social marketing strategies for access to health promotion programs by African Americans was presented by Icard, Bourjolly, and Siddiqui.[24] In early-stage market research, focus group participants identified the need to consider subsegments within the African American community who might need different messages and different channels for dissemination. Although the authors described a primarily promotional strategy approach, the research-based method was utilized prior to full development of the strategy, messages, and channel selection as is done in a market-driven approach.

Although a useful framework for developing communications, the SMW is not a market-driven approach to developing comprehensive social marketing strategies using all elements of the marketing mix.

THE TARGET MARKET AND MARKET SEGMENTATION

A **target market** may be defined as a specific group of customers or individuals that an organization or company wants to attract with its bundle of offerings.[25] This is an alien concept for many healthcare providers. Although the ideal goal may be to ensure the health of "all" individuals in society and to improve everyone's health status, a social marketing program must be targeted to a specific target market to be effective. Albrecht and Bryant appropriately observed that employing segmentation strategies enables social marketers to be sensitive to diversity within a given population and thereby allocate scarce resources more efficiently.[26]

The closer a program is targeted using the four Ps (product, price, place, and promotion) tailored to that particular market's unique characteristics, behaviors, and attitudes, the greater the likelihood of engendering a positive response. It has been shown that consumers respond more favorably to targeted communications when there is **homophily,** or when people assume similarity between themselves and characteristics within the advertisements.[27] Such characteristics can be communicated via the models, language, or symbols (lifestyles) represented.

Persuasion is enhanced when there is a match between the characteristics of the person in an advertisement and the viewer of the ad. In a meta-analysis of targeted print communications and resultant health behavior changes, those programs in which targeted communications were used far outperformed the alternative general message.[28] Although there are several theoretical rationales for these findings, it is the result that leads marketers to focus on a target market strategy. Another study found that reduced levels of persuasion can occur when a member of a majority group views an advertisement featuring a minority member.[29]

For social marketing and population health, the subtleties in this area are significant for communication. In the commercial environment, an effective target marketing strategy would lead an individual to search the Web for an article of clothing or a car. The search engine would promptly display advertisements for these items along with listings of retailers in the area. The more targeted and well defined the marketing, the more refined the social marketing strategies that can be developed.

The basis for making a target market more specific is market segmentation. Market segmentation is the clustering of customers or individuals with similar wants or needs to which an organization can tailor a marketing mix to meet those needs. The ideal market segment is as homogeneous as possible, and there are multiple ways in which segments can be formed. Figure 17-3 shows the hierarchy of a segmentation scheme.

SOCIODEMOGRAPHIC SEGMENTATION

A common way to segment individuals is by sociodemographic factors—age, income, gender, ethnicity. From a population health perspective, segmentation has shown some negative effects, particularly with regard to race (e.g., the food-marketing environment and its likely negative effect on prevention and control of obesity for African Americans). In a macroreview of studies, Grier and Kumanyika reported a less favorable climate for this segment compared to other ethnic or racial segments of the population.[30]

Despite the foregoing, targeted marketing to a sociodemographic segment can be a highly effective social marketing approach for population health. The Balm of Gilead, a community-based organization (CBO) in New York City, developed a target market strategy to improve AIDS education and awareness among African Americans within Black churches.[31] Other sociodemographic segmentation approaches have targeted groups for positive population health purposes; for example, women in lower socioeconomic

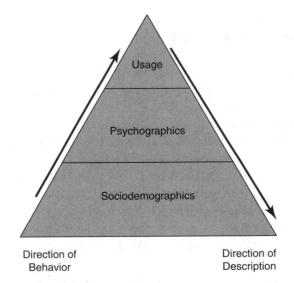

Figure 17-3 Hierarchy of segmentation scheme.

groups were targeted to improve breastfeeding rates with a social marketing effort in the United Kingdom. All four Ps of the marketing mix were utilized, with the product defined as the breastfeeding support service. The price for the target population was low or no cost. The place was at the preferred location for the target population (local children's centers), and the promotion was to raise or "skill up" the midwives (increase their promotional skills regarding breastfeeding).[32]

PSYCHOGRAPHIC SEGMENTATION

This segmentation tactic uses the attitudes, interests, and opinions of individuals to ideally generate lifestyle segments.[33] A **psychographic segmentation** analysis of substance abuse among college-age males and females identified three segments: the safe responsibles, the stoic individualists, and the thrill-seeking socializers. Each psychographic segment had different characteristics and, in some instances, differing behaviors and distinct attitudes.[34] The psychographic approach enables a refined social marketing strategy.

Williams and Flora reported on a psychographic lifestyle segmentation project—the development of a campaign to reduce cardiovascular disease risk among Hispanics. They identified six distinct segments that varied in terms of likelihood to change behavior, newspaper readership, prescription medication usage, and alcohol consumption, among other factors. The distinct differences between segments helped them to refine a social marketing strategy for managing cardiovascular disease among this minority population segment.[35]

BEHAVIOR OR USAGE RATE SEGMENTATION

A third way to segment the market is by behavior or usage rate, often a key factor for segmentation. Frequently, a small group of "heavy half users" account for a disproportionate share of a product's sales or use. This approach is based on **Pareto's rule** or the law of maximum ophelimity, the 80–20 rule. In commercial enterprises, the focus is on defining the 20% of customers that produce 80% of the profits.[36] In a population health management context, one might consider the importance of developing a different social marketing mix strategy for three different behavioral segments:

1. A "heavy" half segment of teenagers, 20% of whom engage in an extremely negative behavior the entire time (e.g., smoking, drug use, alcohol abuse)
2. A significant segment, 60% of whom occasionally engage in the behavior but not on a regular basis
3. A group that does not engage in the adverse behavior at all

Three distinct marketing mix programs are developed for each behavioral segment. These distinct programs may involve different communications and could include other aspects of the marketing mix (e.g., different programming, site locations [place]) and require different efforts on the part of participants. One such behavioral program focusing on alcohol-related crashes among a target market of 21- to 34-year-old males who drove while impaired was developed by the Wisconsin Department of Transportation. Because research indicated that this group disliked admitting to friends that they were too impaired to drive when leaving taverns, the program provided free limousine rides home. Members of the group were then seen as "cool" in exchange for not driving. The measurable program gave 85,000 rides in six communities over 5 years and reduced accidents by 17% in the relevant communities.[37]

The segmentation pyramid and its hierarchy moves from a descriptor level at the base (sociodemographics) to a behavioral level at the apex (usage). Ideally, a marketer wants to affect behavior, purchase, or exchange. Although it is interesting to note gender and race characteristics, these are not relevant unless they affect or relate to behavioral differences. Thus, one might work down the pyramid (i.e., having identified behavioral differences, the marketer might then use attitudinal profiles [psychographics] and sociodemographic profiles to develop a more comprehensive behavioral profile).

DATA MINING AND MARKET RESEARCH

The market-driven approach is founded on robust research that is used to formulate an effective strategy. As shown in Figure 17-3, this research occurs at three stages. Initial research focuses on assessing the needs of the market and establishing a differential advantage relative to competing offerings, behaviors, or programs. The second stage occurs when a program or communication is pretested with a group similar to the intended target market. Stage three research (evaluation) is conducted after implementation.

In the commercial context, the stage three evaluation uses the metrics of market share, sales, and customer repeat purchase and satisfaction. In a social marketing context for population health, program evaluation is more complex. However, systematic, regular feedback and evaluation are essential to modify and improve marketing strategies and tactics on an ongoing basis.[38]

Although the many methodologies used in the conduct of market research are beyond the scope of this chapter, it is essential to recognize that the research at three stages is integral to a market-driven approach. With the advent of large-scale databases in recent years, there have been rather significant advances in analytics that are useful in developing strategies for a target population. Thus, **data mining** is worthy of more discussion.

A chief aim of market segmentation is to identify market segments that are as homogeneous as possible within each segment—and as heterogeneous as possible between the segments—to create more effective strategies. In the ideal environment, the ultimate goal of a commercial or social health marketer would be to develop strategies at the individual level, tailoring programs to the individual's attitudes and behaviors in such a way that the desired exchange (e.g., a purchase, improved health status) is the result. Data mining, the application of specific algorithms for extracting patterns from data,[39] is a new approach to achieving this goal. Data mining is part of a larger process referred to as "**knowledge discovery**," which attempts to ensure that the patterns and correlations observed in the databases are meaningful for the organization in developing an actionable strategy.[40]

The sophistication of computer models designed to identify behavioral patterns has potential for social marketers and population health. One clinical area, diabetes, has received significant attention across many market segments. Using the Oracle Data Miner Software Tool, researchers analyzed data sets of noncommunicable diseases from the World Health Organization regarding Saudi Arabia to identify the effectiveness of specific treatments for different age groups. Among other results, the researchers found that drug treatment appears to be more effective for patients in the older adult age group versus the young group. Although diabetes drugs are usually prescribed for people with type 2 diabetes—along with recommendations to make specific dietary changes and exercise regularly—young patients are advised to concentrate more on other modes of treatment (e.g., diet control, weight reduction, exercise, smoking cessation). Exercise was found to be more beneficial for older diabetic patients than for younger ones.[41] The potential value of data mining in assessing differential treatment approaches across market segments was clearly demonstrated by this analysis of a large data set.

THE MARKETING MIX

As noted earlier in the chapter, the discussion of social marketing has centered on promotion, limiting its potential value when applied to population health issues. The marketing mix and its four Ps (product, price, place, and promotion)[42] are the basis on which an effective marketing plan is developed to affect behavior or attitude change in an individual. Thus, it is important to fully appreciate each element of the marketing mix and its potential applications to population health challenges.

PRODUCT

The **product element** is anything "that can be offered to the market to satisfy a need. It includes physical objects, services, persons, places, organizations, and ideas."[43] Central to the product component is the exchange of dollars for the positive benefits expected from the purchase of a product, service, or interaction with a service provider. The challenge for social marketing and population health is to have the exchange perceived as a positive.

Smith suggests that from a social marketing perspective, the attempt to reduce obesity or alcohol use among pregnant females (whether by educating, instilling fear, or creating inspiration) is a promotional approach rather than one that is both product and exchange based.[44] He notes that HIV/AIDS educational messages have had mixed and short-term success. Yet development of new condom products marketed to make them more sensual and affordable (the price component of the marketing mix) as well as accessible (the place component of the marketing mix) has a greater effect on changing behavior.

The following is an example of targeting a distinct marketing segment: A colonoscopy screening program using African American patient navigators was designed to target African American patients at Mount Sinai Hospital in New York City. Rather than relying on the more common communication or promotional campaign approaches, these researchers opted for a social marketing approach. The product element of the marketing mix was the training of navigators to maximize the likelihood of their identifying with the target market, effectively communicating the benefits of the service and providing necessary assistance.[45]

A significant dimension of the product for commercial marketers is the brand (e.g., consumers willingly engage with popular brand logos). In Chicago, the branding dimension of the product component was considered a key factor of the marketing mix in the creation of the *5-4-3-2-1 Go!* initiative, a branded healthy lifestyle program directed at improving family food choices and promoting physical activity in six targeted communities. The initiative was part of a strategic effort to reduce obesity in a broader social marketing campaign tied to awareness and a website with trusted information and other channel partners.[46]

PLACE

In a traditional marketing context, place refers to how a product is accessed by the consumer—and thus is the product's distribution channel. In a commercial context, this involves questions such as where the product will be distributed—in a retail store, online, or delivered to the home. In a healthcare context, place might pertain to a system's decision to open primary care satellites or to have weekend hours in its clinics.

For a commercial organization marketer, the **channel of distribution** is the "path a product takes as it travels from the manufacturer to the end consumer."[47] Figure 17-4a shows the channel of distribution for a typical consumer product purchased in a supermarket. The manufacturer ships its products to a wholesaler who assembles large amounts of various items from multiple manufacturers and distributes them to retailers who sell products to the end consumers. Effective marketing strategies are developed not only to the end consumer but also for the entities within the channel as manufacturers compete against one another, vying to get their products carried by wholesalers and retailers as well as to the end consumer. This issue is important to consider in social marketing.

The healthcare channel of distribution is represented in Figure 17-4b. In this situation the flow is reversed (i.e., a patient experiencing a clinical issue often begins the process by seeking care from the primary care physician). If the problem requires a higher level of care, the individual is placed in an acute care facility. If it is more serious, the person may be sent to a tertiary facility.

In considering the place element of the marketing mix for social marketing, Lotenberg suggests that it is essential to consider three related questions:

1. Does the target group (market) have the opportunity to *engage* in the desired behavior?
2. Does the target group have the *motivation* to engage in the desired behavior?
3. Does the target group have the *ability* to engage in the desired behavior?[48]

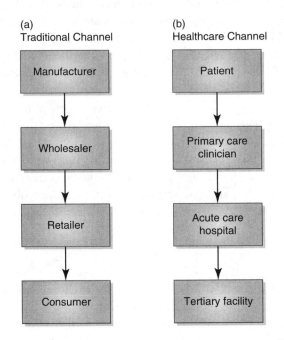

Figure 17-4 Channels of distribution.

Considering these three questions broadens the perspective on place and its relative importance in social marketing for population health. For example, Lotenberg notes that if the issue is trying to reduce obesity, a key component might be better access to nutritious foods.[48] The target market may live in a food desert where access to markets that stock an adequate variety of fresh fruits and vegetables is severely restricted. Thus, while one element of the channel (the end user) might want to change behavior in response to a more desirable end state, other channel entities do not provide the opportunity. The social marketer must target these stakeholders in the key target market to successfully accomplish the ultimate population health outcome.

Motivation is a second factor in the function of the channel. When considering population health around weight management or fitness, a key channel partner may be employers, and strategies should encourage these stakeholders to work toward the established health goal.

Harvard Community Health Plan, a Massachusetts-based health insurer, created employee teams that competed to "walk the most steps." Participants were given pedometers to track each step. The program provided motivation to use stairs rather than an elevator and to walk around the building with coworkers during lunch breaks—an approach that motived employees beyond going to a gym or fitness center after work.

Based on their work in the traditional marketing environment that revealed that consumers react negatively when a desired product is not available, Kreuter and Bernhart posit the same concern in formulating social marketing strategies for population and public health programs. If evidence-based programs are not readily available to a motivated target market, the frustration level of that audience may increase, which could seriously impede implementation.[49]

Finally, there is the aspect of ability. This consideration is best demonstrated by a study that attempted to increase public awareness of hypertension.[50] The results of a mass media campaign to raise hypertension awareness among the general population were disappointing. The authors concluded that it is important to support such messages by utilizing other channel intermediaries (i.e., to "include providers armed with proper educational tools and supports to change hypertension behavior.")[51] This highlights the value of considering other elements of the marketing mix beyond communication. Providers are key elements in most of the critical population health management issues, and social marketing strategies should include sufficient provider products (e.g., proper educational tools).

PRICE

Whether in the commercial or social marketing context, two dimensions of price should be considered. First is the out-of pocket price the individual must exchange for a program, product, or service. Second, is the **opportunity cost** the individual must incur to interact with the organization to partake in the program. The opportunity cost is the amount of effort the individual has to expend to interact with the organization to engage in the program or service. In a systematic review of 13 studies using the price element of the marketing mix for social marketing purposes, lowering price was a frequently used strategy for addressing issues such as sexually transmitted disease and HIV interventions. Reducing the opportunity cost by making it less inconvenient for testing was found in several other instances.[52]

Out-of-pocket price can be an important factor in any context. In one social marketing study, out-of-pocket price was a consideration in attempting to increase the penetration of treated mosquito nets for malaria control among the poor in Tanzania. Retail prices were set at $5.00 for these treated nets in communities where the average monthly income ranged from $77 to $96. This strategy using sales agents (shopkeepers and some health educators) who had educational material resulted in a significant increase in treated net ownership.[53]

Commercial marketers have recognized that price has a psychological component. Consumer research conducted by Population Services International found that many teenagers did not trust free condoms given away by public health agencies, indicating that consumers often see some "value added" benefit in the exchange. If a product is priced "too low," there is a perceptual factor that negatively affects the desired exchange.[54]

PROMOTION

Historically, promotion has meant the traditional media of broadcast (radio, television), publications (brochures, newspapers, magazines and brochures, and other forms of print vehicles), and personal sales. This type of promotion has been used by public health organizations for hundreds of years. Cotton Mather utilized a communication campaign to promote smallpox vaccination in Boston in the early 1700s.[55] Today, a promotional campaign often involves the use of the Internet and other social media and mobile communication devices to reach the intended target market. Consistent positive effects have been reported regarding the use of mass media campaigns to promote positive healthcare interventions or to change lifestyles.[56]

The significant challenge for healthcare marketers is the existence of the Web 2.0 environment, in which all organizations now exist. In the pre–Web 2.0 environment, a healthcare organization would craft a message for population health management purposes and use a particular media vehicle to send it to the market, as shown in Figure 17-5. In this example, the health marketers would craft the message for the intended target audience, and the message would be pretested, as described in a diabetes education program by Thackery and Neiger.[57] The significant advantage of the pre–Web 2.0 environment for health professionals in a social marketing campaign was control. In a meta-analysis of several mass media campaigns to reduce drinking and driving, the advantage of using mass media to control placement of messages (as opposed to the public service announcement [PSA] approach) allowed for targeting and afforded control over placement with maximum exposure.[58] A concern expressed by social marketers as they increasingly turned to paid placement of messages is that broadcast and print media, which once were willing to provide PSAs for public health announcements, would be less willing to provide previous free public service announcements without charge.[59] However, there are distinct advantages to the control provided in the pre–Web 2.0 environment. By paying for the placement of an advertisement, the commercial organization or health organization controlled four key elements:

1. What was said to the market
2. To whom it was said
3. How often it was said
4. When it was said

These advantages were minimized or lost when a PSA was utilized. Although an organization could create a public health message, the company doing the broadcasting or printing decided when the message was broadcast or where it was placed in the printed media vehicle. This critical decision ultimately affected the market that viewed or read the message. Often, the number of times the message ran was out of the control of the organization that wanted to communicate the message. Thus, commercial marketers did not rely on PSAs to get their message out to their market in spite of the positive budget implications.

The healthcare professional crafted, pretested, and refined the message, and selected the media vehicles to, in effect, push the message for diabetes education, cardiac care, or other population health issues. The underlying advantage of this environment was control.

Consider the differences today's health professionals face as they formulate their social marketing strategy promotions in the Web 2.0 environment (Figure 17-6). The challenge in this environment is the lack of control, or the recognition of an implicit "architecture of participation."[60] In a Web 2.0 environment, it is this architecture of participation that has led to the ever-evolving strength of Wikipedia, which allows users to add to and edit

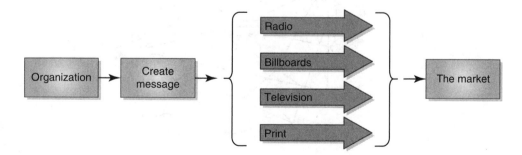

Figure 17-5 Pre–WEB 2.0 environment for social marketing promotion.

content. In fact, Wikipedia's best articles or sources are those that have the greatest participation. Individuals interact through various social media forums, and population health social marketers must develop strategies to participate in these conversations.

It is not the environment displayed in Figure 17-6 of pushing a well developed, pretested message. Although a message can be developed regarding population health today, the healthcare professional must be able to participate in the conversation regarding the behavior or attitude that is to be affected or changed. This new environment and its effectiveness and architecture of participation were demonstrated in Australia with a campaign to raise and stimulate awareness about sun protection barriers among teenagers. Australia has the highest skin cancer rate in the world. A social media campaign was developed titled, "It's a Beautiful Day . . . for Cancer." Featuring a music video, it was posted on YouTube and supported with repostings on Facebook and MySpace. Traditional media were used to help drive viewership to these sites. The hip hop artist in the video contributed updates and conversed with site "friends" on Facebook. Viewers were encouraged to share the content with their friends. The results were impressive:

- The video received more than 250,000 views on YouTube in 4 months.
- Eighteen percent of the viewers were younger than 18 years of age.
- The estimated value of television, press, and radio coverage was more than $1 million.
- Moreover, a quarter of the people surveyed said they shared the video with friends, and positive attitudinal results were reported with the groups that viewed the video.[61]

In recent years, support sites for specific diseases or conditions have become more common. Representative examples include Patients Like Me (http://www.patientslikeme.com/), Ihadcancer.com (http://www.ihadcancer.com/), diabeticconnect.com (http://www.diabeticconnect.com/), and a thyroid support group on Facebook (https://www.facebook.com/ThyroidDiseaseSupportGroup). All of these are representative of this architecture of participation.

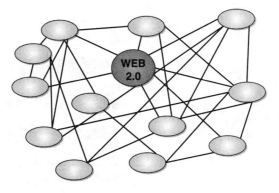

Figure 17-6 The WEB 2.0 environment.
Reproduced from Berkowitz, N. *Essentials of Health Care Marketing,* 3rd ed. Sudbury, MA: Jones & Bartlett Learning; 2011: 348.

From a social marketing perspective—and as part of a population health promotional strategy—clear advantages of this environment have been identified when individuals participate in developing or refining the message. First, it can increase loyalty to the program and increase the likelihood of individuals "purchasing," or going along with, what is being promoted (in a population health context, a behavioral or attitudinal change). Second, inherent in the Web 2.0 environment is interaction with others about the message being conveyed (i.e., the product or service). It is also important to underscore that this form of promotional strategy is inherently more cost effective. Finally, a customer-developed message has a greater likelihood of relating to the target market that participated in its development.[62]

CONCLUSION

Marketing is a consumer-centric, research-based discipline that seeks to affect a voluntary exchange between an individual and an organization. In the commercial environment, marketing focuses on persuading individuals to purchase products. For population health management, effective marketing strategies may result in meaningful, positive outcomes of diabetes control, improved cardiac health, or obesity management. In healthcare settings, the utilization of marketing strategies has been narrowly constrained to one element of marketing, promotion. However, marketing is based on a marketing mix of four key components: product or service, price, place or distribution, and promotion. All four elements are utilized in developing a comprehensive, effective marketing strategy.

A market-driven strategy is based on market research that determines the market's needs and assesses the competition. Even in the population health environment, it is important to recognize that there is competition for programs and services. An effective marketing strategy requires identifying a target market, segmenting that market so that it is as homogeneous as possible, and implementing a marketing mix tailored to that segment. Marketing strategy is now developed and implemented in a Web 2.0 world in which individuals, rather than organizations, are in control. The challenge for population health social marketers is to channel these issues into the constellation of ongoing conversations.

STUDY AND DISCUSSION QUESTIONS

1. Marketing has often been described as a framework for an organization to develop a strategy as opposed to a tool. Describe how this statement could be accurate. If you were to sit in a committee at a health center trying to develop a program around a critical issue for population health management, how might you as a consultant identify whether they were in fact using a marketing framework, or not? What would be the appropriate indicators of the committee's process?

2. Segmentation is a key component of developing an effective marketing strategy. A hierarchy of segmentation scheme was presented in terms of order of power of segmentation and direction of description of market segments. Explain each direction and how it relates to the hierarchy.

3. For many years in social marketing, the perspective of marketing was rather constrained to one element of the marketing mix. Explain this limited view versus the full range of the marketing mix. Identify what the full range of the marketing mix is and how each element might then be applied to population health challenges.

4. Promotional strategy today, unlike like prior years, exists in what has been described as a Web 2.0 world. Describe the pre- and present Web 2.0 environment for healthcare organizations in terms of how it affects their communication programs and promotional challenges. In what way does it affect them in terms of their media choices and ultimate tactics for population health? Do healthcare organizations have to be more cognizant of this Web 2.0 environment in developing population health promotional or communication strategies for particular market segments?

SUGGESTED READINGS AND WEBSITES

READINGS

Andreasen AR. *Social Marketing for the 21st Century*. Thousand Oaks, CA: Sage; 2006.

Berkowitz EN. *Essentials of Health Care Marketing*. 3rd ed. Sudbury, MA: Jones & Bartlett; 2011.

Hillestad SG, Berkowitz EN. *Health Care Market Strategy: From Planning to Action*. 4th ed. Burlington, MA: Jones & Bartlett; 2012.

Lee N, Kotler P. *Social Marketing: Influencing Behaviors for Good*. 4th ed. Thousand Oaks, CA: Sage; 2011.

WEBSITES

Deloitte. Center for Health Solutions: http:// www.deloitte.com/view/en_US/us/Insights/centers/center-for-health-solutions/index.htm

McKinsey & Co. McKinsey Quarterly: http://www.mckinsey.com/insights/mckinsey_quarterly

Pew Research Internet Project: http://www.pewinternet.org/

REFERENCES

1. Maibach E. Explicating social marketing: what is it, and what isn't it? *Soc Mar Q*. 2002;8(4):7-13.
2. American Marketing Association. Definition of Marketing. http://www.marketingpower.com/AboutAMA/Pages/DefinitionofMarketing.aspx. Accessed November 4, 2014.
3. Kotler P, Levy SJ. Broadening the concept of marketing. *J Mark*. 1969;33(1):10-15.

4. Berkowitz EN. *Essentials of Health Care Marketing*. 3rd ed. Sudbury, MA: Jones & Bartlett; 2011.

5. Morris ZS, Clarkson PJ. Does social marketing provide a framework for changing healthcare practice? *Health Policy*. 2009;91:135-41.

6. Gordon R, McDermott L, Stead M, et al. The effectiveness of social marketing interventions for health improvement: what's the evidence? *Public Health*. 2006;120:1133-9.

7. Andreasen A. *Marketing Social Change: Changing Behavior to Promote Health, Social, Development, and the Environment*. San Francisco, CA: Jossey-Bass; 1995.

8. Andreasen A. Social marketing: its definition and domain. *J Public Policy and Marketing*, 1994;13(1) 108-14.

9. Stead M, Hastings G, McDermott L. The meaning, effectiveness and future of social marketing. *Obes Rev*. 2007;8(Suppl 1):189-93.

10. McDermott L, Stead M, Hastings G. What is and what is not social marketing: the challenge of reviewing the evidence. *J Marketing Manag*. 2005;21:545-53.

11. Maibach EW, Abroms LC, Marosits M. Communication and marketing as tools to cultivate the public's health: a proposed "people and places" framework. *BMC Public Health*. 2007;7(88). http:// www.biomedcentral.com/1471-2458/7/88. Accessed November 5, 2014.

12. Rothschild ML. Using social marketing to manage population health performance. *Preventing Chronic Disease: Public Health Research, Practice, and Policy*. 2010;7(5)1-6. http://www .cdc.gov/pcd/issues/2010/sep/10_0034.htm. Accessed November 5, 2014.

13. Adapted from MacFadyen L, Stead M, Hastings G. A Synopsis of Social Marketing. University of Sterling; 1999. http://staff.stir.ac.uk/w.m.thompson/ Social%20Enterprise/Library/Synopsis%20of %20 Social %20 Marketing.pdf. Accessed November 5, 2014.

14. Andreasen A. *Marketing Social Change: Changing Behavior to Promote Health, Social Development, and the Environment*. San Francisco: Jossey-Bass; 1995.

15. Kotler P, Levy S. Demarketing, yes demarketing. *Harv Bus Rev*. 1971;49(6):74-80.

16. Kotler P, Levy S. Demarketing, yes demarketing. *Harv Bus Rev*. 1971;49(6):75.

17. Wansink B, Huckabee M. De-marketing obesity. *Calif Manage Rev*. 2005;47(4):6-18.

18. Mitchell A. Involvement: a potentially important mediator of consumer behavior. *Adv Consum Res*. 1979;6(1):191-6.

19. Mah M, Deshpande S, Rothschild M. Social marketing: a behavior change technology for infection control. *Am J Infect Control*. 2006;34:452-7.

20. Evans WD. What social marketing can do for you. *BMJ*. 2006;332(7551):1207-10.

21. MacFadyen L, Stead M, Hastings G. A Synopsis of Social Marketing. University of Sterling; 1999: 3. http://staff.stir.ac.uk/w.m.thompson/Social%20 Enterprise/Library/Synopsis%20of%20Social%20 Marketing.pdf. Accessed November 5, 2014.

22. Evans WD, McCormack L. Applying social marketing in health care: communicating evidence to change consumer behavior. *Med Decis Making*. 2008;28:781-92.

23. Stead M, Gordon R, Angus K, et al. A systematic review of social marketing effectiveness. *Health Education*. 2007;107(2):126-91.

24. Icard L, Bourjolly J, Siddiqui N. Designing social marketing strategies to increase African Americans' access to health promotion programs. *Health & Social Work*. 2003;28(3):214-23.

25. Berkowitz DN. *Essentials of Health Care Marketing*. 3rd ed. Burlington, MA: Jones & Bartlett; 2010: 24.

26. Albrecht T, Bryant C. Advances in segmentation modeling for health communication and social marketing campaigns. *J Health Commun*. 1996; 1:65-80.

27. Rogers E, Bhowmik DK. Homophily-heterophily: relational concepts for communication research. *Public Opin Q*. 1970;34:23-38.

28. Noar S, Benac C, Harris M. Does tailoring matter? Meta-analytic review of tailored print health behavior change interventions. *Psychol Bull*. 2007; 133(4):673-93.

29. Aaker J, Brumbaugh A, Grier S. Nontarget markets and viewer distinctiveness: the impact of target marketing on advertising attitudes. *J Consum Psychol*. 2000;9(3):127-40.

30. Grier S, Kumanyika S. The context for choice: health implications of targeted food and beverage marketing to African Americans. *Am J Public Health.* 2008;98(9):1616-29.

31. Harris A. AIDS promotion within the black church: social marketing in action. *Soc Mar Q.* 2010;16(71):72-91.

32. Lowry R, Austin J, Patterson M. Using social marketing to improve breast-feeding rates in a low socioeconomic area. *Soc Mar Q.* 2011;17(64):64-77.

33. Wells WD. Psychographics: a critical review. *J Mark Res.* 1975;12(2)196-213.

34. Suragh TA, Burgh CJ, Nehl EJ. Psychographic segments of college females and males in relation to substance use behaviors. *Soc Mar Q.* 2013;19(3):172-87.

35. Williams JE, Flora JA. Health behavior and campaign planning to reduce cardiovascular disease among Hispanics. *Health Educ Behav.* 1995;22(36):36-48.

36. Duboff, RS. Marketing to maximize profitability. *J Bus Strategy.* 1992;6:10-13.

37. Rothschild ML. Using social marketing to manage population health performance. *Preventing Chronic Disease: Public Health Research, Practice, and Policy.* 2010;7(5):A37. http://www.cdc.gov/pcd/issues/2010/sep/10_0034.htm. Accessed November 5, 2014.

38. Walsh DC, Rudd RE, Moeykens BA, et al. Social marketing for public health. *Health Aff.* 1993;12(2):105-19.

39. Fayyad U, Piatetsky-Shapiro G, Smyth P. From data mining to knowledge discovery in databases. *AI Magazine.* 1996;17(3):37-54.

40. Rygielski C, Wang J, Yen DC. Data mining techniques for customer relationship management. *Technol Soc.* 2002;24:483-502.

41. Aljumah A, Ahamad MG, Siddiqui MK. Application of data mining: diabetes health care in young and old patients. *Journal of King Saud University—Computer and Information Sciences.* 2013;25:127-36.

42. Borden NH. The concept of the marketing mix. *J Advert Res.* 1964;4:2-7.

43. Kotler P, Clarke RN. *Marketing for Health Care Organizations.* Englewood Cliffs, NJ: Prentice Hall; 1987: 328.

44. Smith B. The power of the product P, or why toothpaste is so important to behavior change. *Soc Mar Q.* 2009;15(1)98-106.

45. Jandorf L, Cooperman JL, Stossel LM, et al. Implementation of culturally targeted patient navigation system for screening colonoscopy in a direct referral system. *Health Educ Res.* 2013;28(5):803-15.

46. Evans WD, Necheles J, Longjohn M, et al. The 5-4-3-2-1 Go! Intervention: social marketing strategies for nutrition. *J Nutr Educ Behav.* 2007;39:s55-9.

47. Berkowitz EN. *Essentials of Health Care Marketing.* 3rd ed. Sudbury, MA: Jones & Bartlett; 2011:315.

48. Lotenberg LD. Place: where the action is. *Soc Mar Q.* 2010;16(1):130-5.

49. Kreuter MW, Bernhardt JM. Reframing the dissemination challenge: a marketing and distribution perspective. *Am J Public Health.* 2009;99(12):2123-27.

50. Pertella R, Speechley M, Kleinstiver PW, et al. Impact of social marketing media campaign on public awareness of hypertension. *Am J Hypertens.* 2005;18(2):270-5.

51. Pertella R, Speechley M, Kleinstiver PW, et al. Impact of social marketing media campaign on public awareness of hypertension. *Am J Hypertens.* 2005;18(2):270-5.

52. Luca NR, Suggs LS. Strategies for the social marketing mix: a systematic review. *Soc Mar Q.* 2010;16(122):122-49.

53. Nathan R, Masanja H, Mshinda H, et al. Mosquito nets and the poor: can social marketing redress inequities in access? *Trop Med Int Health.* 2004;9(10):1121-6.

54. Grier S, Bryant C. Social marketing in public health. *Annu Rev Public Health.* 2005;39:319-39.

55. Maibach EW, Abroms LC, Marosits M. Communication and marketing as tools to cultivate the public's health: a proposed "people and places" framework. *BMC Public Health.* 2007;7(88):1471-58.

56. Grilli R, Ramsay C, Minozzi S. Mass media interventions: effects on health services utilisation. *Cochrane Database Syst Rev.* 2009;1:1-37. http://www.update-software.com/pdf/CD000389.pdf. Accessed November 5, 2014.

57. Thackery R, Neiger BL. Using social marketing to develop diabetes self-management education interventions. *Diabetes Educ.* 2002;28(536):536-43.

58. Tay R. Mass media campaigns reduce the incidence of drinking and driving. *Evidence-Based Healthcare & Public Health.* 2005;9:26-9.

59. Ling JC, Franklin BAK, Lindsteadt JF, et al. Social marketing: its place in public health. *Annu Rev Public Health.* 1992;13:341-62.

60. O'Reilly T. What Is Web 2.0: Design Patterns and Business Models for the Next Generation of Software. September 30, 2005. http://oreilly.com/pub/a/web2/archive/what-is-web-20.html?page=1. Accessed November 5, 2014.

61. Potente S, McIver J, Anderson C, et al. "It's a Beautiful Day for Cancer": an innovative communication strategy to engage youth in skin cancer prevention. *Soc Mar Q.* 2011;17(3):86-105.

62. Thackery R, Niger BL, Hanson CL, et al. Enhancing promotional strategies within social marketing programs: use of Web 2.0 social media. *Health Promot Pract.* 2008;9(4):338-43.

Chapter 18

RESEARCH AND DEVELOPMENT IN POPULATION HEALTH

R. DIXON THAYER, RAYMOND J. FABIUS, AND
SHARON GLAVE FRAZEE

Executive Summary

Measurements are essential to track the health of people, work sites, and communities.

Research and development in population health is a challenging but potentially rewarding endeavor. Fortunately, those entering the field today can learn from the early efforts of population health pioneers. Seminal works by Dee Edington[1] and John Wennberg and colleagues[2] provide an understanding of the biological tendency toward illness over time as humans age and the effect of variations in care. Yet much work remains to be done before standardized, effective programs and initiatives make significant progress in achieving the Triple Aim of health care:[3] simultaneously improving population health, improving the experience of care, and reducing per capita healthcare costs.

Using the best experimental techniques for research and development—and moving beyond small, controlled studies within academic settings toward more strategic population-based efforts—will add to our understanding of what works and significantly improve the health of our nation.

Learning Objectives

1. Appreciate the different views of population health from the multiple constituencies in health care.
2. Describe key elements and tasks associated with effective research and development processes.
3. Analyze the various approaches to research and measurement in population health.
4. Mitigate the challenges of population health research.

5. Identify emerging and future trends that will affect population health research and development.
6. Discuss the five segments of population health.

Key Terms

bias	regression to the mean
comparative effectiveness	scientific method
double-blind confirmation	secondary research
predictive modeling	systematic process optimization
primary research	trend analysis
proof of concept	Triple Aim

INTRODUCTION

The vision of population health is healthy people, healthy work sites, healthy communities, and, ultimately, healthier nations. Improved population health is one of three components of what we must strive for in health care—improved population health, improved patient experiences with the healthcare system, and reduced per capita healthcare costs. Taken together, these are referred to as the **Triple Aim** of health care.[3] If the health status of a population is to be improved, the objectives for health must be identified, and progress toward these objectives must be measured. The understanding and measurement of population health are supported by work done in the public health arena and in the regulatory space of occupational health.[4] Organizations such as the Centers for Disease Control and Prevention (CDC) and the American College of Occupational and Environmental Medicine have developed community and workplace health metrics in response to legislative and regulatory mandates. Effective measures of progress toward improvements in population health must include various clinical process and outcome indicators, patient and provider satisfaction assessments, functional status and quality of life measures, economic and healthcare utilization indicators, and an evaluation of the effect of initiatives on known population health disparities.

Process measures used to assess the delivery pathway of population health services might include the percentage of health risk assessments completed by a population compared to performance benchmarks or the rate of screening colonoscopies for members of the population who are over age 50. Clinical process indicators may also reflect the pathway of disease, injuries, and population risk factors (e.g., tracking the average number of risk factors within a particular population over time). Measures of patient or provider satisfaction may focus on the consumer's or clinician's perception of the value of a service or the effect of the intervention.

Outcomes measures are quantifiable expressions of the desirable effects of an intervention that are to be achieved by a certain point in time. For example, *Healthy People 2020*, a national initiative to advance a comprehensive health promotion and disease prevention agenda, focuses on measuring 26 leading health indicators such as the rate of medical coverage, suicide prevalence, and percentage of students who graduate with a high school diploma 4 years after entering 9th grade.[5] Although most population health improvement programs may not be as ambitious in terms of measurement and improvement, they do need to focus on the specific outcomes they are attempting to achieve. Accurate assessment of outcomes requires both numerator and denominator data to enable the measurement of baseline health status and incremental improvements over time. Outcome measures might include healthcare costs, percentage of participants who achieve normal blood pressure, or percentage of overweight individuals who reduce their body mass index (BMI). Ideally, outcomes data from one population should be comparable to other populations to facilitate benchmarking and to allow data aggregation at various levels. This requires agreement on the outcomes to be measured and, possibly, the technology to support transparency.

Measurement should be longitudinal, and comparable instruments should be applied across measurement periods to support trend analysis. The frequency at which each measure is collected should be determined by the interval over which meaningful change can be expected and linked to long-term, intermediate, and near-term objectives for health programs. Although counting health events such as illnesses and injuries is a common activity in both medical and public health practice, the systematic use of health data to improve population health requires measuring lifestyle and behavioral risk factors and the burden of chronic diseases in populations as well.[6]

This isn't easy! Efforts to quantify the effect of interventions on the health status of populations have led to the recognition of the magnitude of this challenge as well as a growing awareness of opportunities for improvement. The old adage that "you cannot improve what you do not measure" definitely applies to population health improvement programs.

Population health measurement efforts are often inconsistently applied, thus hampering the ability of researchers to produce generalizable, universally accepted outcomes of population health improvement programs. The importance of producing research that creates evidence of effect or "proof of concept" is of extreme importance, particularly to employers and other payers.

This chapter provides an overview of measurement techniques, the challenges to research, the viewpoints of different constituencies in health care, and research approaches that are applicable across the spectrum of illness. It describes the development techniques and challenges associated with establishing effective population health management programs and introduces emerging technologies that will have a significant effect on future population health research and development.

EFFECTIVE POPULATION HEALTH RESEARCH

Research can be described as any systematic investigation to establish facts. It is carried out to increase understanding of fundamental drivers and responses to drivers of behavior: that is, to isolate cause and effect.[7] In population health, research is usually focused on understanding how different actions affect collective behavior change and how those changes influence population health and wellness. There are two basic kinds of research:

- **Primary research** involves the collection and analysis of original source data, which are collected specifically for the research study.
- **Secondary research** involves the analysis of existing data and prior research information for possible new uses or conclusions.[8]

The scientific method provides a framework for conducting research. The steps of the method include identifying a topic, generating a hypothesis, defining a data collection and analysis strategy, gathering data, testing the hypothesis, and making decisions based on the results.[9] Whether applied to primary or secondary research, the scientific method provides structure for a research project.

Disturbing increases in obesity, sedentary lifestyles, and chronic illness threaten American life expectancy and quality of life[10] and signal a need for additional research in the area of population health. With the upward trend of healthcare costs in the United States challenging the competitive nature of American business,[11] establishing evidence-based solutions that improve the effectiveness and efficiency of care delivery will help advance healthcare delivery for everyone.

RESEARCH DESIGNS

Although there are a number of possible approaches to population health research, studies typically utilize one of four research designs: double-blind confirmation, trend analysis, comparative effectiveness, or predictive modeling.

Double Blind

Double-blind confirmation is the quintessential research approach to establishing a causal link between intervention and outcome based on severity-matched, double-blind study methodology. In this approach, members of a population (cohort) are matched by their relative level of illness and separated into experimental and control groups. A new treatment or service is provided to the experimental group while the control group receives usual care. After a sufficient period of time, determined by the research team, progress of the experimental and control groups is compared. Once the research team controls for external factors, differences can be attributed to the new intervention.

Cohort-matched, double-blind experimental and control studies remain the hallmark of population health; however, these studies are expensive and often impractical. The pharmaceutical industry has traditionally applied this methodology to demonstrate the effectiveness of a new medication compared to placebo or, less frequently, to compare proven drug alternatives. In the pharmaceutical context, such results can support efficacy, superiority to current recommended treatment, or equal potency to standard therapy; the latter example refers to so-called "me too" drugs that provide no distinct advantages over current therapies.

Trend Analysis

Trend analysis is a more common, less expensive, and often more practical approach. This design allows study of the same population cohort over the course of a new treatment or service to determine its effect. The approach is sometimes referred to as "Time 1 versus Time 2" study. Because this is not a double-blind, illness burden–matched design, researchers are less able to establish causality, but associations can be drawn. This method compares a population cohort at two different points in time, generally before and after an intervention (e.g., assessing an obese population before and after participation in a weight management program). Researchers using this method must consider the effect of regression to the mean. Generally speaking, populations of patients who are dealing with significant illness will improve over time even without treatment, thus challenging researchers to prove that the *intervention* produced a greater effect than would have been observed after the normal healing process.

Comparative Effectiveness

Comparative effectiveness studies compare two or more different treatment approaches. For example, researchers have compared clinical indicators and outcomes for three procedures that are commonly performed on patients with coronary artery obstruction: balloon angiography versus arterial stenting versus bypass. This quasi-experimental model approximates the precision and validity of cohort-matched experimental and control methods while utilizing a practical setting. In a population health context, comparative effectiveness is usually ascertained by comparing the effect of a (population health) program or therapy on a group of participants with a severity-adjusted cohort of participants in a different program or treatment pathway.

As the size of the comparative groups increases, the need for severity adjustment decreases. Smaller comparative studies of control and experimental groups require this adjustment, because the burden of illness may be significantly different between groups, thus influencing the outcome. This is particularly true when there is known selection bias between the two groups. To mitigate bias, comparisons can be made between two local organizations—one wherein a new intervention is piloted and the other wherein the traditional approach is taken.

Predictive Modeling

Predictive modeling is an approach that uses existing data to predict future behavior or consequences. This concept can be illustrated by means of asking three primary questions: How are we doing? How can we make this better? What if we did this?[12] The *what if* question can help formulate and pretest hypotheses about improvement. Data analysis is used both to generate mathematical estimates of the current state (how we are doing) and to run possible alternate scenarios (what if). Findings from such modeling exercises allow researchers to anticipate consequences of an intervention on a population. Altering the predicted trend in positive ways is an important goal of population health research and development.

RESEARCH DEVELOPMENT PROCESSES

In the context of this chapter, development is a systematic process to transform research into actions (e.g., programs, procedures, and protocol design and redesign; products and services innovation; behavior change program design). Although there are many different approaches that might be considered, the two primary categories of development processes are new concept development (often applied to the exploration and development of new products and services) and systematic process optimization (often used to reduce the number of defects, or suboptimization, in an existing process):

- The new concept development process consists of five primary steps: (1) *search* for unmet needs, (2) *explore* alternative possible solutions (to the unmet need), (3) *develop* the "best" solution, (4) *apply* and assess the developed solution in the marketplace, and (5) *maximize* the effect and penetration of this new product or service in the marketplace. This process is often referred to by its acronym, the SEDAM process.

- Systematic process optimization (SPO): Existing process improvement can be achieved by means of point-in-time research. Assuring an organizational culture of improvement, however, requires continual process improvement tracking and measurement. Utilizing statistical measurement of current processes and procedures, SPO looks for opportunities to improve them within the current program. This method has proven to be highly effective in reducing defects and error rates in repeatable process steps. Six Sigma, Lean, and TPS (Toyota Production Systems) are well documented SPO approaches to simultaneous improvement of both effectiveness and efficiency, and all of these industry-based approaches have been successfully applied to health care.[13,14]

Development process programs have also demonstrated the power to create common frameworks for continual improvement that translates into three keys to success for effective population health program development. By engaging the entire community in a consistent process and by using these techniques, one can garner:

- Issue ownership (by all core constituents): Research must be compelling and accessible and made relevant to each participant in order to develop true ownership and collaboration.

- Champions for change (by key respected and trusted figures in the specific population, as well as the population at large): This point is best illustrated by the adage "what gets measured gets done or improved." It is important to clearly identify the respected champions and cheerleaders for a population's health in a specific community. It is equally important to be clear about how the champions will measure success. Research efforts must be made clear, compelling, accessible, and relevant to each key champion.
- Convergence of constituencies: Aligned measurement approaches (across patient, provider, payer, purchaser, and supplier constituencies) are key to driving convergent behaviors by each. How each constituent defines success determines what will be measured and how success is determined. This will drive the systems, processes, and behaviors within each constituency. If key definitions and measures are aligned at the outset, measurement and relevant reporting will improve success by driving convergence (as opposed to random divergence).

THE STATE OF THE ART OF POPULATION HEALTH MEASUREMENT

Systematic measurement of improvement in the health status of populations is a key component of research and development. Proof of concept refers to demonstrating the effect of a program or product using measures of effectiveness, efficiency, or both. Efficiency studies are increasingly in demand as global healthcare inflation continues to outpace general inflation. These efforts explore ways to deliver improvements less expensively by using technology or substituting less costly clinical resources (e.g., substituting nurse practitioners for physicians). Examples of outcomes studied include the effect of a specific program on reducing the frequency or cost of hospitalization, reducing absence from work, reducing the cost and frequency of diagnostic services, and effecting a shift to more cost-effective pharmaceuticals or generic drugs. These types of efficiency studies often analyze utilization data such as health and disability claims, laboratory data, or prescription claims.

In contrast to the economic focus of efficiency studies, effectiveness studies seek to determine better ways to improve care outcomes. These studies often rely on the aggregation of data extracted from medical records and frequently include laboratory and pharmacy data. One could argue that there is a sensitive balance between efficiency and effectiveness. Ideally, these two system measures would be aligned (i.e., maximizing efficiency would be associated with greater effectiveness). However, systems that attempt to see too many patients per hour (increased efficiency) will fail to produce the desired results (increased effectiveness).

Assessment of the value of population health efforts includes both return on investment (ROI) studies and measurement of less tangible effects. Increasingly, the comprehensive assessment of population health programs includes the satisfaction of key constituents (i.e., patients, caregivers, providers, and purchasers). Measuring perceived value from multiple perspectives is crucial to the development of lasting, successful programs. Functional status trumps survival rates from the perspective of most patients and purchasers of care, and the ties between health and productivity cannot be denied. Capturing parameters such as absenteeism and disability can augment the research and development of population health products and services.[15]

EMERGING TRANSFORMATIONAL RESEARCH TECHNOLOGIES

Three emerging and intersecting technological developments are beginning to show promise in the evolution and transformation of population health research.

PERSONAL MONITORING, DIAGNOSIS, AND COMMUNICATION TECHNOLOGIES

As mobile communication devices continue to get "smarter," many ventures are experimenting with collecting biometric and clinical data directly from patients or subscribers in real time for electronic integration into personal electronic health records. Wearable devices are able to track blood pressure throughout the day, daily activities such as steps taken, quantity and quality of sleep, and caloric output. The future offers clinicians the ability to track heart rhythms, pulmonary function, and brain activity. As technology develops, the possibilities of accessing real-time, detailed, person- and cohort-specific information in the analysis of population segments will expand the opportunities for health research.[16]

BIOLOGIC MARKERS

As the new fields of genomics, protenomics, and microbiomes develop correlations to health and disease, each will have a significant effect on population health research. Expanding knowledge (e.g., the effect of genetics and its unique direction and production of combinations of proteins in the body, the mapping of individual microbial colonization patterns) will likely require a reassessment of disease and its classification. These new domains will undoubtedly cast new light on treatments and cures as well.[17]

BIG DATA TECHNOLOGIES

The emergence of cloud computing and flexible data collection, storage, and analysis capacities (big data technologies) has recently expanded research possibilities. These technologies enable researchers to manage large volumes and varieties of data in more accessible, affordable, and usable databases for significant mining and correlations. For example, double-blind comparative effectiveness studies can now be generated faster and less expensively than ever before. By identifying matched cohorts on different therapeutic modalities and following their health outcomes (e.g., need for hospitalization or emergency care), comparative effectiveness can be established without the expensive and time-consuming requirements of double-blind studies.[18]

THE VIEW FROM THE FIVE CONSTITUENCIES OF HEALTH CARE

When embarking on the research and development of population health initiatives, it is important to understand the perspectives of the key constituents of healthcare delivery: patients, providers, payers, purchasers, and suppliers. From the *patient's* perspective, ease of access to programs and services that can produce tangible benefits with minimal inconvenience and expense is of greatest interest. Ideally, these programs are delivered or facilitated by trusted, caring clinicians and designed to improve patient self-care and feelings of self-efficacy. *Providers* are most concerned with applying evidence-based guidelines and producing clinical outcome improvements. Their research and product development rely on clinical measures such as biometrics (e.g., weight, blood pressure, lab values, functional capacity) and patient self-report. *Payers* (e.g., health plans) pursue studies utilizing claims data to demonstrate efficiency gains. *Purchasers*, especially employers, increasingly demand evidence of improved functional status and reduced absenteeism, presenteeism, and disability. *Suppliers* (e.g., the pharmaceutical and durable medical equipment industries) apply population health research to demonstrate the value of their drugs and devices by showing decreased medical utilization and costs.

CLASSES OF MEASURES

One of the simplest ways to categorize measures is based on the work of Donabedian, who described a framework of structure, process, and outcomes.[19] Without much difficulty, one can tie structural and process components to better results. Structural and process indicators of improved outcomes are, in fact, easier to measure than are patient outcomes. For example, because the evidence shows that patients cared for by a primary care provider in a trusted relationship over an extended time have better outcomes, it is reasonable to study the effectiveness of programs that drive more members of a population into "medical homes." Additionally, research has demonstrated that improved engagement and retention rates of disease management programs can be used as an upstream process indicator for improved outcomes.[20,21] Another example might be to study the results of a program that improved the rate of colonoscopy, knowing that this will lead to improved outcomes through early identification of colon cancer.

TECHNIQUES OF MEASUREMENT

Generally speaking, research and development in population health draws from a measurement tool kit that contains things such as surveys and health assessments, administrative claims data, personal health records (PHRs) and electronic health records (EHRs), and other types of information.

Surveys and health assessments are often the first tools used to measure baselines, process measures, and health outcomes in population health. One of the easiest tools to deploy is a satisfaction survey. Valuable information can be gained by assessing the perceived value of a program or service from the perspective of as many constituents as possible, but always starting with the patient. Patients can be questioned on many levels, from specific improvement in control of a disease process to a self-assessment of general well-being or a report on improved convenience or functional status. Surveys requesting patients' evaluations of care providers are also being utilized (e.g., patients are asked to comment on the performance of their doctors or their healthcare delivery systems). Providers are also being asked to evaluate their patients' compliance with and adherence to treatment plans. Recently, with the use of health risk appraisals and health and productivity instruments, self-assessment and self-reporting have become fundamental components of population health research and development.

When focusing on efficiency studies, the use of administrative claims data is foundational. If the purpose of a population health research study is to reduce medical expenditures or demonstrate a reduced need for intensive medical services, the data warehouse of claims-based information is a key data source. Health plans and health informatics organizations are expert at evaluating the effect of programs and services based on hospitalization rates, total hospital days, and the use of emergency room resources and specialty services. Analyses of health plan claims data may demonstrate the use of recommended services by a population (e.g., screenings, preventive services) or reveal overuse of questionable treatments. In fact, claims-based studies can even measure the effect of health services that are misused (e.g., knee surgery for patients with arthritis).

Pharmacy benefit management organizations can use their claims information to illuminate the effect of medication use and adherence. Linking of claims, lab, and pharmacy data can produce elegant measurement of the burden of illness on populations. This becomes particularly important when studying the differential effect of programs and services between populations that are not severity-matched control and experimental groupings.

Although the move toward requiring *International Classification of Diseases, Tenth Revision, Clinical Modification/Procedure Coding System* (ICD-10-CM/PCS) level diagnosis code nomenclature will markedly improve the specificity of these analyses, it will increase complexity. The number of diagnosis codes under ICD-10-CM exceeds 171,000 (compared to 17,849 codes in ICD-9-CM). ICD-10-CM/PCS includes clinical modifications of the World Health Organization's ICD-10 system, which incorporates the level of detail needed for morbidity classification and diagnostics specificity in the United States and to capture procedure codes in a more detailed manner than is currently included in the ICD-9-CM (ICD-10-PCS).[22]

In the future, there likely will be increasing reliance on PHRs. These may be tied electronically to EHRs, which capture data in real time and allow for more rapid research analysis. Medical records, whether electronic or paper-based, are a rich source of data that can be used to assess the need for new population-based programs and services. In both cases, interreviewer reliability is very important, especially when data are being extracted from patient records. Aggregate data from EHRs offer great promise for improved accuracy and real-time results.

Tangible clinical results of population-based research and development can be obtained through biometrics, such as urine and blood tests. These results can demonstrate wellness (e.g., a low cholesterol level is a measure of cardiovascular health), identify risks (e.g., high blood pressure readings), or indicate control of a chronic illness (e.g., a hemoglobin A1C test within normal limits for a patient with diabetes).

Other types of information can be useful. For instance, disability reports that track the incidence, cause, and cost of short-term and long-term cases can give employers a measure of the most compromised cohort of their employee populations. From a research and development standpoint, the employee population is particularly attractive because of the potential for significant improvement in functional status and return to work.

Other factors that influence disability include job satisfaction and recent job performance. Job dissatisfaction and poor performance are measures of occupational or career wellness. Robust return to work efforts that include a broad spectrum of modified work options are more likely to return employees with moderate illness to work sooner, reducing the perceived magnitude of the catastrophic or disabled sector. This example emphasizes the multifactorial nature of population health research and development as well as its real-world applications.

CHALLENGES TO SUCCESSFUL RESEARCH

Bias is a form of systematic error in research and presents a formidable challenge. There are legitimate concerns about selection bias in participant cohorts, clinical and administrative bias by those who provide the intervention, and publication bias because journals are more likely to accept manuscripts that demonstrate effectiveness. As discussed previously, double-blind, cohort-matched experimental models offer the best defense against bias. Importantly, reputable journals recognize that publication of negative and nonimpactful efforts contributes to the evidence base for population health and supports continued research and development toward more effective interventions.

Time can present a significant challenge to effective research as well. Demonstrating the true effectiveness of population-based programs often requires several years. Many programs have claimed success in changing people's behavior (e.g., smoking cessation, weight loss); however, the test of true success requires tracking and recording the maintenance of these behavior changes over an extended time. Some disease state complications develop over a period of years, and adequate time is necessary to demonstrate the effectiveness of disease management programs in reducing or delaying their onset.[23]

Confounding influences are difficult to eliminate in population health studies. A health prevention or disease management program is markedly affected by an individual's community or residence, media influences, healthcare professionals providing treatment, economic status, gender, language spoken, and cultural beliefs. Although it is nearly impossible to eliminate these influences, larger sample sizes in both the experimental and the control groups give researchers greater ability to measure and statistically control for their effects.

As discussed earlier, unrecognized or unequal illness severity and regression to the mean are key challenges to conducting credible research and evaluating pilot projects. Using severity adjustment techniques and tracking experimental and control groups over time are the best ways to deal with these issues.

ESTABLISHING GOALS

When conducting population health research or developing programs, it is important to establish clear goals. This is best accomplished by establishing baseline measures and determining what may be possible to change under ideal circumstances. Next, it is important to engage in a crosswalk from that baseline to the predetermined "stretch" or ideal goals. In this way, one can develop a pilot program to test whether the intervention steps were successful in achieving the goals.

Goals can be based on governmental or nationally respected initiatives (e.g., *Healthy People 2020*, the National Quality Forum, or the National Committee for Quality Assurance's Health Effectiveness Data and Information Set [HEDIS] measures). Establishing quantitative benchmarks against which improvement will be measured objectively is an effective approach to goal setting. Benchmarks are derived from three primary sources: history (i.e., measuring participants' personal best), aspiration (i.e., what program designers hope to accomplish), or assigned according to an established goal (such as those contained in *Healthy People 2020*) or another cohort (e.g., a control or best practice).

THE FIVE SEGMENTS OF POPULATION HEALTH STATUS

Research and development in population health can cover the spectrum from wellness to catastrophic illness. The best population health efforts attempt to affect the health status of all segments of a patient, or consumer, community. Such programs try to keep the well free of disease while reducing the illness burden of the others.

Today's broadened view of the first segment—the well—is increasingly holistic. It encompasses its many domains including physical, emotional, spiritual, intellectual, environmental, and social wellness. Increasingly, research and development in the domain of workforce health and productivity provides measures for the multiple dimensions of wellness.

Beyond wellness research and development, population health researchers have studied the at-risk population and efforts that have been exerted to mitigate health risks. The premise underlying such studies is that certain risks can be reduced or eliminated before the onset of disease, especially chronic disease, and that risk mitigation can markedly improve the long-term health status of populations. To accomplish risk reduction, the population health industry has dedicated great effort to developing and refining health risk appraisals and biometric screening. Health coaches and care managers now specialize in assisting cohorts of patients to reduce identified risks such as high cholesterol, obesity, drinking and driving, sedentary lifestyle, and smoking. Research has demonstrated that patients with multiple risks have higher medical expenditures and reduced work performance. The mitigation of health risks can result in lower healthcare costs and improved functionality.

The next segment of population health status—acute illness—is usually defined as sickness that is short lived and typically resolves without complications. Examples include ear infections, sore throats, flu, intestinal infections, and acute low back pain. While acute illnesses receive less attention in population health research than chronic or life-threatening health issues do, they can have a significant effect on the health of a population as evidenced by the preparation undertaken by countries, states, counties, and local employers and institutions to prevent or mitigate pandemic flu.

Efforts to reduce the illness burden of the chronically ill segment have been characterized as disease management (DM). Common chronic illnesses that have been targeted for research and development of population health programs include diabetes, coronary heart disease, asthma, emphysema, congestive heart failure, and depression. Research has demonstrated that a large percentage of people enrolled in disease management programs are living with multiple diseases and conditions and may benefit from a more comprehensive care management program. Programs dedicated to helping those with complex and rare conditions, such as hemophilia and renal failure, provide an important service to patients and their families as they navigate the complex American healthcare system.[24] These programs sometimes include referral to local, regional, or national centers of excellence.

Lastly, population health research and development efforts have been undertaken to ease the burden of illness among the most fragile cohort, those with catastrophic illness (e.g., persons with end-stage cancer, stroke and trauma victims, children with genetic complexes, and others requiring continuous nursing assistance). From an economic standpoint, health plans, insurers, and employers often have defined these population segments by the economic costs associated with their care.

Catastrophic population segments are those whose health care costs exceed some threshold (e.g., $50,000 in a year). They normally comprise only 1% to 2% of a population of covered lives. Individualized case management programs have demonstrated favorable ROI for interventions with catastrophically ill cohorts.

CONCLUSION

Research and development within population health integrates clinical medicine, health informatics, and creative innovation. The research process utilizes a variety of measurement techniques and analytics to demonstrate impact (e.g., satisfaction surveys, self-reported health appraisals, functional status, claims databases, clinical records). When researchers use well respected research approaches such as double-blind or comparative effectiveness methods, it is not difficult to produce proof of concept results. Understanding potential biases and the normal trends of illness within populations can reduce the misinterpretation of outcomes. Increasingly precise and sophisticated biometric analyses can compare the past to the present and validate improvement in future performance against that which was predicted. Such techniques can shorten the window of time required to reach statistical significance and move a project into mainstream production faster.

Pilot efforts can bridge research and development. Those that demonstrate improvements in the effectiveness or efficiency of existing or new population health products or services are worthy of further development and, in some cases, large-scale application in the marketplace. When designing and producing new products and services, great care must be taken throughout the process to appreciate the viewpoint of all constituents.

STUDY AND DISCUSSION QUESTIONS

1. Is it more valuable to assess the effectiveness or the efficiency of population health programs?
2. Compare and contrast the different views of the five constituencies of healthcare delivery. Why is this important to know when conducting research or development in population health?
3. What are the key elements and tasks of the research process and development programs?
4. How can you mitigate the challenges of population health research?
5. What are the five segments of population health? Why is this important to know when conducting research or development in population health?

SUGGESTED READINGS AND WEBSITES

READINGS

Edington, DW. *Zero Trends*. Ann Arbor: University of Michigan Health Management Research Center; 2009.

Kane RL, ed. *Understanding Health Care Outcomes Research*. 2nd ed. Sudbury, MA: Jones and Bartlett; 2006.

Kessler, RC, Stang PE, eds. *Health and Work Productivity*. Chicago: University of Chicago Press; 2006.

Leutzinger J, Sullivan S, Chapman L., eds. *Platinum Book: Practical Applications of the Health and Productivity Management Model*. Omaha: Institute for Health and Productivity Management; 2004.

Solberg LI, Mosser G, McDonald S. The three faces of performance measurement: improvement, accountability, and research. *Jt Comm J Qual Improv*. 1997;23(3): 135-47.

WEBSITES

Employer Measures of Productivity, Absence and Quality (EMPAQ): http://www.empaq .org/

The Health Enhancement Research Organization (HERO): http://hero-health.org/

Healthy People 2020: http://www.healthypeople.gov/2020

Institute for Health and Productivity Management: http://www.ihpm.org

REFERENCES

1. Edington, DW. *Zero Trends*. Ann Arbor: University of Michigan Health Management Research Center; 2009.

2. Wennberg J, Fisher ES, Sharp SM, et al. The Care of Patients with Severe Chronic Illness. 2006. The Center for Evaluative Clinical Sciences: Dartmouth Medical School. http://www.dartmouthatlas.org/ downloads/atlases/2006_Chronic_Care_Atlas.pdf. Accessed November 5, 2014.

3. Steifel M, Nolan K. Measuring the Triple Aim: a call for action. *Popul Health Manag*. 2013; 16(4):219-20.

4. Szreter S. The population health approach in historical perspective. *Am J Public Health*. 2003; 93(3):421-31.

5. U.S. Department of Health and Human Services (HHS). Healthy People.gov. 2020 LHI Topics. Washington, DC. https://www.healthypeople.gov/ 2020/leading-health-indicators/2020-LHI-Topics. Accessed December 30, 2014. Last updated December 30, 2014.

6. Yen L, Schultz AB, Schnueringer E, et al. Financial costs due to excess health risks among active employees of a utility company. *J Occup Environ Med*. 2006;48(9):896-905.

7. Davenport TH, Harris JG. *Competing on Analytics*. Boston: Harvard Business School Press; 2007.

8. Lentz CA. *The Delphi Primer: Doing Real-World or Academic Research Using a Mixed-Method Approach in The Refractive Thinker*. Vol. 2. Las Vegas: The Lentz Leadership Institute; 2006.

9. Wilson, EB. *An Introduction to Scientific Research*. New York: McGraw-Hill; 1952.

10. Hoyert DL, Xu J. Deaths: preliminary data for 2011. *National Vital Statistics Reports*. 2012;61(6). Hyattsville, MD: National Center for Health Statistics. http://www.cdc.gov/nchs/data/nvsr/nvsr61/ nvsr61_06.pdf. Accessed November 5, 2014.

11. Shortliffe EH, Cimino JJ. *Biomedical Informatics: Computer Applications in Health Care and Biomedicine*. New York: Springer Science; 2006.

12. Towers Perrin 2008 Health Care Cost Survey. http://www.towersperrin.com/tp/getwebcachedoc? webc=HRS/USA/2008/200801/hccs_2008.pdf. Accessed November 24, 2009.

13. Lloyd DH, Holsenback JE. The use of Six Sigma in health care operations: application and opportunity. *Academy of Health Care Management Journal*. 2006;2:41-50.

14. Association for Manufacturing Excellence, ed. *Lean Administration: Case Studies in Leadership and Improvement*. London: Productivity Press; 2007:90-105.

15. Change Agent Work Group. Employer Health Asset Management; 2009. http://www.aon.com/attachments/improving_health.pdf. Accessed November 5, 2014.

16. Steinhubl SR, Muse ED, Topol EJ. Can mobile health technologies transform health care? http://jama.jamanetwork.com/article.aspx?articleID=1762473. Accessed November 4, 2014.

17. Agus DB. *The End of Illness*. New York: Free Press; 2011.

18. Kayyali B, Knott D, Van Kuiken S. The big-data revolution in US health care: accelerating value and innovation. McKinsey & Company. January 2013. http://www.mckinsey.com/insights/health_systems_and_services/the_big-data_revolution_in_us_health_care. Accessed November 4, 2014.

19. Donabedian A. *The Definition of Quality and Approaches to Its Assessment*. Chicago: Health Administration Press; 1980.

20. Frazee SG, Kirkpatrick P, Fabius R, et al. Leveraging the trusted clinician: documenting disease management program enrollment. *Dis Manag*. 2007;10(1):16-29.

21. Frazee SG, Sherman B, Fabius R., et al. Leveraging the trusted clinician: increasing retention in disease management through integrated program delivery. *Popul Health Manag*. 2008;11(5):247-54.

22. World Health Organization. International Classification of Diseases (ICD). http://www.who.int/classifications/icd/en/. Accessed November 5, 2014.

23. Knight K. Badamgarav E., Henning JM, et al. A systematic review of diabetes disease management programs. *Am J Manag Care*. 2005;11(4):242-50.

24. Rula E, Sacks R. Incentives for health and wellness programs: strategies, evidence and best practice. *Outcomes and Insights*. 2009;1(3). http://www.healthways.com/WorkArea/showcontent.aspx?id=266. Accessed January 9, 2015.

Chapter 19

THE ROLE OF COMPARATIVE EFFECTIVENESS RESEARCH AND ITS EFFECT ON POPULATION HEALTH

LYNN NISHIDA, HELEN SHERMAN, DAN OLLENDORF, AND STEVEN D. PEARSON

Executive Summary

Comparative effectiveness research can identify treatment options that have the greatest potential for improved health outcomes.

Decisions made about medical treatment and care frequently involve choices among available therapies. Commonly, there are few research studies that directly compare alternative treatments and provide evidence to guide a particular decision. Even less plentiful are studies that compare treatment options to assess which work best in real-world settings; rather, research is conducted under strictly controlled experimental conditions. A greater realization for this type of research has sparked the growing interest and investment in what is known today as comparative effectiveness research (CER).

With the current national focus on improving population health, CER has received substantial attention. In addition, in early 2009, the American Recovery and Reinvestment Act allocated $1.1 billion in new funds to increase the number of new CER studies. Study designs most commonly used to support comparative effectiveness research include randomized controlled trials, systematic reviews, meta-analyses, and observation studies. If conducted well, these types of studies can help build the foundation for which CER can identify selection of treatment options that have the greatest potential for improved health outcomes.

This chapter provides a basic primer on CER concepts that are essential to understand for CER's appropriate and practical application in healthcare decision making. When successfully applied, CER has the potential to fill the knowledge gap with the essential information that can best help healthcare decision makers and patients in selecting the most effective options for treatment and for the overall improvement in population health.

Learning Objectives

1. Introduce the principles of CER.
2. Describe key areas of research methodology needed to conduct or collaborate in CER.
3. Identify specific types of studies that can be used to conduct CER, along with their strengths and limitations for use.
4. Explain the value and effect of CER on population health.
5. Describe best practice approaches used for assessing and interpreting CER.
6. Identify examples today where CER is currently used and how.

Key Terms

comparative effectiveness research
health technology assessment
Institute for Clinical and Economic Review

observational studies
pragmatic clinical trials
randomized controlled trials
real-world data

INTRODUCTION: DEFINITIONS FROM NATIONAL AUTHORITATIVE SOURCES

Comparative effectiveness research (CER) is a type of research that directly compares healthcare interventions to determine which is the most effective or provides the best chances of positive health outcomes. CER is a widely used term within the scientific and healthcare industries. Although many in the public and private sectors are engaged in CER, there is no single, standard definition. Various professional organizations have developed their own definitions to guide their scientific research activities (Table 19-1).

Additionally, the following organizations are involved in or influence CER:

- Center for Medical Technology Policy[1]
- The Cochrane Collaboration[2]
- Institute for Clinical and Economic Review (ICER)[3]
- International Society for Pharmacoeconomics and Outcomes Research (ISPOR)[4]
- National Institutes of Health (NIH)[5]
- National Pharmaceutical Council (NPC)[6]
- New England Comparative Effectiveness Public Advisory Council (CEPAC)[7]
- Patient-Centered Outcomes Research Institute (PCORI)[8]

Although the definitions and standards for CER may vary, certain components of CER are important when applying it to population health. The common CER characteristics across health care and scientific sectors include the following:

CER compares benefits and harms of healthcare interventions. CER compares at least two alternative interventions, each with the potential to be a best practice. Interventions may include medical procedures, drugs, or other treatment modalities. CER highlights research that compares a new treatment or intervention with viable alternatives. For many clinical

Table 19-1 CER Definitions from National Authoritative Sources

Organization	CER Definition
Congressional Budget Office[9]	Rigorous evaluation of the impact of different options that are available for treating a given medical condition for a particular set of patients.
Institute of Medicine (IOM)[10]	The generation and synthesis of evidence that compares the benefits and harms of alternative methods to prevent, diagnose, treat, and monitor a clinical condition or to improve the delivery of care. The purpose of CER is to assist consumers, clinicians, purchasers, and policy makers to make informed decisions that will improve health care at both the individual and population levels.
Agency for Healthcare Research and Quality (AHRQ)[11]	A type of research that compares the results of other approaches. Comparative effectiveness usually compares two or more types of treatments, such as different drugs, for the same disease. Comparative effectiveness also can compare types of surgery or other kinds of medical procedures and tests. The results often are summarized in a systematic review. The direct comparison of existing healthcare interventions to determine which work best for which patients and which pose the greatest benefits and harms. . . . [T]he core question of comparative research [is] which treatment works best, for whom, and under what circumstances.
American College of Physicians[12]	Comparative effectiveness analysis evaluates the relative (clinical) effectiveness, safety, and cost of two or more medical services, drugs, devices, therapies, or procedures used to treat the same condition. Although the use of the term *comparative effectiveness* broadly refers to the evaluation of both the relative clinical and cost differences among different medical interventions, it is notable that most comparative effectiveness research engaged in and used by stakeholders in this country focuses solely on evaluating relative clinical differences to the exclusion of cost factors.
Academy of Managed Care Pharmacy[13]	Recognizes IOM definition.

Data from Center for Medical Technology Policy @ http://www.cmtpnet.org/. Accessed 1/31/2014. The Cochrane Collaboration. http://www.cochrane.org/. Accessed 1/31/2014. Institute for Clinical and Economic Review (ICER) @ http://www.ICER.org. Accessed 1/31/2014. International Society for Pharmacoeconomics and Outcomes Research (ISPOR) @ http://www.ispor.org. Accessed 1/31/2014. National Institutes of Health (NIH) @ http:/www.NIH.gov. Accessed 1/31/2014. National Pharmaceutical Council (NPC) @ http://www.npc.org. Accessed 1/31/2014. New England Comparative Effectiveness Public Advisory Council (CEPAC) @ http://cepac.icer-review.org/. Accessed 1/31/2014. Patient Centered Outcomes Research Institute (PCORI) @ http://www.pcori.org. Accessed 1/31/2014.

decisions, "optimal usual care" reflecting current standards is used as an appropriate potential comparator.

CER identifies what works best when, and for whom, for informed decision making. CER describes results at the population or subgroup level (i.e., it provides a measure of the "average effect" of trial interventions on a specific population). When selecting options from various proven strategies, a good clinician judges whether a particular patient is sufficiently similar to the population studied for that strategy.

CER defines results for subgroups that are often excluded or overlooked in standard clinical trials (e.g., demographics, ethnicity, physiologic and genetic makeup). In this way, CER fills in the information gap for the clinician (and patient) in weighing the options for a more individualized approach. Through subgroup analysis (comparative analysis of interventions in subjects with common clinical characteristics), CER provides information to guide individualized care and selection of options that best suit the demographic, ethnic, physiologic, and genetic characteristics of a particular patient or population.

CER is conducted in settings that are similar to those in which the intervention will be used in practice. CER studies interventions in realistic practice settings rather than in a controlled study environment, enabling collection of **real-world data**. CER should reflect actual practice settings as much as possible to ensure that results are generalizable and applicable. Highly controlled studies designed to prove cause and effect are geared toward proving efficacy and assessing the extent to which an intervention produces a beneficial result under controlled conditions. For example, in **randomized controlled trials** (RCTs), patients are often followed and monitored very closely to ensure up to 100% adherence on study medications. In a realistic practice setting, medication adherence to study medication may be more sporadic.

CER is designed to measure improvement in health outcomes. CER measures outcomes (both benefits and harms) that are important to healthcare decision makers. Harms and risks of unintended consequences are outcomes of interest because these factors influence the net benefits of an intervention (i.e., the balance of harms and benefits). Resource utilization is also important in describing net health benefits in CER. Cost-effectiveness analysis and modeling are important CER tools to evaluate treatment outcomes and their relative differences in cost.

Over the years, there has been much progress toward raising awareness of CER and its value. Ideally, CER should bridge the gap between scientific research and healthcare decision makers. Although common characteristics and concepts in CER are evident, there is a need for authoritative organizations to partner and consolidate this work to achieve meaningful impact on healthcare decision making.

CER lacks full acceptance in today's healthcare purchasing arena. Work is proceeding to improve agreement on methods and standards among all CER sources so that healthcare decision makers will be better able to assess the validity, credibility, and overall application for use of CER results.

IMPORTANCE OF COMPARATIVE EFFECTIVENESS RESEARCH IN POPULATION HEALTH

LIMITATIONS OF RANDOMIZED CONTROLLED TRIALS

All clinical trials are limited by the intrinsic methodologies and circumstances under which they are conducted. While RCTs can study cause and effect, they are not designed to address the vast array of real-world, practical scenarios that come with global, widespread use and introduction of technologies in noncontrolled settings. CER has the potential to fulfill this unmet scientific need.

Viewed as the gold standard for proving efficacy (cause and effect) of an intervention, RCTs are generally designed to control and eliminate biases and confounders that might influence results that are not solely due to the intervention being studied. Thus, the study environment mirrors more optimal conditions than those in real-world settings. CER is not a replacement for efficacy trials but rather an extension of research that addresses the population health question of what option works best and for whom.

QUALITY

By providing evidence that allows greater precision in selecting options with the best relative chances of a positive outcome (e.g., preventing, diagnosing, treating, and monitoring a clinical condition) and minimizing or reducing adverse consequences, CER has great potential for improving healthcare quality and patient outcomes. Broader use and application of CER will help shift the healthcare system toward proven treatment options that lead to higher quality patient care.

FINANCIAL AND ECONOMIC

CER may bring rigor to decision making that is often more influenced by tradition and marketing and eventually bend the health cost curve. Research has estimated that as much as 30% of healthcare spending may be wasted on care that does not improve health.[14] Topping the list were more expensive treatments that were unnecessary or failed to produce better outcomes. For example, from 1992 to 2003, spending on lumbar fusion, a type of back surgery, increased by 500% ($75 million to $482 million) despite a lack of evidence supporting its effectiveness.[15]

TYPES OF COMPARATIVE EFFECTIVENESS RESEARCH

CER aims to produce information that real-world decision makers can use to make informed treatment and coverage decisions. A study's relevance, feasibility, and timeliness of results must be considered in the context of the specific research question being asked by the healthcare decision maker. These considerations help determine the study design and methods most likely to answer the CER question.

Although there continue to be varying perspectives, CER types generally fall into two broad categories—experimental and nonexperimental.

CER data sources most often come from published studies, existing data from the delivery of care (administrative claims, medical charts, electronic health records), clinical registries, and information collected by clinical investigators either retrospectively or prospectively.

EXPERIMENTAL STUDIES

In experimental studies, the investigator manipulates a variable and examines the effect on an outcome. The following are types of experimental trials and their strengths and limitations when used in CER.

Randomized Controlled Trials

Patients are randomized (assigned by chance) to a particular intervention based on a well defined study protocol. Because patients are enrolled prospectively, it may require many years to enroll a sufficient number of study participants and observe effects of treatment. Study protocols are tightly controlled to prevent potential biases and confounders that could influence the results. Usually the intervention under examination is compared with a placebo or with another active treatment for head-to-head comparison.

Cluster Randomized Trials

In cluster randomized trials, patients are assigned to a treatment intervention or to a control group in clusters (e.g., a cluster of patients receiving a specific intervention from the same physician or the same health plan).

Pragmatic (Noncontrolled) Clinical Trials

Pragmatic clinical trials are designed to measure the benefit of an intervention in normal, routine practice (effectiveness) to help guide decisions between options for care.[16,17] Pragmatic trials are designed to test interventions in the full spectrum of everyday clinical settings to maximize applicability, generalizability, and feasibility. These trials are geared toward answering research questions of whether an intervention works in real life, and trial designs tend to favor more heterogeneity (e.g., variability of practitioners, patients, and healthcare delivery) to represent the real-world setting. Because heterogeneity may dilute the observations of a potential outcome, the population must be large enough to detect small effects. To achieve a greater number of study patients, the study must be more feasible to perform, provide follow up, and report outcomes to ensure timeliness of results.

Pragmatic trials are sometimes described as the middle ground between RCTs and **observational studies**. Some well known pragmatic trials are summarized as follows.

ALLHAT[18] The Antihypertensive and Lipid-Lowering Treatment to Prevent Heart Attack Trial was a long-term, multicenter trial conducted on a large group of participants, ages 55 and older, with stage 1 or stage 2 hypertension and at least one other risk factor for cardiovascular disease (CVD). The study was sponsored by the National Heart, Lung, and Blood Institute (NHLBI) and is one of the largest clinical studies to date comparing the effectiveness of medications to treat hypertension. For a subset of these patients, ALLHAT included a cholesterol-lowering study, in which statin drug treatment was compared to usual care. Both of these studies measured mortality as well as cardiovascular events (e.g., fatal and nonfatal myocardial infarction.) The ALLHAT hypertension study results indicated that less costly, traditional diuretics were more effective than newer medicines at lowering high blood pressure and preventing some forms of heart disease. Although both statin and usual care provided substantial decreases in cholesterol levels, the 10% difference in cholesterol levels between the groups was insufficient to produce significant decreases in death and provided only a small, insignificant reduction in heart attacks and strokes.

ACCORD[19]   The Action to Control CardiOvascular Risk in Diabetes study was designed to determine whether a combination strategy (i.e., intensive lowering of blood sugar levels, intensive lowering of blood pressure, or treatment of blood lipids with a fibrate drug plus a statin drug) could decrease the risk of major cardiovascular events in patients with type 2 diabetes who are at especially high risk of CVD. Results from this study indicated that intensively targeting blood sugar to near-normal levels in adults with type 2 diabetes at especially high risk for heart attack and stroke does not significantly reduce the risk of major cardiovascular events (e.g., fatal or nonfatal heart attacks, stroke) but increases risk of death compared to standard treatment.

Key learnings from this study included setting goals with some caution for glucose, blood pressure, and lipid lowering, particularly in older patients with established cardiovascular or other disease. Overaggressive therapy in such people may lead to the development of other problems and may increase mortality without sufficiently reducing their risk.

CATIE[20]   The Clinical Antipsychotic Trials for Intervention Effectiveness Schizophrenia trial was designed to examine the relative effectiveness of second-generation antipsychotic (SGA) medications (i.e., olanzapine, risperidone, quetiapine, and ziprasidone) to a first-generation antipsychotic, perphenazine. Based on study outcomes with time to discontinuation as a measure of effectiveness, patients taking olanzapine experienced a slightly longer time to discontinuation (greater effectiveness) than patients on other agents. The efficacy of the conventional antipsychotic agent perphenazine appeared similar to that of quetiapine, risperidone, and ziprasidone. Cost-effectiveness analysis suggested a significant advantage for perphenazine due to the effect of the high-priced, brand-name SGAs on overall healthcare costs.

STAR*D[21]   The Sequenced Treatment Alternatives to Relieve Depression study is one of the largest real-world studies that examined the comparative effectiveness of several antidepressant medication strategies in the treatment of depression. Consistent with a pragmatic study, the STAR*D trial was designed to examine these strategies under real-world circumstances. To accomplish this, the study employed minimal exclusion criteria, allowed incorporation of patient preferences for treatment options, and had no blinding (i.e., both the patient and the clinician knew what treatment was being provided). Conclusions from this study suggested that a patient with persistent depression can get well after trying several treatment strategies but that the patient's odds of being symptom free lessen as additional treatment strategies are needed.

NONEXPERIMENTAL STUDIES

In nonexperimental studies, the investigator observes the outcome of naturally occurring differences in a variable.[22,23] The following types of studies fall into the nonexperimental category.

Prospective, Observational Studies

Analysis of Patient Registry   Registries can require years to accumulate depending on the condition and outcomes being studied. Because it is difficult to enroll the number of patients generally required under experimental studies, patient registries are particularly valuable for analyzing treatment options for rare diseases over time.

Cohort Study   This type of study examines groups of patients exposed to certain interventions and monitored over time to observe for specific outcomes. The cohort (group of participants) remains together in the same study over time. Outcomes are compared between subsets of the cohort who were exposed or not exposed to a particular intervention. A prospective cohort study identifies and follows them into the future; a retrospective (or historical) cohort study identifies participants from past records and follows them from a previous time point to the present.

Case-Control Study   This usually retrospective study compares individuals with a specific disease or outcome (cases) to individuals from the same population without the disease or outcome (controls). The goal is to identify any associations between the outcome and prior exposure to particular risk factors. This design is particularly useful where the outcome is rare and past exposure can be reliably measured.

Cross-Sectional Study   This type of study examines a characteristic (or a set of characteristics) in a subgroup of participants at a specific time or time period.[23]

Case Series   This type of study simply describes results and outcomes observed for a group of patients receiving a similar intervention (e.g., individuals undergoing a new type of surgery, the users of a new device or medication).

Systematic Reviews

This is a structured literature review conducted in a systematic fashion using preset criteria and a set protocol. Required steps in conducting a systematic review include constructing the specific research question; identifying and acquiring the evidence from the available literature; appraising the evidence for its reliability, validity, and applicability; and summarizing the findings for a qualitative synthesis of the evidence.[23]

Meta-Analysis

This statistical technique is used in a systematic review to combine results from multiple studies for a quantitative synthesis and summary of the data that allows inferences to be made and applied to a population of interest. In CER, the objective of a meta-analysis is to increase the precision and power of the overall estimated effect of an intervention or treatment by producing a pooled estimate for relative comparisons.[22]

Health Technology Assessment

This type of analysis is a form of policy research that examines short- and long-term consequences in the application of new healthcare technology (e.g., new medical procedures or drugs). The **health technology assessment** (HTA) is a method of evidence synthesis that considers evidence regarding clinical effectiveness; safety; cost effectiveness; and, when broadly applied, includes social, ethical, and legal aspects of the use of health technologies. The precise balance of these inputs depends on the purpose of each individual HTA. A major use of HTAs is for guiding reimbursement and coverage decisions, in which case HTAs include benefit and harm assessment and an economic evaluation. In addition to providing policy makers with information on new treatments or interventions, the HTA assesses the effectiveness of medical technologies using either single studies or systematic reviews. Used to evaluate health technologies, including medications, procedures, diagnostics, and other treatment modalities, the purpose of an HTA is to provide a framework for patient-specific healthcare decisions that achieve the best outcomes and value.[24,25]

BEST PRACTICES IN ASSESSMENT AND INTERPRETATION OF COMPARATIVE EFFECTIVENESS RESEARCH

Misleading information can cause harm or false hope. Can we rely with assurance on health outcomes predictions? Highly disciplined, critical appraisal methods are necessary to ensure that the information and conclusions derived from CER studies are valid before they are applied. Thus, misleading information that poses risks or leads to inappropriate decisions and unintended consequences must be eliminated.

IMPORTANCE OF CRITICALLY APPRAISING THE EVIDENCE

Understanding the limitations of the study author's analysis and interpretation of data is important. When evaluating CER information, the decision maker should apply a systematic method to critically appraise evidence for both internal and external validity and identify any confounding variables. Although there are various tools to assess clinical study research, the PICOT technique provides a consistent and simple method for evaluating the quality of scientific research for its validity and applicability.[26] The five areas considered by this technique are described as follows.

Patient Population or Problem

Does the CER study address the target population? Are results from this study likely to be applicable and generalizable to the patient or population of interest? Factors to consider include age, gender, health conditions, medication regimen, and access to healthcare services.

Intervention

Is the intervention defined and does it match the issue of interest? This may include an assessment for the use of a specific diagnostic test, treatment, adjunctive therapy, medication, or procedure for a specific patient or its broad use for a specific population.

Comparison

What are the comparators? Are the comparators reasonable, and do they reflect best practice and standards of care?

Outcome

What is the outcome being measured? Is it a true health outcome (e.g., survival, death, cardiovascular events) or a surrogate measure (e.g., A1C lowering, LDL-cholesterol lowering, or blood pressure reduction)? If outcomes are based on surrogate measures, are these validated and known to correlate with improved health outcomes? Does the manner in which the outcome is measured and described allow for conclusions of comparative effectiveness (either qualitatively or quantitatively)? Outcomes may consist of relieving or eliminating specific symptoms, improving or maintaining function, or enhancing esthetics. When defining the outcome, "more effective" is not acceptable without a description of how the intervention is more effective.

Time Frame

Are the time frame and duration of the study sufficient and appropriate to determine the effect of the intervention in a given population? The period could be brief (e.g., the first 24 hours after surgery) or much longer (e.g., 3 months on a new antidepressant medication). Whatever the time period, the duration should be long enough to observe the effect of the intervention and outcome being measured. (Note: This step may not always apply in all clinical settings and is optional. However, assessing the specific time frame and duration of study is a key step in critically appraising and analyzing results for validity and appropriateness.)

The last step in the critical appraisal of CER studies is to weed out those studies and information that do not pass the litmus test of PICOT. This ensures that potentially misleading information from poor-quality or irrelevant research is not used.

BEST PRACTICES IN SYNTHESIZING A BODY OF EVIDENCE

Synthesizing a body of evidence allows the collation of research and development of practical, evidence-based information that can be used to guide healthcare choices. Central to the structure of CER is the determination of value and probability of net benefit among treatment modalities. For CER to be useful, the information must be presented and summarized in a manner that is understandable to patients, physicians, and health plan policy leaders for use in decision making. If CER information is not communicated in a manner that audiences can easily understand, it is of little value.

The **Institute for Clinical and Economic Review** (ICER) Integrated Evidence Rating matrix combines a rating for comparative clinical effectiveness and a rating for comparative value.[27] The clinical effectiveness rating arises from judgments of the level of certainty provided by the body of evidence and the net health outcomes observed (balance between benefits and harms). Using this matrix for rating the clinical effectiveness of interventions offers a consistent and standard way to communicate conclusions of CER for healthcare decision makers (Figure 19-1).

CONCLUSION: FUTURE DIRECTIONS AND PRACTICAL APPLICATIONS

Investment and collaboration in CER will bring great potential to help improve the quality, outcomes, and value of health care. For CER to affect the healthcare delivery system or outcomes, the results must be integrated into the healthcare delivery system across all stakeholders, from patients and physicians to healthcare policy decision makers and payers. How these data are utilized at the policy level is a matter of continued debate. Some healthcare thought leaders have raised concerns that CER will inappropriately limit access to care,[28] while others believe that CER can help in making more appropriate coverage decisions, based on "better" information available.[29]

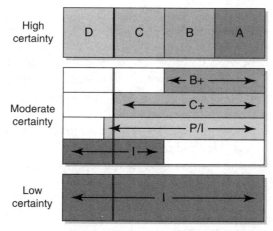

Figure 19-1 ICER evidence rating matrix and application.
Reproduced from Institute for Clinical and Economic Review. Synthesizing a Body of Evidence. A Collaboration of the Academy of Managed Care Pharmacy, the International Society for Pharmaeconomics and Outcomes Research, and the National Pharmaceutical Council. Comparative Effectiveness Research Tool. http://cercollaborative.org. (Last accessed 10/13/2014).

Despite ongoing controversy, there are signs that CER is taking shape with the emergence of value-based insurance designs (VBIDs). VBIDs incentivize health plan enrollees with lower cost shares when they opt for treatments and services that provide better value and positive net health outcomes. VBIDs have been popular with employers and health plans as a way to use financial incentives to encourage medication adherence, improve health outcomes, and reduce overall healthcare costs associated with unnecessary spending. VBIDs align insurance incentives (e.g., copays, deductibles) with the goals of consumer health behavior (e.g., adhering to wellness and prevention guidelines, following guidelines for managing chronic conditions). At the heart of VBID, CER provides the foundation and necessary information to guide decisions about which options and services are best under which circumstances and for whom.

Value-based purchasing is an additional strategy used by the federal government as well as employers to leverage marketing power to promote healthcare services that provide quality and value. Using this strategy, buyers are able to hold healthcare providers accountable for their performance in providing high-quality, cost-effective care according to best practices based on scientific research (including CER). Key elements of value-based purchasing include:

- Measuring and reporting comparative performance
- Paying providers differentially based on performance
- Designing value-based insurance designs that complement health benefit strategies and incentives to encourage individuals to select services and providers of health care that demonstrate higher value

Investment in CER use for practical healthcare decision making has the potential to improve the quality, outcomes, and value of health care in the United States. In areas where few studies have been done to directly compare different treatment options or examine their effect on different subpopulations (e.g., age, sex, ethnicity, or comorbid conditions) in real-world settings, CER helps fill the knowledge gap. With a strong push by both public and private sectors for more CER activities, consistent standards, methodologies, and applications must be more firmly established. In particular, continued education must be provided for end users, who ultimately analyze and apply information from CER studies to make the best treatment decisions. Success in these endeavors will strengthen CER and ensure its use for years to come.

STUDY AND DISCUSSION QUESTIONS

1. What is the primary goal of comparative effective research?
2. What are examples of key areas of research methodology needed to conduct or collaborate in CER?

3. What specific types of studies can be used to conduct CER? What are the strengths and limitations of their use?
4. How does CER provide value for positive effect on population health?
5. Identify examples today where CER is currently used and why.

SUGGESTED READINGS AND WEBSITES

READINGS

Chalkidou K, Tunis S, Lopert R, et al. Comparative effectiveness research and evidence-based health policy: experience from four countries. *Milbank Q.* 2009;87(2):339-67.

Garber A, Tunis S. Does comparative-effectiveness research threaten personalized medicine? *N Engl J Med.* 2009;360(19):1925-7.

Gibson TB, Ehrlich ED, Graff J, et al. Real-world impact of comparative effectiveness research findings on clinical practice. *Am J Manag Care* 2014;20(6):e208-20.

Higgins, JP, Altman DG, Gøtzsche PC, et al. The Cochrane Collaboration's tool for assessing risk of bias in randomised trials. *BMJ.* 2011;343:d5928.

Luce BR, Paramore LC, Parasuraman B, et al. Can managed care organizations partner with manufacturers for comparative effectiveness research? *Am J Manag Care.* 2008;14(3):149-56.

Pignone M, Saha S, Hoerger T, et al. Challenges in systematic reviews of economic analyses. *Ann Int Med.* 2005;142(12):1073-9.

Sackett DL, Straus SE, Richardson WS, et al. *Evidence-Based Medicine: How to Practice and Teach EBM.* London: Churchill-Livingstone; 2000.

Schneeweiss S, Gagne JJ, Glynn RJ, et al. Assessing the comparative effectiveness of newly marketed medications: methodological challenges and implications for drug development. *Clin Pharmacol Ther.* 2011;90(6):777-90.

Viswanathan M, Ansari MT, Berkman ND, et al. *Assessing the Risk of Bias of Individual Studies in Systematic Reviews of Health Care Interventions. Agency for Healthcare Research and Quality Methods Guide for Comparative Effectiveness Reviews.* March 2012. AHRQ Publication No. 12-EHC047-EF. http://www.effectivehealthcare.ahrq.gov/ehc/products/322/998/MethodsGuideforCERs_Viswanathan_IndividualStudies.pdf. Accessed November 6, 2014.

WEBSITES

Academy of Managed Care Pharmacy: http://www.amcp.org

Agency for Healthcare Research and Quality (AHRQ). Effective Health Care Program: http://www.effectivehealthcare.ahrq.gov

Center for Medical Technology Policy: http://www.cmtpnet.org

The Cochrane Collaboration: http://www.cochrane.org

Comparative Effectiveness Research Collaborative Initiative (CER-CI), a joint initiative of the Academy of Managed Care Pharmacy, the International Society of Pharmacoeconomics and Outcomes Research, and the National Pharmaceutical Council: http://www.npcnow.org/issue/cer-collaborative-initiative

Emergency Care Research Institute (ECRI): http://www.ecri.org

Institute for Clinical and Economic Review (ICER): http://www.icer-review.org/

International Society for Pharmacoeconomics and Outcomes Research (ISPOR): http://www.ispor.org

National Institutes of Health (NIH): http://www.nih.gov

National Pharmaceutical Council (NPC): http://www.nationalpharmaceuticalcouncil.org/

New England Comparative Effectiveness Public Advisory Council (CEPAC): http://cepac.icer-review.org

Patient-Centered Outcomes Research Institute (PCORI): http://www.pcori.org

REFERENCES

1. Center for Medical Technology Policy. http://www.cmtpnet.org/. Accessed November 6, 2014.
2. The Cochrane Collaboration. http://www.cochrane.org/. Accessed November 6, 2014.
3. Institute for Clinical and Economic Review (ICER). http://www.icer-review.org/. Accessed November 6, 2014.
4. International Society for Pharmacoeconomics and Outcomes Research (ISPOR). http://www.ispor.org. Accessed November 6, 2014.
5. National Institutes of Health (NIH). http://www.nih.gov/. Accessed November 6, 2014.
6. National Pharmaceutical Council (NPC). http://www.nationalpharmaceuticalcouncil.org/. Accessed November 6, 2014.
7. New England Comparative Effectiveness Public Advisory Council (CEPAC). http://cepac.icer-review.org/. Accessed November 6, 2014.
8. Patient-Centered Outcomes Research Institute (PCORI). http://www.pcori.org. Accessed November 6, 2014.
9. A CBO Paper: Research on the Comparative Effectiveness of Medical Treatments. Congress of the United States Congressional Budget Office. Pub. No. 2975. December 2007. http://www.cbo.gov/sites/default/files/12-18-comparativeeffectiveness.pdf. Accessed November 6, 2014.
10. Sox HC. Defining comparative effectiveness research: the importance of getting it right. *Med Care*. 2010;48(6):S7-S8.
11. Agency for Healthcare Research and Quality (AHRQ). http://www.effectivehealthcare.ahrq.gov. Accessed November 6, 2014.
12. American College of Physicians. Improved Availability of Comparative Effectiveness Information: An Essential Feature for a High-Quality and Efficient United States Health Care System. Philadelphia: American College of Physicians; 2008. http://www.acponline.org/advocacy/current_policy_papers/assets/healthcare_system.pdf. Accessed November 6, 2014.
13. Academy of Managed Care Pharmacy. http://www.amcp.org. Accessed November 6, 2014.
14. Fisher E. More Care Is Not Better Care. National Institute for Health Care Management Expert Voices. January 2005. http://www.nihcm.org/pdf/ExpertV7.pdf. Accessed November 6, 2014.

15. Weinstein JN, Lurie JD, Olson PR, et al. United States' trends and regional variations in lumbar spine surgery: 1992-2003. *Spine.* 2006;31:2707-14.

16. Schwartz D, Lellouch J. Explanatory and pragmatic attitudes in therapeutical trials. *J Chronic Dis.* 1967;20:637-48.

17. Zwarenstein M, Treweek S, Gagnier JJ, et al. Improving the reporting of pragmatic trials: an extension of the CONSORT statement. *BMJ.* 2008;337:a2390.

18. ALLHAT Collaborative Research Group. Major cardiovascular events in hypertensive patients randomized to doxazosin vs. chlorthalidone. *JAMA.* 2000;283:1967-75.

19. *Action to Control Cardiovascular Risk in Diabetes (ACCORD) Trial. NHLBI Biological Specimen and Data Repository Information Coordination Center.* https://www.accordtrial.org/public/index.cfm. Accessed November 6, 2014.

20. Lieberman JA, Stroup TS, McEvoy JP, et al. Effectiveness of antipsychotic drugs in patients with chronic schizophrenia. *N Engl J Med.* 2005; 353:1209-23.

21. Rush AJ, Trivedi MH, Wisniewski SR, et al. Acute and longer-term outcomes in depressed outpatients requiring one or several treatment steps: A STAR*D report. *Am J Psychiatry.* 2006;163:1905-17.

22. The Cochrane Collaboration. Glossary of Terms. http://www.cochrane.org/glossary. Accessed November 6, 2014.

23. Institute of Medicine. *Finding What Works in Health Care: Standards for Systematic Reviews.* Washington DC: The National Academies Press; 2011. http://www.iom.edu/Reports/2011/Finding-What-Works-in-Health-Care-Standards-for-systematic-Reviews.aspx. Accessed November 6, 2014.

24. Berger ML, et al. *Healthcare cost, quality and outcomes: ISPOR book of terms.* Lawrenceville, NJ: International Society for Pharmacoeconomics and Outcomes Research; 2003.

25. Luce BR, Drummond M, Jönsson B, et al. EBM, HTA and CER: clearing the confusion. *Milbank Q.* 2010;88(2):256-76.

26. Sackett DL, Richardson WS, Rosenberg W, et al. *Evidence-Based Medicine: How to Practice and Teach EBM.* New York: Churchill-Livingston; 1997.

27. ICER Collaborative. Comparative Effectiveness Research Tool. https://cercollaborative.org/global/default.aspx?RedirectURL=%2fhome%2fdefault.aspx. Accessed November 6, 2014.

28. Gottlieb S. Congress wants to restrict drug access: a bill in the House could tie your doctor's hands. *Wall Street Journal,* January 20, 2009. http://online.wsj.com/news/articles/SB123241385775896265. Accessed November 6, 2014.

29. Garber AM, Meltzer DO. Setting Priorities for Comparative Effectiveness Research. Paper presented at Implementing Comparative Effectiveness Research: Priorities, Methods, and Impact, Engleberg Center for Health Care Reform at Brookings: Washington DC. http://www.brookings.edu/~/media/research/files/papers/2009/6/09%20cer%20mclellan/0609_health_care_cer.pdf. Accessed November 6, 2014.

Chapter 20

THE FUTURE OF POPULATION HEALTH AT THE WORKPLACE: TRENDS, TECHNOLOGY, AND THE ROLE OF MIND–BODY AND BEHAVIORAL SCIENCES

DEE W. EDINGTON, ALYSSA B. SCHULTZ, AND JENNIFER S. PITTS

Executive Summary

Population health plays on many stages, the workplace being an important one. Each person has membership in several overlapping populations—community, workplace, healthcare providers, and family and friends—and individuals may receive very different, sometimes conflicting, messages from within and across the contexts of each of these populations. At the workplace, the population health message and expected outcomes typically have focused on behavior change and the positive effect of healthy lifestyles on healthcare and disability costs, time away from work, and performance. Today, this singular focus on behavior change is giving way to broader strategies that incorporate the role of environmental and cultural effects, the introduction of technology innovations involving real-time communications, and participatory activities (e.g., games, fun, and recognition). Social–emotional and other determinants of health are gaining recognition as critical factors that affect overall health. Outcome measures will continue to focus on health behaviors, risks, and disease prevention but will expand to include the effect of additional elements (e.g., wellness and well-being, psychology, organizational health, lifestyle medicine) on the health of individuals and populations.

The signers of the U.S. Declaration of Independence stated as an objective "life, liberty and the pursuit of happiness." Clearly, the pursuit of happiness has been overlooked in the new American model of success. The population health strategies incorporated in future practices will become part of a global solution for shifting the measures of success from pure economics to include a balanced focus on health, well-being, and happiness.

In recognition of these ideas, this chapter focuses on the future of population health in the workplace. Perhaps because of the current financial climate, population health at the workplace is more important than ever for healthy, thriving, high-performing, and sustainable individuals, organizations, and countries.

INTRODUCTION

In recent years, it has become clear that the level of worker participation in wellness programs was insufficient to support desired population health objectives. To increase participation, program leaders turned to financial incentives as a form of behavioral economics (e.g., money, prizes), making participation rates the primary outcome measure. Although financial incentives effectively increased participation, they have demonstrated a limited effect on health risk reduction or sustained positive behavior change. Current programs seldom address basic environmental and cultural issues at the workplace. Because annual increases in financial incentives have been necessary to maintain high levels of participation, wellness program outcomes have come under increasingly greater scrutiny.

The winds of change are beginning to move the field, albeit slowly, toward our original view of the future: that of supportive workplace environments, cultures, and climates coupled with supportive communities. Slowly but gradually, the environment and culture are being viewed as the next steps toward improving the health of workplace populations.

Population health at the workplace faces a critical choice: (1) the field can continue to define population health in terms of biometric screenings, preventive services, and wellness programs with the objective of reducing healthcare and disability costs and time away from work or (2) the field can broaden the current strategy to include social–emotional and other determinants of total health in the context of a supportive workplace environment, culture, and climate.

An organization's vision and expected outcome measures should be the drivers of the strategies and objectives of a population health initiative. To advance the objectives of population health, the health of populations must be the primary focus, with emphasis on assessing the current health needs of the workforce, encouraging those at low risk to remain there, and encouraging those at risk to engage in behaviors that will mitigate their risks and prevent complications. This implies a fundamental shift in the objectives and strategies shown in Table 20-1.

SELECTED CURRENT TRENDS AFFECTING POPULATION HEALTH

Several trends could either promote or derail the movement toward an effective population health strategy at the workplace. The recently approved Patient Protection and Affordable Care Act (ACA) is a positive force in the eyes of most health-related

Table 20-1   Two Options for the Future of Population Health

Options	Objective	Population Health Strategies	Outcome Measures
Current emphasis	Decrease the cost of health care, disability, and time away from work	Decrease health risks and behaviors	Reduced healthcare and disability costs; higher employee performance and decreased time away from work
Adopt population strategies	Increase the total health of the population and of the organization	Increase values-shared results, help the healthy stay healthy, and decrease health risks and behaviors	Appropriate healthcare and disability costs, happiness, engagement, and higher values-shared results

professions. More mention was made of population health, wellness, and prevention in the congressional debates around this law than the sum of all the years leading up to its passage. The following are some of the trends that are affecting the future of population health at the workplace.

PUBLICITY SUPPORTING POPULATION HEALTH STRATEGIES

Nearly every health-related issue of every magazine and newspaper contains an article supporting healthy lifestyles or discussing population health programs in organizations or communities. Many articles also discuss the use of wellness programs as employee recruiting and retention tools for organizations and as a cost-effective way to maintain a healthy and high-performing workplace and workforce.

HEALTH CLINICS

Health clinics have been growing at a rapid pace (e.g., blood pressure screenings at grocery stores, miniclinics at pharmacy chains, mobile units provided by heath systems, and public health units). Some companies have set up workplace clinics to service as few as 200 or even fewer employees. These workplace clinics effectively remove barriers for employees who are seeking preventive services or treatments for relatively minor ailments.

ENVIRONMENT AND CULTURE

One of the most significant trends of the past several years is the recognition of the importance of integrating health into the environment and culture. Although industry leaders such as Judd Allen (culture) and Thomas Golaszewski (environment) have been promoting these areas, others have just begun to recognize the role of the environment and culture at the workplace. Some studies indicate that the culture of an organization has the potential to have a larger effect on the health of an employee population than the health promotion programming offered by that organization.[1,2,3]

FINANCIAL INCENTIVES PROMOTING EXTRINSIC MOTIVATION

Although there is increasing recognition of the importance of intrinsic motivation, the current trend is to favor approaches that use extrinsic motivators, such as financial incentives for participation and biometric or behaviorial outcomes. As noted previously, financial incentives alone may be unsustainable because of the ever-increasing financial resources required to get the same level of participation over more than the initial 1 or 2 years. It is also commonly known that high levels of extrinsic motivation can decrease intrinsic motivation. In addition, high levels of financial incentives could be construed as discriminatory against lower wage employees: the high incentive-to-wage ratio effectively coerces these individuals to participate.

GAMES, COMPETITION, AND COLLABORATION

"Gamification" is the new buzzword of wellness and population health management, and the use of games and challenges has dramatically increased over the past few years.[4] *Games for Health*, a recently launched peer-reviewed journal, is dedicated to "the development, use, and applications of game technology for improving physical and mental health and well-being."[5] Gamification takes an ordinary activity (e.g., jogging, smoking cessation) and adds game characteristics, such as rewards, leader boards, competition between players, and collaboration. Social marketing and online health promotion campaigns can be used on mobile devices to encourage healthy behaviors. One of the very positive outcomes of these campaigns is the resulting increase in social networks. Individuals and organized groups can be mobilized into competitive or collaborative teams to work toward goals and expand workplace social networks. Typically, there is an end goal, and new objectives or games must be organized to maintain interest and motivation. Because gamification is relatively new to population health, its long-term effectiveness in promoting health behavior change is still uncertain.

USE OF TECHNOLOGY, APPS, AND SMARTPHONES

Thoreau once observed that "we become the tools of our tools" and "the more complex our tools become the more complex our lives become."[6] Regardless of whether technology has driven the complexity of our lives or has been a result of it, it is increasingly being used in programs and initiatives designed to affect population health. Integrated databases (now referred to as big data) have been around for decades, but the 24/7 nature of information exchange made possible by thousands of new smartphone applications has taken big data to a new level. Our phones and other devices can be programmed to provide 24/7 biometric information and other outgoing data about us and receive incoming recommendations in real time about what we should do to maintain an algorithmically determined health goal. As the databases and algorithms become more sophisticated, there are endless ways to categorize populations and individuals by the patterns of their health risks, behaviors, and conditions. A constant barrage of improvement messages may eventually become unmanageable even to the youngest of the working generations. Time will tell whether this constant monitoring of individuals will make a positive contribution to global and sustainable health improvements.

NUMBER OF PROGRAMS

The growing numbers of interventions are typically convenient tactics designed to change specific behaviors, often one behavior at a time. Frequently, the intervention is applied regardless of the presence or absence of other diseases, risks, or behaviors (comorbidities). This is similar to many of the single-focused pharmaceutical solutions employed by the medical profession to treat certain symptoms or diseases in isolation.

FUTURE OF POPULATION HEALTH AT THE WORKPLACE: SHORT TERM

The existing model for population health at the workplace will continue to evolve (i.e., more integrated medicine, public health, psychology, organizational health, wellness, well-being, and other individual fields of studies). Although this mix came about by parallel advancements in each of the independent fields rather than by design, the model seems to meet the intuitive needs of the population in terms of health promotion, disease prevention, reduced healthcare costs, and decreased employee time away from work.

Continued growth of wellness programs under the current medical model will be tied to intuition and the discovery of new evidence related to the precursors of disease for the short-term future—a strategy employing quantitative evidence-based programs, which are slow to develop and limited to restrictive rules. As observed in the first decade of the 21st century, best practices and programs are accepted or rejected on the basis of adherence to evidence-based guidelines. The field has progressed from prevention to health promotion to wellness to well-being to population health, all of which continue to be necessary for overall population health; however, a comprehensive concept of individual and health remains elusive.

Within the next couple of years, population health at the workplace will continue to improve, but it is unclear whether the current medical model will remain or a new model that incorporates emerging knowledge will replace it.

PROGRAMS

To the credit of population health professionals, the field still strives for continual improvement and growth. However, programs remain focused on behavior change, and improvements have occurred at the margins. Insufficient attention has been given to core motivational stimulation of individuals, social–emotional decision making, and social interaction at the workplace. On the positive side, a few innovative strategies have been attempted using social media and social interactions to stimulate participation and supportive populations.

HEALTH RISK ASSESSMENTS AND APPRAISALS

An initial version of the health risk appraisal (HRA) was developed in the late 1950s and 1960s, and the Centers for Disease Control and Prevention introduced a computer version in 1980. The HRA has risen to be the leading tool for the early steps in most population health initiatives; over its 35-year history, the University of Michigan's Health Management Research Center has processed more than 12 million HRAs.

Traditional HRAs focus on identifying health risks and behaviors as precursors to disease, high healthcare costs, and time away from work. Because these relationships are now well established, an expanded health assessment is needed to take into account additional determinants of health, new research findings, expanded definitions of health and performance, and new technological advancements. At a minimum these assessments will explore social connectiveness and individual productivity, performance, and fulfillment.

INCENTIVES, PENALTIES, AND MANDATES

Frustration with participation rates has driven program managers to take the easy way forward: financial incentives. Many program administrators have adopted financial incentives and rewards, but it takes increasing rewards each year to keep similar levels of participation. What began with hats and T-shirts gradually increased to $50 to $100 incentives for participation. Today, it is not uncommon for programs to offer incentives totaling $300 to $900. At the extreme end of the spectrum is a program offering $2,000 in exchange for participation or improved biometrics. These high financial extrinsic motivators can result in lower intrinsic motivation, which most would agree is the preferred outcome. A few companies are using penalties rather than rewards (e.g., higher deductibles for employees who do not meet objectives or refuse to participate in offered programs). Even fewer are mandating that their employees achieve their objectives to improve health to receive the most comprehensive health benefits. Through research and application, future approaches will rebalance these tools based on the best evidence of effect. Also it is likely that many of these approaches will be utilized by employers and organizations seeking cultures of health.

MEASUREMENT FOR EMPLOYER RESULTS

Although the health of individuals and populations is the stated goal of wellness programs, lower healthcare and disability costs and reductions in time away from work have been the more frequent goals. The emphasis on economic outcome measures of medical costs, pharmacy costs, and performance measures creates an organizational expectation of a high return on investments (ROI). When challenged, the defense of the financial calculations has often been sparse and relatively weak.

Recognizing that current measurements are focused on the economic value of wellness programs to the employer, employees have raised the question of why they should participate in these programs just so the company they work for is more profitable. Until employers and employees agree on shared values and shared results, low participation in programs and diminishing employee loyalty will continue. This may have been particularly true within represented workforces now and in the past, and recently the nonrepresented part of the workforce is becoming more disillusioned.

The future of population health in the workplace must include true measures of health, vitality, and quality of life that translate into motivated, happy individuals working together to achieve shared results.

BEST PRACTICES TO NEXT PRACTICES

Although quantitative and randomized controlled studies are the gold standard for evidence-based best practices, they are of limited value for population health outcomes at the workplace. The employer–employee relationship typically precludes randomized, controlled, blinded studies. Moreover, populations and the world change too fast to rely solely on evidence-based best practices. Advancing the field and meeting the needs of society require visionaries who can formulate next practices. Next practices can be defined as disruptive innovations based on experiences with best practices, knowledge of the literature, intuition, a high-level vision, and clearly articulated outcomes.

FUTURE OF POPULATION HEALTH AT THE WORKPLACE: LONGER TERM

The health of Americans continues to deteriorate relative to the rest of the world regardless of the criteria applied and the measures used. The longer term (3- to 5-year) prospects provide some encouragement given the successes in implementing the following initiatives.

ADVANCED DEFINITIONS OF HEALTH

The World Health Organization (WHO) in 1946 defined health in this way: "a complete state of physical, mental and social well-being, and not merely the absence of disease or infirmity."[7] During the Ottawa Charter for Health Promotion in 1986, the WHO said that health is "a resource for everyday life, not the objective of living. Health is a positive concept emphasizing social and personal resources, as well as physical capacities." Neither of these definitions has been universally accepted, and many critics call the WHO's definition "utopian" and "unrealistic."[8-10]

Defining population health solely in terms of the medical model takes a very limited view of health. When the definition of population health is expanded to include the determinants of health outside of the medical model, the opportunities for success will broaden as well. Factors that affect health (e.g., positive psychology, positive organization psychology, social–emotional, workplace, workforce, family, friends, and communities) must be incorporated into any successful population health initiative. Health is constrained by the boundaries of the medical model (i.e, waiting for risk factors or disease to be identified through screening, preventive medicine, or clinical examinations). Moving the population to thriving, healthy, high-performing and sustainable outcomes requires earlier and more comprehensive interventions.

The notion of health being much more than the absence of disease has been overlooked for more than 60 years. Perhaps this is because illness and injury are relatively easy to measure and quantify, or perhaps it is because population health professionals have been enmeshed in the medical model of illness or precursor treatment. Whatever the reasons, now is the time to fully embrace the idea of health as a state of well-being, vitality, performance, and a high quality of life. Researchers have done much in the past few decades to identify the constructs that comprise health and well-being and to develop tools for measuring them. McDowell lists dozens of rating scales and questionnaires used to measure different aspects of health.[11] Subject areas include physical ability, disability and handicap, social health and belonging, psychological well-being and resiliency versus anxiety and depression, mental status and motivation, pain measurements, and general health status and quality of life.

ANXIETY AND STRESS AS THE EPIDEMIC OF THE 21ST CENTURY

The WHO Global Burden of Disease Survey estimates that depression and anxiety disorders, including stress-related health conditions, will be second only to ischemic heart disease in the scope of disability experienced by sufferers by the year 2020.[12] According to one estimate, stress-related disorders cost the United States $300 billion per year in absenteeism; turnover; diminished performance; and medical, legal, and insurance costs.[13] There is much evidence to suggest that current work demands are creating unprecedented levels of anxiety and stress among American working adults; for example, one-third of U.S. employees report being chronically overworked.[14] The National Institute for Occupational Safety and Health reports that 40% of workers view their job as very or extremely stressful, 25% believe their job is the number one stressor in their life, and 26% of workers say they are often or very often burned out or stressed by their work.[15]

What can employers do to reduce stress levels among employees and avoid its many negative effects? For years, the same advice has been given to employees: Get enough sleep, exercise regularly, consume a sensible diet, and participate in activities that give employees a sense of autonomy and purpose as well as provide social support. In the near future, innovative employers are likely to go beyond the annual staff retreat or team-building experience and begin addressing stress reduction as a part of the organization's climate and culture. Things that make an employee's day-to-day work less stressful include:

- Setting guidelines for meetings (e.g., a clearly defined agenda, a firm start and end time, and actionable outcomes rather than free-flowing discussion that leaves people feeling their time was wasted).
- Fostering connections between new and long-term employees with mentoring relationships. These sessions get people thinking in new ways, help bring new staff up to speed more quickly, engender professional respect, and promote helpful attitudes when high-pressure situations arise.
- Celebrating successes on a regular basis in a way that demonstrates how each member of the team helped the company to achieve a goal and shows employees how their work is meaningful.[16]
- Allowing flexible schedules can go a long way toward reducing stress. Employees can choose the best time of day to do their work, which may be early morning for some and late night for others. Flexible schedules can also reduce the conflict between job and family demands.
- Teaching employees how to use technology to their advantage (e.g, managing interruptions, avoiding the tendency to become slaves to their e-mail).
- Involving supervisors in managing employees' stress by regularly reviewing team workloads and dynamics and sharing values and results.

All of these factors are part of a larger organizational culture that values and supports employee health and well-being.

STRESS AND ANXIETY AS A RESULT OF 24/7 EXPECTATIONS

International competition and the rise of the global company have created a 24/7 economy, and companies have come to expect many employees to be on call in a similar protocol. The number of stress- and depression-related lost workdays and attrition of valued employees have led some companies to seek solutions such as barring e-mail messages and other forms of communication in the evenings and on weekends. To be effective, an overall conceptual model must be designed and then implemented to reduce anxiety and depression in individuals and lost time for organizations. The human body's stress response system is designed to respond to and resolve acute stressors; the chronic levels of stress experienced by many adults today take an incredible toll on their physical and emotional health in a variety of ways. A renewed emphasis on work–life integration can have positive effects for individuals and organizations, and it is an important component of an organization's population health strategy.

BALANCING SHARED VALUES AND SHARED RESULTS

Two of the major barriers to growing population health successfully are the general perceptions of conflicting values and unequal results. The economic status of many countries continues to favor investment institutions, banks, and employers at the expense of the workers and other lower income populations. As the economic advantage for organizations continues to grow, the employer–employee gap in conflicting values may continue to grow, and the resulting dissatisfaction will likely reduce participation in any employer-sponsored program regardless of its good intentions or potential benefits to individuals.

Employee and employer results come in many shapes and forms. Currently, employer-sponsored health and wellness programs tend to be focused on employer financial outcomes (including reduced benefit costs and increased productivity, absenteeism, presenteeism, worker's compensation and disability, and return on investment). Until employees feel that the most important program outcome is their improved health and well-being, wellness programs will be met with skepticism. This is especially true for companies that have decreased employee numbers or compensation in the face of being increasingly profitable. Recognizing employees on an individual basis for the important work they do is one way of accomplishing this with no added cost to the employer.

Ensuring that employees feel they are valued and doing meaningful work goes a long way toward building loyalty to and enthusiasm for the employer. It is critical that employees feel their values are aligned with those of the employer. Job satisfaction for most individuals is greatly influenced when employees feel they are doing meaningful work whether in the mailroom or in the executive office.

STRATEGIC, SYSTEMATIC, SYSTEMIC, AND SUSTAINABLE

Most population health strategies or programs in organizations and communities are behavior change or tactical in orientation. Major enterprise initiatives typically begin with an enterprise vision (strategic) and plan (systematic). To achieve the goals of population health, visionaries must develop conceptual models to focus on the major objectives of the health of populations. The approach that the organization uses to promote cultures of wellness advocates the use of a conceptual framework modeled on four steps: strategic, systematic, systemic, and sustainable.

RECOGNIZING ADDITIONAL DETERMINANTS OF HEALTH

Over the past several decades, population health interventions have more commonly focused on decreasing the health risks that are demonstrated precursors of illness and directly associated with high costs to employers in terms of healthcare utilization, absences, and disability claims. These risks include body measures (e.g., weight, blood pressure, cholesterol values, and blood glucose levels).[17–21] Unhealthy lifestyle behaviors, including smoking, excessive alcohol use, poor diet, and inactivity, are among the risks that affect costs and are commonly targeted by health interventions. It follows that employers remain focused on the effect of programs on healthcare costs and consider ROI to be the primary metric for demonstrating the value of their programming efforts. Even so, after decades of employer wellness programs, there is limited evidence of reliable long-term improvements in risks or better outcomes in terms of chronic health conditions.[22] For this to happen, population health must move from a singular focus on health risks and behaviors and costs toward a stronger focus on other important determinants or precursors of health and thriving, including attitudes and outlook, environment, and culture.

NEW KNOWLEDGE DRIVING FUTURE TRENDS IN POPULATION HEALTH

Many areas of scientific study have fostered exciting new evidence that may be useful to population health in achieving its full potential. Some future trends for population health management will be driven by new discoveries, whereas others will be driven by older knowledge used in new ways. As the study switches from understanding illness to understanding and promoting wellness, breakthrough findings within the social sciences (including positive psychology, positive organizations, sociology, anthropology, and philosophy) will be important to incorporate. Neuroscience and biology are also yielding important new insights into how the mind and body interact and how the brain and body shape our emotions, thoughts, and well-being. Many of the new discoveries will expand our definitions of wellness and well-being for the 21st century.

THE SCIENCE BEHIND THRIVING

In 1998, Martin Seligman and Mihaly Csikszentmihalyi described a new branch of psychology.[23] Positive psychology is defined as "the scientific study of positive human functioning and flourishing on multiple levels that include the biological, personal, relational, institutional, cultural, and global dimensions of life." In the intervening years, scientific inquiry into characteristics of human flourishing has yielded findings with tremendous implications for population health.

It has become increasingly clear that there is far more to health than the absence of physical illness. The evidence is mounting that factors such as resilience, optimism, gratitude, and mindfulness help individuals to flourish and live creative, satisfying, and meaningful lives. There is evidence that people who embody these positive characteristics are more motivated to act and be productive[24-27] and to have less stress and anxiety,[28] are less likely to become ill and bounce back more quickly from disease,[29,30] and ultimately cost employers less in healthcare spending and lost performance.[31-34]

It comes as no surprise that these concepts resonate with employers and are gaining the attention of health management vendors. What company wouldn't want to have optimistic, creative, resilient employees? CEOs have no trouble seeing the connection between these employee characteristics and better products and services and ultimately the company's bottom line. Key questions emerge such as, "Is the organization committed to doing what is necessary to achieve the vision?" and, "Can you generate a workforce to be optimistic, resilient, gracious, and mindful?"

INFLUENCING A POSITIVE OUTLOOK

It was commonly believed that our dispositions are relatively hard wired—that people have a set tendency toward pessimism or optimism, a positive or negative outlook, or happiness or melancholy—and it is not possible to make substantial changes in these dispositions. An important finding from this relatively new area of inquiry is that although disposition does have a genetic component, with effort and attention one can develop a stronger positive attitude and disposition.[35,36] Simple practices such as recalling three good things that happened during the day or taking the time to express gratitude to someone can lead to increases in happiness and optimism.[37]* Research is ongoing into the conditions, interactions, and practices that effectively increase a positive outlook. Studies of positive leadership have found that manager optimism is positively related to employee optimism, engagement, and project performance.[38] The population health field should remain open to evidence from these and any other areas that may expand our understanding and creativity when applying knowledge to new approaches.

NEW INSIGHTS ABOUT THE MIND–BODY CONNECTION

The relationship between the mind and body has been debated by great philosophers since long before Descartes outlined his dualistic notions of mind and body. Although most modern characterizations of the mind–body relationship hold that they are inseparable, we still do not fully understand "the ghost in the machine."** Most current theories characterize the mind as having an important effect on the body; however, recent research has also demonstrated that the human mind and body have a greater reciprocal effect than was once believed. Some evidence of this comes from research in embodied cognition, an outgrowth of the fields of social and cognitive psychology. This field is providing valuable information about the directional relationship between the body (motor system) and how a person feels (emotionally, spiritually). Studies have shown that the manner in which we carry ourselves, the facial expressions we make, the energy we give out, and how we receive the energy of others and our surroundings can influence our emotions and attitudes. In one classic study, participants holding pencils in their teeth (i.e., forcing them to use the muscles of a smile) were quicker to understand positive sentences than negative sentences. The reverse was true when they held the pencils between their noses and upper lips (i.e., forcing more of a frown).[39]

---

*Seligman, Steen, Park, and Peterson (2005) have suggested that there are at least 100 strategies for increasing happiness, a class of positive psychology students identified more than 1,000 happiness-increasing strategies, and an amazon.com search for books about happiness yields more than 4,000 hits.

**The British philosopher Gilbert Ryle described René Descartes's ideas about mind–body dualism as "the ghost in the machine." He used the phrase to reflect what he thought was Descartes's fallacy in proposing that mental and physical activity occur in parallel without describing the nature of their interaction.

The importance of the mind–body relationship is being embraced by researchers in business education. The research of Amy Cuddy, a Harvard Business School professor, is improving understanding of the link between body language and physiology, emotions, and behavior. Her work provides evidence that faking body postures that mimic positions of power (she calls these "power poses"), even for short periods of time, can affect levels of testosterone and cortisol, increase performance in some situations, and improve coping skills in stressful situations.[40] This work and other research into the reciprocal relationship between mind and body have important implications for the practice of population health management particularly in employer settings (e.g., self-esteem, self-efficacy, and resilience in the individual and in work teams). Producing a resilient workforce would be helpful to any corporation or organization.

ADVANCES IN BRAIN SCIENCE

Modern research has discovered that the brain is much more malleable, or "plastic," throughout life than was once thought. Brain plasticity runs counter to the longheld belief that the brain cannot change substantially after a critical period in childhood except to deteriorate with age. This belief has shaped notions about the structure and function of the brain itself, human nature, brain injury, and aging. New discoveries about the brain have led to some of the most revolutionary and important ideas in science.

Of particular relevance to population health is an improved understanding of how attention physically shapes the brain. There are two basic rules governing neuroplastic changes in the brain:

- The first rule, "use it or lose it," refers to the "competitive nature of brain plasticity."[41] If one does not regularly use a skill or perform a behavior, the area of the brain responsible for that activity will be taken over by brain activity for other skills that are practiced.
- The second rule is that "neurons that fire together wire together." This refers to the tendency of brain cells that are active at the same time to chemically connect, resulting in a greater tendency for one cell to fire when the other is active.

These two basic rules can guide practical application as we strive to achieve population health and well-being.

FORMING GOOD HABITS—REPLACING BAD ONES

Many of the behaviors we undertake on a daily basis are a result of habits formed early in life. William James wrote, "We are what we repeatedly do." Although the brain is indeed more plastic in the early years, research on neuroplasticity is shedding some light on how individuals can effectively shape their brains and rewire old unhealthy habits throughout their lives.

Following the principles of brain plasticity, instead of working to "break" bad habits, we can work to replace them with better ones. This requires an awareness of the habit and its triggers, and a concerted effort to actively shift attention to something pleasurable rather than the old habit, thereby strengthening the brain circuitry and triggering dopamine release, which rewards the new activity. Over time, and with repeated effort, old bad habits can be replaced with new, healthier ones.

The rules of brain plasticity can also work to help build more positive dispositions. As one prominent neuropsychologist Dr. Rick Hanson puts it, "If you point your attention toward the good in life, the better your brain will get at fostering goodness, and the healthier it will become."[42] An increasing body of evidence supports the idea that practicing gratitude and mindfulness meditation, and reframing negative thoughts into positive affirmations work to change the physical structure of the brain and strengthen positive states of mind. This has important implications for any individual or program intending to improve health and well-being.

THE EFFECT OF CONTEXT: ENVIRONMENT, CULTURE, AND SOCIAL SUPPORT

Many of the influences on flourishing described earlier can be moderated by factors related to our context, and we don't have to look far for examples of how our physical and social surroundings can either hinder or bolster our creativity and optimism. The physical and social environments and cultures at home and work and in the community can influence mood, stress levels, creativity, performance, and, ultimately, health. There is research that supports a strong correlation between one's ZIP code and one's perception of health.[43]

Because employed Americans spend more than half of their waking hours at work,[44] the workplace environment, climate, and culture can play a significant role in health and well-being. Although population health vendors are beginning to adopt methods to help employers improve their cultures with respect to health, a company culture is not something that can be "fixed" solely by a program. The Centers for Disease Control and Prevention defines a culture of health as follows:

> Culture of Health is the creation of a working environment where employee health and safety is valued, supported and promoted through workplace health programs, policies, benefits, and environmental supports. Building a Culture of Health involves all levels of the organization and establishes the workplace health program as a routine part of business operations aligned with overall business goals. The results of this culture change include engaged and empowered employees, an impact on health care costs, and improved worker performance.[45]

Although culture of health has become a buzz phrase over the past several years, wellness and population health vendors generally sought to affect culture by means of isolated programs and relatively superficial tactical changes. Effectively and purposefully redirecting a culture requires clear vision and a strategy set forth by senior leaders and embraced by all stakeholders in the company. It takes courage and commitment from leaders to live the vision, dedicate sufficient resources, and participate in the alignment of all stakeholders throughout the organization. It also requires persistence and patience from everyone involved. Like any evolution, culture change takes time—to create a shared vision, to communicate and live the vision consistently, to evolve a shared accountability, to build trust—and the patience and acceptance to persist while the evolution unfolds. Most benchmark culture of health companies will tell you that the building process took a decade or more and that it needs constant cultivation to maintain it.

CULTIVATING INTRINSIC MOTIVATION

Motivating humans to make and maintain health behavior changes to preserve health or to reduce their risks is a complex endeavor. However, to achieve population health, collective behavior change is foundational. Although the relative importance of intrinsic motivation over extrinsic motivation is broadly acknowledged by behavior change professionals, many in the population health field still rely on the use of external rewards or incentives to motivate individuals to initiate and maintain behavior changes—a tactic that has not achieved the level of engagement necessary to reduce risks and improve health long term. In fact, some psychological constructs challenge the notion that humans will respond rationally to extrinsic motivation. For example, the theory of psychological reactance holds that if a person believes that limits, rules, or regulations are being placed on his or her behavioral freedoms, the resulting behavior may be contrary to the initial intentions of the enticement or directive. Miller and associates found that strongly persuasive health appeals can sometimes have the opposite effect.[46] They concluded that using concrete, "low-controlling language" and ensuring individual autonomy with a "choice-emphasizing postscript" may result in less ambiguity and reactance than more overtly persuasive health appeals or corporate mandates.

Another psychological construct, cognitive dissonance, has relevance to understanding the effect of monetary or other extrinsic incentives or rewards on human motivation. According to the theory of cognitive dissonance, we experience discomfort when we hold contradictory or incongruent beliefs, or behave in a manner that is dissonant with the beliefs that we hold. Cognitive dissonance drives individuals to reduce the associated discomfort by adjusting dissonant beliefs and behaviors to be more "consonant." There is evidence that giving a person an extrinsic incentive or reward for performing a behavior that should be intrinsically motivating can serve to undermine that motivation. A related process is involved when giving a person an extrinsic reward to initiate a new behavior or discontinue an old one. Paying the person for the behavior can diminish the intrinsic motivation to sustain the behavior in the long term. This was demonstrated in the General Electric study that paid employees to stop smoking. Although a much smaller control group stopped smoking than those paid to do so, there was a much higher persistence rate 15 to 18 months out in that group. Those intrinsically motivated to stop smoking were more likely to quit for good (72% versus 64%).[47]

Edward Deci and Richard Ryan pioneered the self-determination theory (SDT),[48] which examines motivation from a humanistic perspective. SDT focuses on how individuals become motivated to begin new health-related behaviors and maintain them over time. The theory holds that human motivation is rooted in a basic need to develop self-competence, skills, and self-control and to build connections with others and the environment. Research in this area has generated evidence that once basic human needs have been met (i.e., Maslow's hierarchy[49]), tangible rewards (e.g., money, prizes) can actually undermine our intrinsic motivation. SDT argues that autonomy and competence are crucial components for developing the intrinsic motivation required to both initiate and maintain healthy lifestyle behaviors. In the future, population health programs will foster a sense of autonomy and provide support and opportunities for confidence building. To truly internalize an attitude or behavior, it is also important that approaches foster a sense of relatedness: "People are more likely to adopt values and behaviors promoted by those to whom they feel connected and in whom they trust."[50] Future efforts in well-being will recognize the importance of making positive social connections that support health and well-being at work and in personal life. In fact the research conducted by Christakis and Fowler demonstrated that your health can be determined by your friends' collective health and that obesity may be a consequence of a communicable disease.[51]

DECISION MAKING

Lifestyles are largely composed of the decisions (whether minor or important) made from moment to moment on a daily basis. Ideally these choices are rational, the result of information gathered and acted upon in a logical manner. However, the sheer amount of information available to guide decision making is often overwhelming and difficult to process fully. As a result, people often rely on mental shortcuts and biases to help organize information, screen out irrelevant or inconsistent data, and guide decisions and actions. Although these shortcuts, or heuristics, can save time and sometimes make decisions easier, they can also influence thinking in ways that aren't always useful and can sometimes lead to choices that are less than optimal or even irrational.

Daniel Kahneman won the Nobel Prize in economics in 2002 for his pioneering research with Amos Tversky on human judgment and decision making under uncertainty (behavioral economics). This gave birth to the field of behavioral economics. Their work led to a better understanding of the role of emotions and intuitions in shaping decision making. Although intuition and emotions can serve important functions, they also can bias decisions in a number of important ways:

- We aren't always right when judging how a decision will make us feel at a later time.
- We don't always include or completely process all relevant information at the time of the decision.
- The emotions we feel during decision making can make it harder to reason well, which can affect our choices.
- When we are emotional, we are especially sensitive to the effect of the mental shortcuts and biases that can lead to irrational choices.

These insights from the field of behavioral economics have particular relevance for the future of population health. By understanding the social, cognitive, and emotional influences on decision making and behavior, it will be possible to develop more effective initiatives and approaches.

EXPERIENCING-SELF AND REMEMBERING-SELF

Writing about the important distinction between experience and memory with regard to happiness,[52] Kahneman characterizes humans as having something akin to two distinct selves: an "experiencing-self" and a "remembering-self." The experiencing-self lives in a continuous flow of moments and experiences, one after the other. The remembering-self is a storyteller—creating an almost immediate narrative about experiences. There is an important distinction between the experiencing-self being happy "in" life and the remembering-self being happy "about" life. The experiencing-self is nearly silent in decision making, and the remembering-self has a far stronger voice. The remembering-self is the one who makes choices, whereas the experiencing-self has little say in the decision. According to Kahneman, "[W]e don't choose between experiences, we choose between memories of experiences. Even when we think about the future, we don't think of it in terms of experiences, we think of it in terms of anticipated memories."[53]

The notion of having two selves has important implications for the future of population health, especially with respect to interventions designed to strengthen the precursors of health (positive psychology, positive organizational psychology, social–emotional, workplace, workforce, family, friends, and communities). Improving happiness and well-being can take two very different courses. The experiencing-self finds happiness in things like building connections and spending time with friends, whereas the remembering-self thrives on more tangible things like accomplishments and goals.

Population health must embrace an eclectic array of concepts within and beyond the usual comfort zone and develop approaches that target both "selves." For approaches that help experiencing-selves better experience the moments of life both at home and at work, see the preceding sections within The Effect of Context: Environment, Culture, and Social Support and the work of Mihaly Csikszentmihalyi on flow[54,55] and creativity.[56] Incorporate principles from positive psychology, brain science, and behavioral economics to help remembering-selves develop stronger tendencies toward positive yet realistic narratives about those experiences.

NEW METHODS, MEASURES, AND METRICS

To evolve, the field of population health must embrace a new set of measures and metrics for success (measure what matters) and apply better methods for measuring the effect of initiatives. Although sometimes hotly debated, the more traditional indicator of a program's value has been ROI, which often includes worker performance (absenteeism and on-the-job productivity), healthcare service utilization, and cost savings in the return portion of that calculation. ROI can indicate whether a prescribed program or tactic has saved the employer money by its effect on participating employees. However, an improved understanding of what works best and for whom is dependent upon better measures of the overall value of more comprehensive population-level strategies. This will require adopting a thoughtful framework for understanding the environmental and cultural factors that can influence all individuals across a population (including programs, policies, norms, and rituals). It will also require a new set of metrics that help connect the dots between the environment and culture and the leading and lagging indicators of the effect on health and well-being.

To carry the field forward, employers should continually assess the support for health in their workplace environments and cultures (influences), track both participation and engagement in programs, and measure self-directed behavior change (leading indicators). The value of traditional health assessments (or health risk assessments) can be improved by adding measures of positive outlook (e.g., resilience, optimism, perceived control) and by regularly measuring changes in these important precursors to health. Advances in technology make it possible to more frequently monitor and report on these and other important outcomes with minimal burden on the population. Finally, we recommend better demonstrating the relationships and interactions (mediators and moderators) between the workplace environment and culture, and the short-, moderate-, and longer-term outcome indicators and lagging indicators.[57]

CONCLUSION

Population health, in general, has benefited greatly from several general trends in society. Among the significant population trends are the amount of popular press devoted to wellness and performance, significant advances in technology, use of smartphones, and new research in mind–body and behavioral sciences. In addition, and specific to population health at the workplace, there is a trend to recognize the environmental and cultural determinants of health; increasing installations of health clinics at the workplace; and widespread adaptation of games, competition, and collaboration to drive toward healthy populations.

During the next 1 to 3 years, we expect an updating of the popular health risk assessment to a more inclusive health assessment that takes into account additional determinants of health and performance: the new advances in technology, use of smartphones, and new research.

In 3 to 5 years, we expect major transformational changes, from tactical programmatic offerings to a more enterprise-based wellness and performance strategy; incorporation of a much wider recognition of the value of thriving, healthy, high-performing, and sustaining organizations and individuals; and a much greater attention to stress and anxiety in response to the new economics of 24/7 operations, fewer employees, and cost shifting.

Beyond 5 years, we would expect the pursuit of sophisticated employer–employee relationships, with shared values and shared results within enlightened and successful companies and high-performance organizations.

REFERENCES

1. Hoebbel C, Golaszewski T, Swanson M, et al. Associations between the worksite environment and perceived health culture. *Am J Health Promot.* 2012;26(5):301-4.

2. Pronk NP, Allen CU. A culture of health: creating and sustaining supportive organizational environments for health. In: Pronk NP, ed. *ACSM's Worksite Health Handbook: A Guide to Building Healthy and Productive Companies.* 2nd ed. Champaign, IL: Human Kinetics; 2009:224-30.

3. Golaszewski T, Allen J, Edington D. Working together to create supportive environments in worksite health promotion. *Am J Health Promot.* 2008;24(4):1-10.

4. Ferguson B. The emergence of games for health. *Games for Health Journal.* 2012;1(1):11-17.

5. Mary Ann Liebert, Inc., Publishers. *Games for Health Journal.* http://www.liebertpub.com/overview/games-for-health-journal/588/. Accessed November 6, 2014.

6. Thoreau, HD. *Walden.* New York: Oxford University Press; 1854.

7. WHO. Preamble to the Constitution of the World Health Organization as adopted by the International Health Conference, New York, 19-22 June 1946, and entered into force on 7 April 1948. http://www.who.int/about/definition/en/print.html. Accessed November 6, 2014.

8. Jadad AR, O'Grady L. How should health be defined. *BMJ.* 2008;337:a2900.

9. Larson JS. The conceptualization of health. *Med Care Res Rev.* 1999;56:123-36.

10. Huber M, Knottnerus JA, Green L, et al. How should we define health? *BMJ.* 2011;343:d4163.

11. McDowell I. *Measuring Health: A Guide to Rating Scales and Questionnaires.* 3rd ed. New York: Oxford University Press; 2006.

12. Murray CJL, Lopez AD, eds. *The Global Burden of Disease.* Cambridge, MA: Harvard School of Public Health; 1996.

13. Rosch PJ. The quandary of job stress compensation. *Health and Stress.* 2001;3:1-4.

14. Galinsky E, Bond JT, Kim SS, et al. Overwork in America: When the way we work becomes too much. Families and Work Institute. 2005. http://familiesandwork.org/site/research/reports/OverWorkInAmerica.pdf. Accessed November 6, 2014.

15. U.S. Department of Health and Human Services. National Institute for Occupational Safety and Health. Stress … at Work. http://www.cdc.gov/niosh/docs/99-101/pdfs/99-101.pdf. Accessed November 6, 2014.

16. Helm B. Three ways to reduce employee stress. *Inc.* http://www.inc.com/burt-helm/3-ways-to-reduce-employee-stress.html. Accessed November 6, 2014.

17. Yen LT, Edington DW, Witting P. Corporate medical claim cost distributions and factors associated with high-cost status. *J Occup Med.* 1994;36(5):505-15.

18. Yen L, Edington D, Witting P. Associations between health risk appraisal scores and employee medical claims costs. *Am J Health Promot.* 1991;6(1):46-54.

19. Yen L, Edington D, Witting P. Prediction of prospective medical claims and absenteeism costs for 1284 hourly workers from a manufacturing company. *J Occup Med.* 1992;34(4):428-35.

20. Anderson DR, Whitmer RW, Goetzel RZ, et al. The relationship between modifiable health risks and group-level health care expenditures: Health Enhancement Research Organization (HERO) research committee. *Am J Health Promot.* 2001;15(1):45-52.

21. Yen L, Schultz AB, Schnueringer E, et al. Financial costs due to excess health risks among active employees of a utility company. *J Occup Environ Med.* 2006;48:896-905.

22. Mattke S, Liu H, Caloyeras J, et al. *Workplace Wellness Programs Study: Final Report.* RAND Corporation.

Santa Monica: CA; 2013. http://www.dol.gov/ebsa/pdf/workplacewellnessstudyfinal.pdf. Accessed November 6, 2014.

23. Seligman MEP, Csikszentmihalyi M. Positive psychology: an introduction. *American Psychologist.* 2000;55(1):5-14.

24. Schulman P. Applying learned optimism to increase sales performance. *The Journal of Personal Selling and Sales Management.* 1999;19(1):31-7.

25. Kamen LP, Seligman MEP. Explanatory Style Predicts College Grade Point Average. Unpublished Manuscript. University of Pennsylvania, Philadelphia; 1985.

26. Nolen-Hoeksema S, Girgus JS, Seligman MEP. Learned helplessness in children: a longitudinal study of depression, achievement, and explanatory style. *J Pers Soc Psychol.* 1986;51:435-42.

27. Peterson C, Barrett LC. Explanatory style and academic performance among university freshmen. *J Pers Soc Psychol.* 1987;53:603-6.

28. Sharot T. The optimism bias. *Current Biology.* 2011;21(23):R941-5.

29. Maruta T, Colligan RC, Malinchoc M, et al. Optimists vs pessimists survival rate among medical patients over a 30-year period. *Mayo Clin Proc.* 2000;75(2):140-3.

30. Schou I, Ekeberg O, Ruland CM. The mediating role of appraisal and coping in the relationship between optimism-pessimism and quality of life. *Psychooncology.* 2005;14:718-27.

31. Nyce S, Grossmeier J, Anderson DR, et al. Association between changes in health risk status and changes in future health care costs: a multiemployer study. *J Occup Environ Med.* 2012;54(11):1364-73.

32. Burton WN, Chen CY, Conti DJ, et al. The association between health risk change and presenteeism change. *J Occup Environ Med.* 2006;48(3):252-63.

33. Edington DW, Musich S. Associating changes in health risk levels with changes in medical and short-term disability costs. *Health and Performance Management.* 2004;3(1):12-15.

34. Edington D, Yen LT, Witting P. The financial impact of changes in personal health practices. *J Occup Environ Med.* 1997;39(11):1037-46.

35. Seligman MEP. *Helplessness: On Depression, Development, and Death.* 2nd ed. New York: W.H. Freeman; 1991.

36. Lyubomirsky S, King L, Diener E. The benefits of frequent positive affect: does happiness lead to success? *Psychol Bull.* 2005;131(6):803-55.

37. Seligman MP, Steen TA, Park N, Peterson C. Positive psychology progress. *American Psychologist.* 2005. 60(5):410-421.

38. Arakawa D, Greenberg M. Optimistic managers and their influence on performance and employee engagement in a technology organisation: implications for coaching psychologists. *International Coaching Psychology Review.* 2007;2(1):78-89.

39. Glenberg AM, Havas D, Becker R, et al. Grounding language in bodily states: the case for emotion. In: Pecher D, Zwaan RA, eds. *Grounding Cognition: The Role of Perception and Action in Memory, Language, and Thinking.* Cambridge: Cambridge University Press; 2005:115-28.

40. Carney DR, Cuddy AJ, Yap AJ. Power posing: brief nonverbal displays affect neuroendocrine levels and risk tolerance. *Psychol Sci.* 2010; 21(10):1363-8.

41. Doidge N. *The Brain That Changes Itself: Stories of Personal Triumph from the Frontiers.* New York: Penguin Books; 2007.

42. Hanson R. *Buddha's Brain: The Practical Neuroscience of Happiness, Love & Wisdom.* ReadHowYouWant.com; 2011.

43. Sathyanarayanan S, Brooks A, Hagen SE, et al. Multilevel analysis of the physical health perception of employees: community and individual factors. *Am J Health Promot.* 2012;26(5): e126-36.

44. Bureau of Labor Statistics. American Time Use Survey. Time use on an average work day for employed persons ages 25 to 54 with children. http://www.bls.gov/tus/charts/. Accessed November 6, 2014.

45. Centers for Disease Control and Prevention. Workplace Health Promotion Glossary Terms. http://www.cdc.gov/workplacehealthpromotion/glossary/index.html#C3. Accessed November 6, 2014.

46. Miller CH, Lane LT, Deatrick LM, et al. Psychological reactance and promotional health messages: the effects of controlling language, lexical concreteness, and the restoration of freedom. *Hum Commun Res.* 2007;33:219-40.

47. Volpp KG, Gurmankin Levy A, Asch DA, et al. A randomized, controlled trial of financial incentives for smoking cessation. *N Engl J Med.* 2009;360:699-709.

48. Deci EL, Ryan RM. Self-determination theory. In: Van Lange PAM, Kruglanski AW, Higgins ET, eds. *Handbook of Theories of Social Psychology.* Vol. 1. Thousand Oaks, CA: Sage; 2012:416-437.

49. Maslow AH. A theory of human motivation. *Psychol Rev.* 1943;50(4):370-96.

50. Ryan RM, Patrick H, Deci EL, Williams GC. Facilitating health behaviour change and its maintenance: Interventions based on Self-Determination Theory. *The European Health Psychologist.* 2008;10:2-5.

51. Christakis NA, Fowler JH. The spread of obesity in a large social network over 32 years. *N Engl J Med.* 2007;357:370-9.

52. Kahneman D. *Thinking Fast and Slow.* New York: Farrar, Straus and Giroux; 2011.

53. Kahneman D. The riddle of experience vs. memory. Comment made in a TED Talk. February 2010. http://www.ted.com/talks/daniel_kahneman_the_riddle_of_experience_vs_memory.html. Accessed November 6, 2014.

54. Csikszentmihalyi M. *Flow: The Psychology of Optimal Experience.* New York: Harper & Row; 1990.

55. Csikszentmihalyi M. *Finding Flow: The Psychology of Engagement with Everyday Life.* New York: Basic Books; 1998.

56. Csikszentmihalyi M. Creativity: *Flow and the Psychology of Discovery and Invention.* New York: Harper Perennial; 1996.

57. Pawson R, Tilley N. *Realistic Evaluation.* Thousand Oaks, CA: Sage; 1997.

CASE STUDY: MICHIGAN PRIMARY CARE TRANSFORMATION PROJECT (MIPCT) AND THE ROLE OF MULTIPAYER PRIMARY CARE INITIATIVES IN ACHIEVING POPULATION HEALTH

MARIANNE UDOW-PHILLIPS AND
DIANE L. BECHEL MARRIOTT

OVERVIEW

In June 2010, the U.S. Department of Health and Human Services released a solicitation for the formation of the Multi-Payer Advanced Primary Care Practice Demonstration. The project was designed to bring Medicare into partnership with health plans and other payers who were experimenting with the implementation of patient-centered medical homes (PCMHs). The demonstration was designed to test whether advanced primary care practices can improve quality, safety, efficiency, and effectiveness of care as well as increase patient involvement in decision making and enhance care in underserved areas. The project is overseen by the Centers for Medicare and Medicaid Innovation. Now, several years into the project, several emerging trends are relevant to the goal of improving population health.

Michigan was one of eight states selected in November 2010 to participate in the demonstration. The Michigan initiative, called the Michigan Primary Care Transformation (MiPCT) Project, has at its core a focus on the effective and extensive use of care managers supported by a common clinical model, rapid-cycle performance feedback, and best practices training and sharing. The care managers are affiliated with one of 35 physician organizations (POs), broad groupings of physician practices throughout the state of Michigan.

To be eligible to participate in the MiPCT, practices were required to demonstrate that they had either National Committee for Quality Assurance (NCQA) level 2 or 3 certification or PCMH designation through the Blue Cross and Blue Shield of Michigan Physician Group Incentive Program (PGIP).[1]

The MiPCT aims to improve overall population health, the value of care, and patient experience through reducing risks for healthy individuals, managing disease and symptoms with self-management support for patients with moderate chronic disease, and coordinating care for patients with complex chronic diseases including end-of-life care. The project is expected to be budget neutral (i.e., the amount spent on care for MiPCT patients will be equal to or less than the amount spent for similar patients not in the demonstration).

The state of Michigan partnered with the University of Michigan to coordinate the statewide project. Coordination support includes learning collaboratives, community governance through multistakeholder committees and advisory groups, organizing opportunities for patient representation on project and practice operations, annual in-person summits to share best practices, a project website, regular communication and educational material, and a data collaborative that provides electronic member lists to identify patients eligible for care management services. The data collaborative also produces PO and practice dashboards that identify performance on key metrics such as:

- Percentage of high-, medium-, and low-risk patients in each practice
- Overall and avoidable (ambulatory or primary care sensitive) emergency room and inpatient visits
- Performance on quality measures for diabetes, well-child, asthma, and other metrics
- Standardized costs

Participating practices are required to have at least one care manager per 2,500 eligible MiPCT patients. Participating payers fund three payment components as follows:

- Care management payment: $3.00 per member per month (PMPM) ($4.50 for Medicare)
- Practice transformation payment: $1.50 PMPM ($2.00 for Medicare)
- Performance incentives: $3.00 PMPM

Although some payers reimbursed practices or POs for practice transformation and incentive components prior to 2012, neither Medicare nor Medicaid reimbursed for these components prior to the demonstration. No payers reimbursed POs or practices for care management prior to the MiPCT; thus, all care management funding was new for all POs and practices.

MAGNITUDE

The MiPCT is the largest PCMH demonstration project in the nation, serving more than 1 million patients (one-tenth of the state of Michigan's population). Seventeen hundred primary care providers in 377 practices statewide partner with more than 400 trained care managers to provide team-based advanced primary care, manage population health, and coordinate care.

Perhaps the most important advantage of the program's large scale is the ability to leverage the influence of five large payers in the state who are aligned on a common approach. This multipayer aspect of the project serves to focus the attention of POs and practices around the central clinical and financial model. The magnitude of the MiPCT also allows for the cost of project infrastructure to be shared among project funders.

EFFECT OF THE MIPCT ON POPULATION HEALTH

In 2014, the MiPCT demonstration entered its third year, and final program outcomes from national and state evaluations will not be available until 2016. However, preliminary results suggest that the project has produced quarter-to-quarter improvement in Medicare PMPM payment and hospital admissions compared to a control group. Primary care–sensitive emergency department (ED) visits have also been reduced by almost 4% statewide in the program's first year.

Care manager self-reporting indicates improvement on the extent of physician engagement and championship in identifying and servicing patients most likely to benefit from care management and self-management to reduce health risks, prevent disease, and manage symptoms. This is key to building the infrastructure that will allow population health management to be a focus throughout primary care practices in the state.

Additionally, the MiPCT has expanded the linkages among medical neighborhood partners. In 2013, electronic admission, discharge, and transfer notifications were piloted to provide real-time notification of hospital ED visits and discharges to care managers in primary care practice offices. Work is underway on an electronic directory to allow messaging between MiPCT care managers and care managers in health plans, hospitals, extended care facilities, and specialty offices. The project has enabled the Michigan Department of Community Health to supplement information it provides to primary care practitioners with maternal and child health, mental health and substance use programs, and services information across the state.

CRITICAL SUCCESS FACTORS AND BUILDING BLOCKS

The MiPCT's large statewide reach is unique in its scale and breadth. Although the project continues to evolve, the following factors have been critical to the program's ability to contribute to robust population health management in Michigan:

- POs as partners to practices in program contracting, reporting, and program operations

- Standardized care manager training
- Shared community governance with central project support and coordination
- Multipayer support

Each is described in greater detail in Table I-1.

IMPLICATIONS FOR POPULATION HEALTH

The patient is central to the PCMH and population health. A key article defines PCMH as "focused on improving the health of whole people, families, communities and populations, and on increasing the value of healthcare."[2] Thus, patient-centered care serves as a necessary component of an integrated population health infrastructure.

TABLE I-I MiPCT Critical Success Factors and Building Blocks

Key Success Factor/ Building Block	Rationale/Example
Physician organizations (POs) as partners to practices in program contracting, reporting, and program operations	Annual participation agreements POs responsible for implementing yearly MiPCT participation agreements and communicating with their practices Program reporting POs help practices collect required self-reported metrics on care management activity and practice infrastructure to support team-based care POs had access to practice and PO dashboards for claims, eligibility, and registry-based measures to facilitate results sharing with practices Program operations Some POs serve as the employers of practice-based care managers, and some organize information sharing with practice team members
Standardized care manager training	To ensure a common approach to implementation of the clinical model, training and continuing education of complex care managers was provided centrally by the MiPCT staff. A select set of available self-management and training programs were approved for moderate care management training.
Shared community governance with central project support and coordination	Stakeholders were encouraged to participate in community project governance to foster achievement of project goals over self-interest. A management team coordinated efforts across stakeholders and facilitated communication via a central e-mail server, a website, webinars, and leadership meetings.
Multipayer support	Payer alignment permits the leveraging of a common voice among participating health plans toward the achievement of common project goals. The greater the alignment of payers, the more likely the achievement of project goals.

To achieve population health goals, the primary care practice continues to serve as a gateway and foundation, facilitating coordination among the medical neighborhood partners. Multipayer, coordinated programs to build practice capability and spread best practices are essential to achieving population health goals. But, like the promise of population health itself, it will take time and sustained effort to develop and embed the processes that are integral to identifying and effectively addressing risks, symptoms, and conditions and improving the health of individuals and populations.

REFERENCES

1. Share DA, Mason MH. Michigan's Physician Group Incentive Program offers a regional model for incremental "fee for value" payment reform. *Health Aff.* 2012;31(9):1993-2001.

2. Stange KC, Nutting PA, Miller WL, et al. Defining and measuring the Patient-Centered Medical Home. *J Gen Intern Med.* 2010;25(6):601-12.

CASE STUDY: ASSESSING ORGANIZATIONAL READINESS FOR POPULATION HEALTH

KEITH C. KOSEL

OVERVIEW

Today, there is widespread agreement that the current structure of health care in the United States is outdated, inefficient, and inequitable and does not optimize the patient experience. When these shortcomings are combined with the fact that the current system's heavy reliance on a fee-for-service payment mechanism is rapidly pushing healthcare to the brink of financial insolvency, it becomes clear that a new focus is required. This new focus is population health. Where our current system focuses on care of the individual, population health widens that lens to include care of populations of individuals. Where our current model emphasizes the delivery of acute care services once an illness or condition presents itself, population health takes a more progressive approach by emphasizing health promotion in the form of preventive and wellness services. By its very design, population health brings with it the potential for meaningful cost management and improved patient outcomes.

Passage of the Patient Protection and Affordable Care Act (ACA) opened the door for organizations to move more aggressively into population health by promoting the concept of accountable care under the Medicare Shared Saving Program (MSSP). Central to the MSSP is the notion of keeping the target population healthy and minimizing the use of inpatient care. Accountable care organizations (ACOs) that are able to do this can share in savings with the Centers for Medicare and Medicaid Services (CMS). As more organizations move into accountable care contracts with CMS or commercial payers, the need to proactively address the health needs of their populations will take center stage and drive much of the transformation of today's health care.

THE CHALLENGE

Managing the health of a population of individuals, many of whom are healthy or without discernable disease, is a major challenge for even the most sophisticated healthcare provider systems. For providers without experience in population health or adequate resources, the challenge can be overwhelming. Several factors combine to make the transition to population health a daunting prospect.

- First, population health isn't traditionally taught in medical schools or hospital administration programs. This means that many of today's leaders are learning about population health at the same time they are being tasked with leading population health initiatives for their organizations. Although many nursing programs include elements of community health, most don't include the detailed data analytics and financial considerations (e.g., physician alignment) necessary to seamlessly implement a population health delivery model.
- Second, moving to a population health model requires that the health system redesign its care delivery systems and undertake new models of payment, many of which are risk based. Although simple in concept, these changes are very difficult to bring about, particularly in a short period of time. Development of an integrated medical record across all entities in the network, identifying at-risk individuals, and gaining patients' engagement in their self-care all pose substantial barriers to those embarking on a population health journey.
- Finally, building the necessary network to deliver a wide array of services seamlessly across the care continuum is a major undertaking. In many cases, the realization that acute care hospitals, physician practices, and postacute community-based provider organizations each have different—and in many cases conflicting—needs and incentives comes only after substantial time and resources have been committed.

What all these challenges have in common is the need for leaders to understand an organization's readiness to undertake a population health model well before implementing it.

RATIONALE FOR A READINESS ASSESSMENT

A good population health readiness assessment helps leaders to do the following: (1) understand how population health differs for their current practice, (2) identify the critical elements that all population health programs have in common, and (3) identify the organization's current level of preparedness across these critical elements. Although many population health readiness assessments are available,[1-4] it is essential that organizations select one that is both comprehensive in scope and designed to elicit meaningful data to inform the discussion and planning.

In 2012, VHA Inc., a national alliance of more than 1,300 hospitals and some 90,000 postacute provider entities, began working with a small number of member hospitals and health systems that were interested in moving into the population health arena. Preliminary conversations revealed that most of these organizations were unsure about what it would take to become proficient in population health and uncertain that they had the necessary resources and infrastructure in place to succeed. Additional questioning revealed that the first step in the population health journey was to do a critical assessment of organizational preparedness. With that objective in mind, VHA developed the Population Health Organizational Assessment (PHOA), a tool that was easy for hospitals to complete yet provided the level of detail necessary for a reasoned decision about whether to pursue a population health strategy. VHA's organizational approach to population health creates an assessment that pinpoints an organization's strengths and opportunities and enables leaders to gain valuable insights around infrastructure, partnerships, and community collaboration.

In building the PHOA, VHA made use of the lessons learned by developing the Patient Safety Organizational Assessment (PSOA), a tool that proved popular with VHA member institutions and gained the endorsement of the American Hospital Association.

THE NUTS AND BOLTS OF POPULATION HEALTH

The PHOA is an easy-to-use tool that assesses six domains that are the recognized building blocks or success factors for population health. These domains include: (1) organization and leadership, (2) care delivery and management, (3) physician integration and alignment, (4) community health promotion, (5) information technology and informatics, and (6) patient and family involvement. Each of the six domains contains two to four key aspects of population health, which highlight critical strategies required in population health (Table II-1).

Within each key aspect are four to seven activities that support the strategic aspects and provide detailed operational requirements. In effect, the PHOA provides a comprehensive look at what is required to be a competitive player in the population health arena.

TALKING TOGETHER

Although the nature and scope of the information used to fashion the domains, key aspects, and activities are critical to the comprehensiveness of the assessment, how the assessment is administered and how the results are interpreted are of equal importance. Drawing on its past experience in developing organizational assessments, VHA recommended that each organization completing the PHOA create a team of six or seven

Table II-1 PHOA Domains and Key Aspects of Population Health

Domain	Key Aspect of Population Health
Organization and leadership	Strategic plan Leadership and governance Workforce Financial position and scale
Care delivery and management	Continuum of care Chronic care and disease management programs
Physician integration and alignment	Physician leadership Physician availability and coordination Risk and financial arrangements Physician collaboration
Community health promotion	Coordination with nonclinical community Entities Prevention and screening Educational programs
Information technology and informatics	Electronic health record Data warehouses and clinical registries Analytics and decision support Patient-centric technology
Patient and family involvement	Patient activation and engagement Patient-centric care Self-care/self-management

individuals (including hospital and physician leaders, ambulatory care and postacute services administrators, and internal staff with expertise in risk contracting, epidemiology, and patient experience). It was specified that team members have experience and awareness of the organization's strategic plan and its resources and capabilities as well as market dynamics, competition, and physician relations. Knowledge of population health, while beneficial, was not a prerequisite for participation.

After each member of the team had reviewed and completed the assessment independently, the team assembled as a group. Each activity was reviewed and scored based on team consensus. Responses were categorized in a hierarchy based on the levels of activity, rated from 1 (low/no readiness) to 5 (fully prepared):

1. There has been no discussion around this activity.
2. This activity is under discussion, but there is no implementation.
3. This activity is under development, but there is no implementation.
4. This activity is partially implemented.
5. This activity is fully implemented.

Final scores, along with demographic information about the organization, were entered into the electronic tool and sent to VHA for processing.

DEPLOYMENT

Because this was the first time the PHOA would be used in a widespread assessment campaign, a decision was made to deploy the PHOA first to VHA partner and shareholder institutions (i.e., 400 large organizations that form the core controlling membership of VHA). A subset of these partner and shareholder organizations comprises the board that governs VHA's 12 regions. It was decided that the regional board meetings, held quarterly, would provide appropriate opportunities to deploy the PHOA.

The entire assessment process was structured around two board meetings held approximately 12 weeks apart. At the first board meeting, the PHOA was introduced and its intended purpose was discussed. Emphasis was placed on the strategic importance of assessing organizational readiness for population health. After the board meeting, the PHOA was distributed to the chief executive officers with instructions to assemble a team, complete the assessment, and return it to VHA within 4 weeks; most CEOs took between 3 and 7 weeks to complete the instructions. The initial deployment of the PHOA was in five of the 12 regions. Response rates across the five regions varied from a high of nearly 90% to a low of 40%. Once the surveys were returned, VHA analyzed the data using both quantitative and qualitative methods and produced hospital-specific reports for the respondents. At the next board meeting, VHA subject matter experts reviewed the collective responses with the entire board and discussed the implications of findings for individual organizations and the industry.

FINDINGS

QUANTITATIVE FINDINGS: DEMOGRAPHICS

Analysis of the data provided insights into how well prepared hospitals and health systems were for undertaking population health. As part of the demographic section, respondents were asked two fundamental questions: "How would you rate your organization's commitment to population health?" (Q1) and "How would you rate your organization's ability to provide population health?" (Q2) (Table II-2).

Table II-2   Level of Commitment vs. Capability

Q1: Commitment	Q2: Ability to Provide
High—35%	High—4%
Moderate—46%	Moderate—58%
Low—15%	Low—34%
None—4%	None—4%

Participant responses confirmed that although there is widespread interest in population health and how it can help position an organization for accountable care, most have little strategic or tactical expertise about how to do this.

The demographic questions also shed light on how health systems deliver essential services. Table II-3 shows that although most of the essential inpatient and ambulatory care services are already in place, hospitals and health systems generally lack the services typically delivered by community-based, postacute provider entities (e.g., long-term acute care, skilled nursing, hospice) and expect to acquire these through a partnership arrangement. Interestingly, the majority of hospitals and health systems reported owning resources related to behavioral health and home health, two components necessary to deliver fully integrated care across the continuum. Long-term acute care and skilled nursing care were the two service areas that were likely to be lacking or not currently available from a partner.

QUANTITATIVE FINDINGS: ACTIVITIES

Table II-4 illustrates the overall responses across the six domains along with the range of scores recorded. The grand mean was 3.2 out of 5, indicating that most of the elements assessed were under development but not yet implemented. The domain that received the highest score was community health promotion (3.8), and the lowest, as expected, was patient and family involvement (2.8). We were somewhat surprised to find that the highest scoring domain was community health promotion; it is possible that respondents equated this domain with the community needs assessments that are required in some areas and the associated community outreach services tied to those needs assessments. It is worth noting that the range of scores across the six domains was highly variable from organization to organization. This likely represents a combination of factors including differential

Table II-3 Availability of Key Services

Service	Owned by Hospital	Provided by Partner	Not Provided
Primary care	60%	35%	5%
Specialty care	56%	37%	7%
Behavioral care	49%	25%	26%
Outpatient imaging	81%	17%	2%
Skilled nursing	25%	31%	44%
Long-term acute care	9%	42%	49%
Home health	49%	30%	21%
Hospice	32%	52%	16%
Outpatient physical rehabilitation	89%	11%	0%
Outpatient cardiac rehabilitation	84%	9%	7%

Table II-4   Respondent Scores by Domain

Domain	National Average	Minimum–Maximum
Organization and leadership	3.0	1.8–4.9
Care delivery and management	3.7	1.7–4.9
Physician integration and alignment	3.3	1.2–4.8
Community health promotion	3.8	1.7–4.8
Information technology and informatics	3.2	1.4–4.9
Patient and family engagement	2.8	1.8–4.6

level of actual preparedness, misunderstanding of the question, or lack of actual knowledge of one's current resources.

Drilling down from the domains, the key aspects that received the highest scores represented an interesting mix of competencies. The three highest scoring key aspects were (1) delivering services across the continuum (3.8), (2) physician leadership (3.8), and (3) community health promotion (3.8). Although these are not typically considered core competencies for most healthcare systems, substantial progress in advancing these areas has been made by those with an eye on becoming an ACO or undertaking risk-based payer contracts.

At the other end of the spectrum, the key aspects that received the lowest scores were (1) patient engagement (2.5), (2) lack of population health champion (2.7), and (3) patient self-care for chronic conditions. It is interesting that two of the three lowest scoring competencies involve patients. As we have learned from recent studies, patient activation and engagement is central to success with population health and accountable care. As providers become more attuned to the need for partnering with their patients, strong gains are expected in this area. Also telling was the fact that respondents had difficulty identifying universal support for population health and lacked an executive champion. Clearly, an organization must have the support of its key players both within and outside the organization, and it must be able to identify an executive champion to lead this work.

QUALITATIVE FINDINGS

In responding to questions regarding what the CEOs found most helpful about the PHOA, many reported that the most valuable element of the assessment was the process by which their teams completed it. Specifically, most commented that while they found their individual scores and comparison to the national norms interesting, what added value was the group discussion that preceded the assigning of the final response score. Many realized that they had fewer resources than they initially thought, whereas others were pleasantly surprised to find out that their assets were greater than they believed. Many of the executives commented that having a wide variety of participants helped provide perspective and insight that many of the leaders lacked. Several noted that including frontline staff on the assessment team was instrumental in arriving at a more realistic assessment than would have been possible otherwise. These comments parallel those received from individuals completing the PSOA many years earlier.

NEXT STEPS

Providing the PHOA to approximately 100 VHA hospitals and health systems should not be construed as adequately describing the entire VHA membership, nor the state of the entire healthcare industry. However, the responses generated are likely representative of the vast majority of those organizations that have yet to complete the assessment. To that end, several actions will be taken to further strengthen the PHOA and broaden the insights that can be gleaned from the resulting data.

First, the PHOA will be deployed to all VHA member organizations in the remaining seven regions to increase the sample size and strengthen the reliability of the findings. The focus will be on those organizations that are underrepresented in terms of demographic characteristics in this first deployment. Second, the questions will be validated through factor analysis and other statistical methods. Third, the breadth and depth of the questions used in the PHOA will be reviewed continually. Questions may be added or removed to make the assessment more comprehensive and meaningful to users. At the same time, efforts will be made to achieve an optimal balance between the total number of questions and the time required to complete the assessment.

Fourth, and most importantly, the findings represented by the PHOA may be subject to intentional or unintentional manipulation. We know with a high degree of certainty that respondents tend to overestimate their experience and capabilities when completing self-assessments. To address this potential shortcoming, review teams will be dispatched to organizations that complete the PHOA with scores of 5 (activity fully implemented) across one or more domains. The teams will review the activities underlying the scores of 5 to determine whether they were accurately assessed. This process will also provide important insights into the correlation between high-scoring organizations and how fully developed their population health programs are. These insights will be especially valuable to organizations beginning the population health journey.

CONCLUSION

Completing an organizational readiness assessment is a crucial first step for organizations contemplating a population health model. The VHA Population Health Organizational Assessment (PHOA) provides a tool that allows organizations to evaluate their level of preparedness across six foundational areas. Feedback from users confirmed that most organizations are in the early discussion stages of preparing for population health. Further, respondents indicated that the conversations among the group completing the PHOA were by far the most valuable part of the exercise.

REFERENCES

1. Objective Health, a McKinsey Solution for Healthcare Providers, 2013. http://www.objectivehealth.com/. Accessed November 6, 2014.
2. Population Health Management: Organizational Self-Assessment. Sg2, 2013. https://www.sg2.com/wp-content/uploads/2014/05/PHM_Organizational-Self-Assessment.pdf. Accessed November 6, 2014.
3. Hospital Readiness for Population-Based Accountable Care. Health Research and Educational Trust, Chicago, 2012. http://www.hpoe.org/resources/hpoehretaha-guides/804. Accessed November 6, 2014.
4. Safety Net Accountable Care Organization (ACO) Readiness Assessment Tool. University of California, Berkeley School of Public Health, 2012. http://www.law.berkeley.edu/files/bclbe/Mar6_FINAL_combined.pdf. Accessed November 6, 2014.

CASE STUDY: THE POWER OF COMMUNITY IN POPULATION HEALTH: POWERUP FOR KIDS

MARNA CANTERBURY, NICO PRONK, THOMAS E. KOTTKE, AND DONNA ZIMMERMAN

OVERVIEW

Population health improvement efforts often focus on adults; however, increasing rates of childhood obesity have resulted in a growing emphasis on health improvement efforts for children.[1] The food and physical activity environments have a strong influence on youth behavior and contribute to the sobering prediction that without change, today's children will lead shorter, less healthy lives than the previous generation did.[2] To have a positive effect on children's health, population health improvement efforts must engage the community and address the multiple determinants of health, including medical care; health behaviors; and the physical, social, and economic environments.[3] Involving and engaging the community requires trusted leadership to convene multiple sectors and bring together diverse community stakeholders around the goal of improving children's health.

HealthPartners is a Minnesota-based, consumer-governed, nonprofit, integrated health system serving 1.4 million members. Committed to a population health improvement strategy since the early 1990s, the organization adopted a community health business model to focus on macrosocial determinants of health in 2010. To achieve its mission—"To improve health and well-being in partnership with our members, patients, and community"—health improvement initiatives must reach beyond clinic and hospital walls and include collaboratives with community partners. The case study presented here is one such example of HealthPartners becoming a trusted convener of a multisectoral childhood obesity prevention initiative in the St. Croix River Valley area of western Wisconsin and eastern Minnesota.

POWERUP FOR KIDS

PowerUp is a regional, community-wide initiative with a goal to *make better eating and active living easy, fun, and popular so that youth can reach their full potential.* PowerUp focuses on children ages 3 to 11 and the adults who influence their food and physical activity choices. This initiative requires a broad approach that goes beyond individual behavior change to encompass the community-level changes necessary to increase access to healthy foods, reduce access to foods of low nutritional value, and develop physical activity–friendly environments.[4,5] PowerUp is designed to work in partnership with community stakeholders in a comprehensive approach to population health improvement for youth. The initiative reflects a 10-year commitment by HealthPartners and Lakeview Health (part of the HealthPartners family of care, located in Stillwater, Minnesota, and including Lakeview Hospital, Lakeview Foundation, and the Stillwater Medical Group) to create community-level change with a focus on childhood obesity prevention.

The PowerUp Health and Wellness Advisory Committee of the Lakeview Foundation comprises representatives from a variety of sectors including businesses, schools, healthcare providers, health plans, nonprofit organizations, community leaders, families, civic leaders, the faith community, and public health organizations. In addition, a PowerUp Steering Committee and numerous work groups help guide the effort. Strong partnerships have formed, and these community advisers support strategy development, set priorities, and hold the initiative accountable for results. Advisers also serve as key agents of change in the community by seeking opportunities to improve the food and physical activity environment for children.

A FOCUS ON CHILDREN

Following extensive review and discussion of the evidence pertaining to community health, the need for early prevention, and the importance of positive messaging for childhood obesity, the advisory groups agreed to focus their efforts on children. Obesity and lifestyle issues were identified as a top community health priority in community health assessments performed by local county health departments.[6,7] Local data were considered (e.g., results from the Minnesota Student Survey indicating that the majority of children do not meet recommendations for fruits and vegetables, physical activity, sugar-sweetened beverages, or screen time and that by 8th grade, more than one in five boys and nearly one in seven girls are obese or overweight).[8] The focus on childhood obesity prevention was also supported by the Community Health Needs Assessment (CHNA) completed by Lakeview Hospital, a requirement for all nonprofit hospitals.[9] In essence, PowerUp is a strategy to meet these obligations for Lakeview Hospital and deliver a positive message to the community while working toward achievement of the overall mission of HealthPartners.

A GEOGRAPHIC FOCUS

The PowerUp initiative serves the St. Croix River Valley, a collection of smaller communities in Minnesota and western Wisconsin that are considered the most rapidly growing section of the Minneapolis and St. Paul metropolitan area. Initially (2013), efforts were concentrated in Stillwater and Mahtomedi, Minnesota, and Somerset, Wisconsin. In 2014, efforts expanded to include another part of the HealthPartners care system (i.e., Hudson and New Richmond, Wisconsin, in partnership with Hudson Hospital and Clinic and Westfields Hospital and Clinic). This local focus is instrumental in developing partnerships and relationships with key stakeholders by drawing on the community's shared values and identity.

COMMUNITY INITIATIVE FRAMEWORK

The PowerUp initiative is guided by a multilevel, multistakeholder, community-based framework designed to bring about environment change, community engagement, targeted programs, and clinical interventions. The framework is informed by the socioecological model, but accepted among all stakeholders as a simplified approach for various audiences. The resulting PowerUp Initiatives Framework Pyramid (Figure III-1) has five sections. The top two sections represent the greater reach and lower intensity of interventions focused on environment change and community engagement. The bottom two

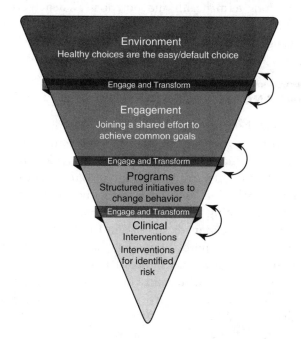

Figure III-1 PowerUp initiative framework for multilevel, multisector community change.

sections represent programs of higher intensity and clinical interventions that reach smaller numbers of children and families. The "engage and transform" zones between the various levels represent the ongoing efforts for relationship and partnership building. Each level of the pyramid is linked to measurement, and reporting objectives and goals of each level are stated as follows:

1. Food and physical activity environment: The community supports and integrates healthy food, beverage, and physical activity options.
2. Community engagement: The community joins a shared effort to establish better food, beverage, and activity choices.
3. Programs: The target audience improves food, beverage, and physical activity behaviors.
4. Clinical interventions: The clinic provides resources and referrals to youth and families with identified risk.
5. Engagement and transformation zones between each level of the pyramid illustrate the importance of developing community relationships and partnerships to generate support and create sustainability for the initiative.

All five levels of intervention are necessary for a comprehensive approach that recognizes the vital importance of community involvement, engagement, and adoption for success and sustainability and that requires common goals among all stakeholders to improve children's long-term health and potential. When the community is engaged, change can be contagious—when one restaurant, school, child care facility, or neighborhood makes a change, others see the benefits and are more likely to change themselves.

COMMUNICATIONS AND MESSAGE STRATEGY

Nutrition and exercise behaviors are rooted in early childhood.[10] A key to the success of the PowerUp initiative is a strong message and communication strategy that includes branding, name, logo, visual look, and main messages. Communications are developed to be relevant to children ages 3 to 11 years, and thus relevant to the adults who influence their food and activity behavior. PowerUp uses positive, simple, and fun messages through multiple channels, including print materials, advertising, a website (http://www.powerup4kids.org), and social media sites (e.g., Facebook, Twitter).

Kid-friendly, PowerUp Countdown messages are consistent, positive, and fun—more like a conversation with a peer rather than a lecture about health (Figure III-2). The Countdown is also consistent with, and complementary to, the nationally recognized 5-2-1-0 messages for childhood obesity prevention.[11] The Countdown has been well received by adults and children alike. One father reported, "My two girls ask for four colors on their plates at dinner. That means we need to offer more fruits and vegetables, but it's become really fun!"

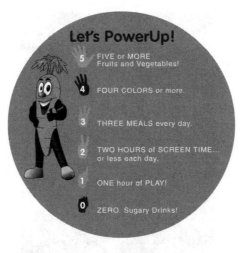

Figure III-2 The PowerUp countdown key messages.

A POWERUP SUPERHERO

Recognizing that it would have to compete with cartoon characters endorsing sweet treats and advertisements illustrating the power of energy drinks to effectively reach children, PowerUp developed Chomp, a giant carrot superhero. Chomp is an integral part of all PowerUp communications and the Chomp mascot makes personal appearances as well (Figure III-3). Children strongly identify with Chomp, who receives messages from kids at his own e-mail address.

ADULTS INFLUENCED TO CHANGE ON BEHALF OF CHILDREN

Although focused on change for children, PowerUp expends significant effort engaging and educating adult influencers (e.g., parents, teachers, food service staff, youth leaders, community members) to do what is best for kids. PowerUp encourages adults to consider how to be role models of positive behaviors and how to support the changes necessary for creating a better food and physical activity environment for kids. This call to action for adults has been well received by parents and community leaders in multiple sectors.

COMMUNITY OUTREACH

Community outreach has significantly raised the visibility of PowerUp with the target audience. Publically launched with a community leadership kick-off in the summer of 2012, PowerUp engaged more the 120 community leaders from numerous sectors. On May 4, 2013, PowerUp held a large community-wide launch for families, including an official world

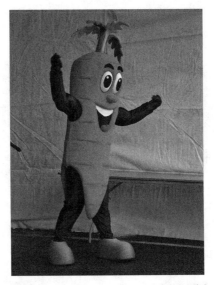

Figure III-3 Chomp, the PowerUp superhero mascot, visits with children at an early childhood center.
Courtesy of PowerUp.

record attempt for the most people doing the Cha Cha Slide. More than 750 people attended despite the cold and rainy weather. In keeping with the fun PowerUp brand, the games, food options, and community vendors were consistent with the PowerUp Countdown message. Overall, a strong PowerUp presence at more than 150 community events has reached more than 35,000 families and children with PowerUp resources since mid-2012.

KEY POWERUP PROGRAMS AND PARTNERSHIPS

As a multilevel intervention, PowerUp works across a wide variety of community sectors. Following are examples of effective partnerships and programs.

POWERUP SCHOOL CHALLENGE

This 4-week, classroom-based, elementary school program was developed in partnership with the HealthPartners yumPower School Challenge—another community-based program focused on healthy eating and active living (http://www.yumpower.com). The challenge kicks off with a high-energy student assembly featuring Radio Disney to generate excitement about increasing fruit and vegetable intake and physical activity. Students track their fruits and vegetables on weekly trackers. Teachers, parents, and school food service personnel all participate to reinforce lessons and activities. In addition, schools receive incentives for high participation rates in the form of PowerUp bucks, which can be used to purchase wellness-related items for the schools. Data from student trackers and parent and school surveys indicate that students are more interested in fruits and vegetables and are increasing their intake as a result of the challenge.

SCHOOL CHANGE

The primary local school board issued a PowerUp proclamation in support of PowerUp, and better food and physical activity priorities are incorporated into the districts' 5-year strategic plans. After-school programs have replaced many processed foods with fruits and vegetables, food service offers fruit and veggie snacks, and sugary beverages and foods at school carnivals and concessions have decreased.

OPEN GYM EVENTS

Open gyms have been a highly successful intervention to increase physical activity. PowerUp partnered with local schools in three communities to provide more than 30 free or low-cost open gyms during cold weather months to give families an opportunity to be active. Hundreds of kids and families attended, with up to 120 people attending a single session, exceeding school district officials' expectations.

FOOD SHELF CHANGE

In an innovative attempt to reach underserved populations, PowerUp partnered with the local Valley Outreach food shelf. Working collaboratively to revise food lists, inventory, and layout, more fruits and vegetables are now available to clients, at least five a day for each family member for the days food comes from the food shelf. Positive promotion has made fruits, vegetables, and whole grains the easy choice. Food shelves and hunger organizations from across the region have toured Valley Outreach to learn from this model and create change at their own food shelves.

MEASURING PROGRESS

PowerUp uses multiple internal and external measures to evaluate progress, including program surveys and data from the clinics, health plans, counties, and school districts. Reporting is summarized in an evaluation dashboard and organized around two types of measures as follows:

- What we are doing: Process measures include outreach and marketing efforts, programs, trainings, and community-sector engagement.
- What difference it makes: Outcome measures include community response; environment or policy change; changes in attitude, awareness, or behavior; long-term health; and body mass index (BMI) trends.

Results are reported at multiple levels of the PowerUp Pyramid Framework, and results to date for key PowerUp activities are summarized in Table III-1. The consistent growth of community outreach is illustrated in Figure III-4. The evaluation approach also includes a family survey tool that measures child and family behaviors, attitudes, and

Table III-1   PowerUp: Intervention Results Summary: 2013–Q1 2014

PowerUp Key Intervention/ Resource	Reach (January 2013–First Quarter of 2014)	Results
Community Outreach Activities, games, and information at local community fairs and events	More than 35,000 people reached at more than 150 events	Majority of target audience aware and value PowerUp after 1 year of outreach. Requests for PowerUp at events is growing rapidly.
Open Gyms Offered in partnership with three school districts as an alternative for family physical activity in cold-weather months	30 open gyms in three communities; attendance ranges from 45–120	Surveys indicate great appreciation by families for low-cost physical play options. Attendance continues to grow.
PowerUp Kids Cooking Classes Offered for two age groups in partnership with local cooking school and hospital dietitians	18 classes with a total of 325 attendees	75% of attendees indicate that they will make a specific food behavior change as a result of the class
The PowerUp Pledge A call to action for a family, a person, or an organization to PowerUp (http://www.powerup4kids.org/pledge)	Pledge included at events and website	700 have taken the pledge
PowerUp Food Coach Training Training food service and child care staff on methods to increase and positively promote fruits and vegetables offered	205 staff trained	More than 9,000 children are exposed to positive messages about fruits and vegetables.
PowerUp Sports Nutrition Playbook Developed at request of local coach to provide athletes and parents with information about better food and beverage choices for athletes	300 athletes, coaches, and parents reached	Sports teams no longer provide sugar-sweetened sports drinks to athletes but rather provide and encourage water. Parent volunteers lead changes in concessions at school events to reduce sugary foods and beverages and provide better choices.
PowerUp School Challenge A 4-week, classroom-based, elementary school program with an assembly to generate excitement about fruits and vegetables. Students track fruits and vegetables daily. Teachers, parents, and school food service personnel participate with lessons and activities.	2013: 5,300 students, two school districts, three other schools 2014: 8,200 students, four school districts, four other schools	Data from student trackers and parent and school surveys indicate that students are more interested in fruits and vegetables and are increasing intake as a result of the challenge.

Website and Social Media Powerup4kids.org (https://www.facebook.com/#!/ PowerUpKids)	14,762 unique website visitors; 813 Facebook and 75 Pinterest followers	Community response on website and social media grows consistently. Popular content includes recipes, "Veggie Voting," and letters to Chomp.

awareness. Households with young children were randomly selected to receive the survey in five communities in January 2014. The survey will be repeated at 2-year intervals over the course of the intervention to measure progress. Early survey results indicate very high awareness and perceived value of the initiative, with three out of four being aware of PowerUp and 95% indicating that the initiative is important or very important. Responses related to intake of fruits, vegetables, and sugar-sweetened beverages; screen time; and physical activity are being analyzed and will be compared over time.

The PowerUp initiative is an excellent example of engaging the local community to affect a large population and working collaboratively toward sustainable change and improved population health. The initiative also demonstrates how a health system can work in partnership with the community as a trusted convener of multiple stakeholders— a role that is paramount for successful community initiatives. Importantly, this initiative targets both individual behavior change and the relevant social, physical, and economic environments, thus changing the social norms that affect overall health.

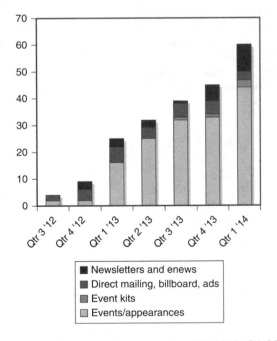

Figure III-4 PowerUp community outreach by quarter, Q3 2012–Q1 2014.

REFERENCES

1. Centers for Disease Control and Prevention. Childhood obesity in the United States, 2010. http://www.cdc.gov/about/grand-rounds/archives/2010/download/GR-062010.pdf. Accessed May 30, 2014.

2. Olshansky SJ, Passaro DJ, Hershow RC, et al. A potential decline in life expectancy in the United States in the 21st century. *N Engl J Med.* 2005;352:1138-45.

3. Isham G, Zimmerman D, Kindig D, et al. HealthPartners adopts community business model to deepen focus on nonclinical factors of health outcomes. *Health Aff.* 2013;32(8):1446-52.

4. Glickman D, Parker L, Sim L, et al., eds. *Accelerating Progress in Obesity Prevention: Solving the Weight of the Nation.* Committee on Accelerating Progress in Obesity Prevention, Food and Nutrition Board. Institute of Medicine. Washington, DC: National Academies Press; 2012.

5. Keener D, Goodman K, Lowry A, et al. *Recommended Community Strategies and Measurements to Prevent Obesity in the United States: Implementation and Measurement Guide.* U.S. Department of Health and Human Services. Centers for Disease Control and Prevention; 2009. http://www.cdc.gov/obesity/downloads/community_strategies_guide.pdf. Accessed November 7, 2014.

6. Washington County, Minnesota, Community Health Board. *Washington County 2008 Community Health Assessment: Community Health Improvement Plan 2009–2014.* http://www.co.washington.mn.us/DocumentCenter/View/6. Accessed November 7, 2014.

7. Healthier Together—St. Croix County: Community Health Improvement Plan, 2009–2014. http://www.co.saint-croix.wi.us/vertical/Sites/%7BBC2127FC-9D61-44F6-A557-17F280990A45%7D/uploads/Healthier_Together_-_St__Croix_County_Plan_FINAL_6-15-11.pdf. Accessed November 7, 2014.

8. 2010 Minnesota Student Survey. Washington County Tables. http://www.health.state.mn.us/divs/chs/mss/countytables/washington10.pdf. Accessed November 7, 2014.

9. Minnesota Hospital Association. Community health needs assessment. http://www.mnhospitals.org/policy-advocacy/priority-issues/community-benefitactivities/communityhealth-needs-assessment. Accessed November 7, 2014.

10. Cunningham SA, Kramer MR, Venkat Narayan KM. Incidence of childhood obesity in the United States. *N Engl J Med.* 2014;370:403-11.

11. Childhood Obesity Action Network: Expert committee recommendations on the assessment, prevention and treatment of child and adolescent overweight and obesity, 2007. http://obesity.nichq.org/resources/expert%20committee%20recommendation%20implementation%20guide. Accessed June 1, 2014.

GLOSSARY

A

absenteeism—employee is absent from work; typified when an employee is not at work for a wide range of issues including chronic or acute illness, injury, health risks, short- or long-term disability, poor morale, or outside obligations (e.g., child care or parent care).

access—the right or opportunity to use or benefit from something.

accountable care organization (ACO)—refers to a network or organization that assumes responsibility for coordinating the continued care of postacute care patient referrals. The patient-centered medical home will ideally become the accountable care organization in the future.

acute care—a branch of secondary health care whereby a patient receives active but short-term treatment for a severe injury or episode of illness or for an urgent medical condition, or during recovery from surgery.

administrative data—result from administering healthcare delivery, enrolling members into health insurance plans, and reimbursing for services. The primary producers of administrative data are the federal government, state governments, and private healthcare insurers. Although the clinical content of administrative data includes only the demographic characteristics and diagnoses of patients and codes for procedures, these data are often used to evaluate the quality of health care.

Affordable Care Act—The Patient Protection and Affordable Care Act (PPACA), commonly called the Affordable Care Act (ACA), is a U.S. federal statute whose goals are to increase the quality and affordability of health insurance, lower the uninsured rate by expanding public and private insurance coverage, and reduce the costs of health care for individuals and the government.

alert fatigue—user insensitivity to pop-up alerts and reminders in electronic health records when there are too many "trivial" alerts, such as minor drug–drug or drug–food interactions; users develop the habit of clicking through trivial alerts without carefully considering each one, which can result in missing an important alert.

alignment of constituencies—the bringing together of all stakeholders, in this case collaborating with organizations, health plans, health delivery systems, foundations, and governmental agencies to pursue a culture of health.

American Recovery and Reinvestment Act (ARRA)—passed by Congress on February 13, 2009 to stimulate the economy by creating new jobs and saving existing ones, spurring economic activity, investing in long-term economic growth, and fostering accountability and transparency in governmental spending. This act also enacted expansions to the Health Insurance Portability and Accountability Act (HIPAA) and includes the provisions of the Health Information Technology for Economic and Clinical Health (HITECH) Act.

apology laws—laws that prevent admissibility of comments made by healthcare providers when expressing an apology or extending sympathy regarding an unanticipated medical outcome in a court of law.

B

behavioral economics—the science of understanding financial and nonfinancial elements that influence human decision making.

behavioral intervention—the use of various conditioning methods to positively or negatively reinforce or modify one's behavior.

benchmark performance—benchmarks are established within a given field to quantify the level of performance (poor, fair, good, excellent). Benchmarks are used to compare one organization's performance with others in the same field.

best practice—a method or technique that consistently achieves superior results and is used as a benchmark for others.

bias—a systematic error in research; a deviation from the "true" finding based on the strategy used to select study participants and administer the intervention.

big data—data sets that are too large and complex to manipulate or interrogate with standard methods or tools.

biometrics—the analysis of biological data using mathematical and statistical methods.

Blue Button initiative—a national program that allows patients to view and download personal health information. The program includes pledges of support from many stakeholders to make it easier for individuals and their caregivers to have secure, timely, and electronic access to their health information.

breach notification rules—the federal requirement to notify individuals of breaches of their protected health information (PHI); established by the Health Information Technology for Economic and Clinical Health (HITECH) Act.

bundled payment—a single payment to providers or healthcare facilities (or jointly to both) for all services to treat a given condition or provide a given treatment.

C

care coordination—a part of the primary care practice that involves deliberately organizing patient care activities and sharing information among all of the participants concerned with a patient's care to achieve safer and more effective care.

care coordinator—the individual responsible for providing care coordination to a patient.

care transitions (also transitions of care)—the coordination and continuity of health care during a movement from one healthcare setting or practitioner to another or to the home setting, or when a patient's condition and care needs change during the course of an episode of illness.

carve-out—a service or benefit not covered in a health insurance contract (e.g., mental health services); usually reimbursed according to a different arrangement or rate formula than those services specified under the contract umbrella. Term also refers to a population subgroup for whom separate healthcare arrangements are made.

case management—the coordination of services on behalf of an individual person in different settings such as health care, nursing, rehabilitation, social work, disability insurance, employment, and law.

centers of excellence—highly specialized health delivery units that cater to specific patient cohorts and produce benchmark results.

channel of distribution—the network of individuals and organizations involved in the process of moving a product or service from the producer to the end user.

chronic care—providing or concerned with long-term medical care lasting usually more than 90 days, especially for individuals with chronic physical or mental impairment.

chronic care management—coordination of care focused on reducing fragmentation and unnecessary use of resources, preventing avoidable conditions (complications), and promoting independence and self-care to improve the quality of care and self-management, clinical information systems, evidence-based clinical decision support, redesigned healthcare delivery, clinical and community systems, and policies.

Chronic Care Model (CCM)—an organizing framework for improving chronic illness care at both the individual and population levels. The model is based on the assumption that improvement in care requires an approach that incorporates patient-, provider-, and system-level interventions.

claims data—data sets created for third-party payers that contain data from health insurance claims. Claims data are structured, by definition, because billing standards dictate the data content, format, and code sets (terminology systems) for claims.

clinical data—data pertaining to or founded on actual observation and treatment of patients.

clinical decision support—tools that provide clinicians or patients with clinical knowledge and patient-related information, intelligently filtered and presented at appropriate times, to enhance patient care. These are often implemented as context-specific pop-up alerts or reminders in electronic health records (EHRs), e-prescribing, computerized provider order entry systems, or convenient links to reference materials appropriate to the clinical situation.

clinical guidelines—include recommendations that are intended to optimize patient care and are informed by a systematic review of evidence and an assessment of the benefits and harms of alternative care options.

CMS quality initiatives—implemented by the Department of Health and Human Services and the Centers for Medicare and Medicaid Services (CMS) to ensure quality health care for all Americans through accountability and public disclosure. Initiatives focus on publicly reporting quality measures for nursing homes, home health agencies, hospitals, kidney dialysis facilities, and ambulatory care providers. The information is available for consumers to assist them in making healthcare choices or decisions.

comparative effectiveness—the assessment of the relative merits of two active therapeutic approaches by direct comparison.

comparative effectiveness research (CER)—a type of research that directly compares healthcare interventions to determine which is the most effective or provides the best chances of positive health outcomes.

computable data—an alternative term for structured data; it can be used by computer algorithms for clinical decision support, in contrast to information stored in an unstructured form such as a free-text narrative.

computerized physician order entry (CPOE)—computer-based systems for ordering medications; they share the common features of automating the medication ordering process.

consumer-driven health plan (CDHP)—the broad term for health benefit plan designs that require employees to spend more of their own money in the form of a deductible or coinsurance before the plan pays benefits. CDHPs are often linked to various forms of medical savings accounts. More narrowly defined, a consumer-driven health plan is a high-deductible health plan that has deductible and coverage levels that comply with the Internal Revenue Service's requirements and so allows the individual to establish a tax-advantaged health savings account.

controlled vocabulary—a set of terms or codes for expressing information within a certain domain of interest, including industry-standard systems such as SNOMED-CT and "local" code sets that may be adopted for use within a provider organization.

core competencies—fundamental knowledge, ability, or expertise in a specific subject area or skill set.

cost accounting—the recording of all the costs incurred in a business in a way that can be used to improve its management.

cost effectiveness—the cost of a program or intervention associated with a given level of effectiveness.

culture of health—Defined in terms of outcomes, a culture of health and wellness is characterized by an overall improvement in quality of life with a compression of morbidity. Cultures of health and wellness surround people with an environment and policies and cues that lead regularly to healthy choices on both a conscious and unconscious basis.

D

data mining—the application of specific algorithms for extracting patterns from data.

data warehouse—a repository of electronically stored data, either within an organization or across organizations, designed to facilitate reporting and analysis. Typically integrates data from multiple transaction systems with defined processes for periodic updates and data validation.

demographic transition—the transition from high birth and death rates to low birth and death rates as a country develops from a preindustrial to an industrialized economic system.

diagnosis-related groups (DRGs)—a set of approximately 500 categories used to classify hospital stays, based primarily on the patient's diagnoses and surgical procedures developed and used mainly for prospective payment. Several variants of DRGs take different approaches to accounting for severity of illness.

disability-adjusted life years (DALY)—a measure of overall disease burden, expressed as the number of years lost due to ill-health, disability or early death.

discrete field—a data element that stores a specific concept or piece of information.

One aspect of structured data. (The other aspect is a controlled vocabulary or code set for expressing the information.)

disease management (DM)—a system of targeted, coordinated, population-based healthcare interventions and communications for specific conditions in which patient self-care efforts are significant; it seeks to reverse the skyrocketing incidence and prevalence of serious, costly, chronic illness through improving patient outcomes with quality and cost-effective care that includes the patient-centered medical home.

disease registry—an electronic system that aggregates information about all of an organization's patients who have a particular disease or condition for surveillance and tracking at the population level. Enables proactive identification of patients who may be overdue for screening, periodic testing, or follow-up care but have not scheduled an appointment. Typically supports patient outreach via phone calls, e-mail, and so on and allows documentation of patient interactions. (*See also* **patient registry**.)

double-blind confirmation—a research approach that establishes a causal link between intervention and outcome by matching participants based on the severity of their illness and designating an experimental group (receives intervention) and a control group (receives normal care).

E

effectiveness—whether an intervention works in routine clinical care.

efficacy—whether an intervention works under ideal conditions.

efficiency—the measure of cost of care or resource utilization associated with a specified level of care quality.

electronic health record (EHR)—an electronic record of health-related information on an individual that conforms to nationally recognized interoperability standards and can be created, managed, and consulted by authorized clinicians and staff across more than one healthcare organization. An electronic medical record (EMR) is defined similarly, but within a single healthcare organization.

Emergency Medical Treatment and Labor Act (EMTALA)—passed by Congress in 1986 to ensure public access to emergency services regardless of ability to pay.

Employee Retirement Income Security Act of 1974 (ERISA)—federal law that sets minimum standards for health and retirement plans sponsored by employers. It provides protections available to plan participants and their families.

enterprise master patient index (EMPI)—a database that is used across a healthcare organization to maintain consistent, accurate, and current demographic and essential medical data on the patients seen and managed within its various departments.

episode of illness—sequential and temporally associated healthcare services that are either requested by the patient or provided to treat a specific illness. Often used in conjunction with bundled (episode-based) payments in which reimbursement of care providers (e.g., physicians, hospitals) is calculated on the basis of expected costs for clinically defined episodes of care.

evidence-based medicine—a systematic approach to clinical problem solving that allows the integration of the best available research evidence with clinical expertise and patient values.

expected years of life—the number of years researchers expect a person to live.

F

fee-for-service—a payment mechanism by which a provider is paid for each individual service rendered to a patient.

G

gaps in care—the differences between what we know and what we do; and between achievable and actual outcomes.

Genetic Information Nondiscrimination Act of 2007 (GINA)—a law that limits health insurer and employer access to Americans' health records to protect against discrimination based on genetic information.

genomic profile—a set of genetic markers present in a given patient. Specific genomic and molecular (proteomic) markers or combinations of markers may indicate a patient's risk of developing certain diseases or how a patient will respond to certain drugs. The number of markers that are clinically useful is rapidly expanding, providing greater opportunities to tailor prevention and treatment to an individual patient, often called "personalized medicine."

gross domestic product (GDP) per capita—the monetary value of all of a nation's goods and services produced within its borders and a particular period of time, such as a year; serves as the official measure of the U.S. economy.

gross national income—the sum of a nation's gross domestic product (GDP) plus net income received from other countries.

grouper—the software that assigns cases to diagnosis-related groups (DRGs).

H

health advocacy and navigation—direct service to an individual or a family as well as activities that promote health and access to health care in communities and the larger public.

health advocate—an independent professional with broad or focused knowledge of the medical care delivery system and benefits environment who provides assistance to individuals facing health or benefits issues. Health advocates may work in a variety of for-profit and nonprofit settings and business structures.

health and wealth connection—the emerging evidence that health generates wealth and wealth generates health on individual, community, national, and global levels.

health and wellness program—a program that is intended to improve and promote health and fitness that's usually offered through the workplace, insurance plans, or a private company.

health determinants—the wide variety of interacting proximate and distal influences on the health of individuals and populations, including, but not limited to, political contexts; policies; distribution of power and wealth; physical and social environments; health systems and services; and genetic, biological, and cultural–historical characteristics.

health disparities—differences in the incidence, prevalence, mortality, and burden of diseases, as well as other adverse health conditions or outcomes that exist among specific population groups and have been well documented in subpopulations based on socioeconomic status, education, age, race and ethnicity, geography, disability, sexual orientation, or special needs.

health information exchange (HIE)—the electronic movement of health-related information among organizations according to nationally recognized standards. The goal of HIEs is to facilitate access to and retrieval of clinical data to provide safer, timelier, efficient, effective, equitable, patient-centered care.

health information technology (HIT)—a variety of electronic means for managing information about the health and medical care of patients.

Health Information Technology for Economic and Clinical Health Act (HITECH)—a component of the American Recovery and Reinvestment Act (ARRA), which aims to advance the use of health information technology (HIT) to allow a nationwide electronic exchange for use of health information to improve quality and coordination of care, to encourage use of HIT by doctors and hospitals to exchange patient information, to provide resources to improve quality and coordination, and to strengthen laws to secure patient information.

Health Insurance Portability and Accountability Act (HIPAA)—(1996) provides protection of personal health information at the federal level.

Health Level Seven (HL7)—a set of messaging standards widely used for exchanging data such as orders, results, and patient registration information among disparate healthcare information systems. Newer HL7 standards address clinical document architecture and a reference information model for health care. The term refers to the seventh, or highest, layer of an international standard for open systems integration, the layer where "content" is transmitted. Also refers to the international organization that maintains the HL7 standards.

health policy—a field of study and practice in which the priorities and values underlying health resource allocation are determined and supported by government policy makers.

health promotion, prevention, and screening—the process of enabling people to increase control over their health and its determinants and thereby improve their health.

health risk assessment (HRA)—a tool used to evaluate health and identify potential risks.

health services research—the multidisciplinary field of scientific investigation that studies how social factors, financing systems, organizational structures and processes, health technologies, and personal behaviors affect access to health care, the quality and cost of health care, and ultimately our health and well-being. Its research domains are individuals, families, organizations, institutions, communities, and populations.

health status—a measure of wellness compared to ideal or norms.

health technology assessment (HTA)—a form of policy research analysis that examines short- and long-term consequences in the application of new healthcare technology (e.g., new medical procedures or drugs).

healthcare consumerism—an approach to health care whereby educated patients make informed decisions about healthcare options, with a particular focus on preventive care.

Healthcare Effectiveness Data and Information Set (HEDIS)—a tool used by more than 90% of America's health plans to measure performance on important dimensions of care and service. HEDIS consists of 71 measures across eight domains of care.

healthcare quality—the degree to which health services for individuals and populations increase the likelihood of desired health outcomes and are consistent with current professional knowledge.

healthy life expectancy—a term based on one's life expectancy minus one's current age. The result indicates the number of years of healthy life that one can reasonably expect to live if free of disease and disabilities.

heuristics—the study or practice of learning or problem-solving techniques that are based on experience and may or may not be optimal for a particular situation. Examples include rules of thumb, educated guesses, or intuitive judgments.

homophily—A theory in sociology that people tend to form connections with others who are similar to them in characteristics such as socioeconomic status, values, beliefs, or attitudes.

hospital quality improvement—the degree to which hospitals are improving over time, and how they achieve and sustain that improvement.

hotspotting—using data analytics and mapping to identify high utilizers of the emergency department and healthcare resources.

I

Institute for Clinical and Economic Review (ICER)—a trusted, nonprofit organization that evaluates evidence on the value of medical tests, treatments, and delivery system innovations and moves that evidence into action to improve patient care and control costs.

interdisciplinary (or interprofessional) team—a group of individuals from different disciplines who contribute their knowledge, skill sets, and experience and work closely to optimize care for patients. Throughout this text, the term is used to describe the collaboration among students from different disciplines in education.

K

knowledge discovery—the process of discovering useful knowledge from a collection of data.

lobbying—the act of attempting to influence political decisions through various forms of advocacy directed at policy makers on behalf of another person, organization, or group for your or your organization's benefit.

longitudinal patient record—administrative data that reflect all covered services that a patient received, from any provider, and the sequence of billable events.

M

mandatory spending—budget authority provided and controlled by laws other than appropriation acts and the outlays that result from that budget authority.

marketing mix—a term used in business and marketing that incorporates the controllable elements of a product's marketing plan, commonly termed the four Ps: product, price, place, and promotion.

meaningful use—a term that refers to the provision of financial incentives for providers who "meaningfully use" certified electronic health record technology to improve results over time.

medical–legal partnership—a healthcare delivery model that integrates legal care into the healthcare setting to address the social determinants of health.

medically homeless—the segment of the population that lacks trusted relationships with the healthcare provider community.

Medicare Advantage (MA)—a comprehensive plan for Medicare beneficiaries, which is privately run by a health insurance organization with extra benefits and lower copayments than traditional Medicare.

Millennium Development Goals (MDGs)—a set of aims to improve human well-being by reducing poverty, hunger, child and maternal mortality; ensuring education for all; controlling and managing diseases; tackling gender disparity; ensuring sustainable development; and pursuing global partnerships.

models of care delivery—a multifaceted concept, which broadly defines the way health services are delivered.

multiple behavior changes—the interrelationships among health behaviors and interventions designed to promote change in more than one health behavior at a time. Evidence suggests that the potential for multiple-behavior interventions has a greater effect on the population's health than single-behavior interventions.

N

National Priorities Partnership (NPP)—Convened by the National Quality Forum, NPP has a vision for world-class, affordable health care and transforming the U.S. healthcare system. The 28 organizations in the partnership, all committed to improving health care, have collaboratively developed National Priority Goals targeted at proven ways to eliminate harm, waste, and disparities in care.

national provider identifier (NPI)—a system of unique identifiers for all individual and institutional healthcare providers in the United States, mandated by administrative simplification provisions of the Health Insurance Portability and Accountability Act of 1996.

National Quality Forum (NQF)—a nonprofit organization dedicated to improving the quality of health care in the United States. NQF embodies a three-part mission: to set goals for performance improvement, to endorse standards for measuring and reporting on performance, and to promote educational and outreach programs.

National Quality Strategy—Established as part of the ACA, the National Quality Strategy serves as a catalyst and compass for a nationwide focus on quality improvement efforts and approach to measuring quality. The National Quality Strategy is guided by three aims: to provide better, more affordable care for individuals and the community.

natural language processing (NLP)—a field of computer science, artificial intelligence, and linguistics concerned with the interactions between computers and human (natural) languages.

negligence—failure to exercise the care that a reasonably prudent person would exercise in like circumstances.

noncommunicable disease (NCD)—a chronic disease (e.g., cardiovascular disease, cancer, chronic respiratory disease, and diabetes) that is not transmitted through personal contact.

Nurse Licensure Compact—licensure reciprocity that permits nurses licensed in states where the compact has been adopted to practice in other states that have also adopted the compact.

O

observational data—gathered by watching behavior and events, or noting physical characteristics in their natural setting.

observational study—a study in which a researcher simply observes behavior in a systematic manner without influencing or interfering with the behavior.

Office of the National Coordinator for Health Information Technology (ONC)—an office within the U.S. Department of Health and Human Services charged with coordination of nationwide efforts to implement and use advanced health information technology (HIT) and promotion of the electronic exchange of health information. Coordinates policy and standards relating to HIT.

online tools—enable consumers to manage their health, health care, and healthcare costs. Online tools may be independently hosted or tethered to an electronic medical record or health plan database.

ontology—a terminology system that provides names for concepts within a certain domain and defines relationships among the concepts; used loosely for any controlled vocabulary.

opportunity cost—the value of the best alternative forgone when a choice must be made between several mutually exclusive alternatives given limited resources.

outlier—frequently used in statistics, it is an observation point that is distant from other observations.

P

Pareto's rule (80–20 rule)—a theory maintaining that 80% of the output from a given situation or system is determined by 20% of the input.

patient attribution—a physician's patient population.

patient behavior—the way in which a patient acts or conducts herself or himself.

patient centeredness—a partnership among practitioners, patients, and their families that ensures that decisions respect patients' wants, needs, and preferences and that patients have the education and support they need to make decisions and participate in their own care.

patient engagement—any effort to involve a person in his or her own health or health care.

patient engagement framework—a construct describing an expanding partnership between the patient and his or her care team.

patient portal—a secure online website that gives patients convenient 24-hour access to personal health information from anywhere with an Internet connection.

Patient Protection and Affordable Care Act (PPACA)—*See* **Affordable Care Act.**

patient safety organization (PSO)—a group, institution, or association that improves medical care by reducing medical errors.

patient registration—patient-specific data collected by an organization to identify, catalog, and cross reference information regarding medical records, healthcare services, and billing.

patient registry—a collection of secondary data related to a patient with a specific diagnosis, condition, or procedure (*see also* **disease registry**).

patient self-management—the management of chronic illness taught to patients, including diet, exercise, self-monitoring, and medication compliance and involving teaching skills, building confidence, self-assessment, and referrals.

patient-centered medical home (PCMH)—a concept that integrates patients as active participants in their own health and well-being. Patients are cared for by a physician who leads the medical team that coordinates all aspects of preventive, acute, and chronic needs of patients using the best available evidence and appropriate technology. These relationships offer patients comfort, convenience, and optimal health throughout their lifetimes.

pharmacovigilance—detection, assessment, understanding, and prevention of adverse long-term and short-term effects of medications, biological products, herbal preparations, and other medicines. Involves collecting, monitoring, assessing, and interpreting data from healthcare providers and patients, plus developing methods for "signal" detection in large databases assembled from multiple sources.

pharmacy benefit manager (PBM)—a company under contract with managed care organizations, self-insured companies, and/or government programs to administer pharmacy network operations, monitor drug utilization, review outcomes, and participate in chronic disease management.

physician behavior—the way in which a physician acts or conducts himself or herself.

population health—a cohesive, integrated, and comprehensive approach to health care that considers the distribution of health outcomes within a population, the health determinants that influence distribution of care, and the policies and interventions that affect and are affected by the determinants.

population health management—the process of addressing population health needs and controlling problems at a population level.

population management systems—an administrative transaction system designed for physician practices that typically provides several patient financial applications: patient registration, appointment scheduling, billing (including insurance claims), and patient accounts receivable management (collections).

practice management system—the provision of healthcare services by three or more physicians who are formally organized as a legal entity in which business and clinical facilities, records, and personnel are shared.

practice redesign—the intentional efforts to improve practice processes (e.g., workflow) and patient outcomes.

pragmatic clinical trials—studies that evaluate the effectiveness of interventions in real-life routine practice conditions and produce results that can be generalized and applied in routine practice settings.

predictive modeling—a research approach that uses existing data to predict future behavior or consequences.

preemption—a doctrine that indicates federal law takes precedence over state law.

preferred provider organization (PPO)—a health benefit program that encourages the use of a network of contracted "preferred" physicians and other providers. Unlike health maintenance organization (HMO) plans, PPOs offer coverage for out-of-network care, usually with a higher copayment.

presenteeism—employee is present for work, but not optimally productive because of health conditions or health risks; health-related productivity loss while at work, including time not on task (e.g., at work, but not working), decreased quality of work, increased injury rates, negative effect on work teams, employee turnover, and replacement costs.

Preston curve—the concept that increased wealth leads to increased health.

prevention—interlocking and mutually supportive strategies and interventions aimed at deterrence, early detection, and minimization or cessation of disease and injury at a population level.

prevention paradox—a measure that brings much benefit to the population but offers little to each participating individual.

primary research—the collection and analysis of "source" data or data collected for the purpose of a study.

process redesign—approach to reviewing and redesigning the patient journey to meet demand and ensure that care is safe, effective, and efficient.

processes of change—experiential and behavioral activities that individuals use to progress through the stages of change.

product element—anything that can be offered to the market to satisfy a need; it includes physical objects, services, persons, places, organizations, and ideas.

proof of concept—evidence that establishes that an idea, invention, process, or business model is feasible.

prospective payment—a payment mechanism for reimbursing hospitals for inpatient healthcare services in which a predetermined rate is set for treatment of specific illnesses. The system was originally developed by the U.S. federal government to use in treatment of Medicare recipients.

protected health information (PHI)—identifiable information about health status, provision of health care, or payment for health care that can be linked to a specific individual.

psychographic segmentation—a marketing strategy in which customers are divided into various groups based on lifestyle; used to help marketers understand what influences purchase decisions, such as different attitudes and expectations, particularly of a good or service.

public choice model—a construct describing how the costs and gains from political activity that influence legislation and regulation do not affect all citizens equally.

public health—the science of protecting and improving the health of communities through education.

purchasing power parity—an economic theory that estimates the amount of adjustment needed on the exchange rate between countries in order for the exchange to be equivalent to each currency's purchasing power.

Q

quality-adjusted life year (QALY)—a year of life lived in less than perfect health compared to a year of life in perfect health.

R

randomized controlled trial (RCT)—a study in which participants are allocated at *random* (by chance alone) to receive one of several clinical interventions.

readmission rules—Section 3025 of the Affordable Care Act meant to lower hospital readmissions.

real-world data—data that are collected outside the controlled constraints of conventional randomized clinical trials.

regression to the mean—a statistical phenomenon that causes natural variation to appear as a real change.

retail clinic—a walk-in medical facility located inside pharmacies and retail chains where care is delivered by nurse practitioners, often without a physician on the premises.

return on investment (ROI)—size of a return relative to an investment.

revenue cycle—all administrative and clinical functions that contribute to the capture, management, and collection of patient service revenue.

risk adjustment—statistical methods used to account for patient factors that cause some patients to be at greater risk of certain outcomes.

risk management—the approach to developing and implementing safe and effective patient care practices, preserving financial resources, and maintaining safe working environments.

risk reduction—altering the likelihood of an untoward event by means of evidence-based interventions (e.g., not smoking, maintaining a normal weight).

risk stratification—a systematic process for identifying and predicting patient's risk levels relating to healthcare needs, services, and care coordination with the goal of identifying those at the highest risk and managing their care to prevent poor health outcomes. Risk stratification enables a clinical practice to maximize use of limited time and resources to prioritize needs of their patient population. The process incorporates algorithms and registries, payer data, physician/provider judgment/input, and patient self assessments and experiences.

road map—a plan of action over a time line to deliver a result.

S

scientific method—a framework for conducting research that includes identifying a topic, generating a hypothesis, defining a data collection and analysis strategy, gathering data, testing the hypothesis, and making decisions based on the results.

secondary research—a research strategy that involves analysis of existing data and prior research to determine new methods for using the information and drawing conclusions.

segmentation—a marketing strategy that identifies consumers with common needs and who are likely to respond similarly to a marketing action.

self-determination theory—is a theory of motivation that is concerned with supporting humans' intrinsic tendencies to behave in effective and healthy ways.

self-insured—employers (usually larger) who operate their own health plans as opposed to purchasing a fully insured plan from an insurance carrier.

semantic interoperability—the ability of computer systems to exchange data with unambiguous, shared meaning.

social marketing—an approach used to develop activities aimed at changing or maintaining people's behavior to improve their personal welfare and that of society.

stages of change—a categorization of population segments based on where individuals are in the process of change.

structured data—data stored in discrete fields (separate data element for each distinct concept) using a controlled vocabulary or standard code set (also called computable data).

systematic process optimization (SPO)—a strategy used to reduce the number of defects in an existing process.

T

target market—a group of customers toward which a business aims its marketing efforts.

tax-exempt status—a special designation under federal law provided to many hospitals and other charitable organizations to enable the organization to avoid the payment of federal income tax in return for provision of charitable services.

third-party administrator (TPA)—an organization that provides claims processing services to self-insured companies. Typically, TPAs affiliate with a network administrator to provide their clients with access to discounted contracts with hospitals, physicians, and other providers.

tort system—a collective reference to the process of bringing an action, defending it, and the deliberations of the trier of fact under state or federal law. Torts, under the law, are defined as private or civil wrongs or injuries that are independent of contract rights. Usually, a tort is a violation of a duty owed by one to another.

transaction system—an IT system within a typical healthcare provider organization that is focused on the level of the individual patient.

transparency—making available to the public, in a reliable and understandable manner, information on the healthcare system's quality, efficiency, and consumer experience with care, which includes price and quality data, to influence the behavior of patients, providers, payers, and others to achieve better outcomes (quality and cost of care).

transtheoretical model of behavior change (TTM)—a framework for using stages to integrate processes and principles of change across major theories of intervention.

trend analysis—an analytic design used to study the same population cohort over the course of a new treatment or service to determine whether the new intervention had an effect.

Triple Aim—an initiative of the Institute for Healthcare Improvement (IHI) that provides a framework for accountability by focusing on improving population health, per capita cost, and the care experience.

U

U.S. Supreme Court—the highest federal court in the United States.

V

value—worth, utility, or importance in comparison with something else.

value-based insurance design (VBID)—an evidence-based approach to designing health benefits to foster healthy lifestyles and better health outcomes.

W

wellness—the quality or state of well-being.

wellness champions—individuals designated to promote health within a group.

workplace environment—the place where employees spend the majority of their waking hours.

Y

years lived with disability—*see* **disability-adjusted life years**.

INDEX

Note: Page numbers followed by *b*, *f*, and *t* indicate material in boxes, figures, and tables respectively.

A